Conceiving Israel

Divinations: Rereading Late Ancient Religion

Series Editors: Daniel Boyarin, Virginia Burrus, Derek Krueger

A complete list of books in the series is available from the publisher.

Conceiving Israel
The Fetus in Rabbinic Narratives

Gwynn Kessler

University of Pennsylvania Press
Philadelphia

Copyright © 2009 University of Pennsylvania Press

All rights reserved. Except for brief quotations used for purposes of review or scholarly citation, none of this book may be reproduced in any form by any means without written permission from the publisher.

Published by
University of Pennsylvania Press
Philadelphia, Pennsylvania 19104-4112

Printed in the United States of America on acid-free paper

10 9 8 7 6 5 4 3 2 1

Library of Congress Cataloging-in-Publication Data

Kessler, Gwynn.
   Conceiving Israel : the fetus in rabbinic narratives / Gwynn Kessler.
     p. cm. — (Divinations: rereading late ancient religion)
   Includes bibliographical references and index.
   ISBN 978-0-8122-4175-4 (alk. paper)
   1. Fetuses in rabbinical literature. 2. Rabbinical literature—History and criticism. I. Title.
BM509.F48K47 2009
296.1'208612647—dc22

2009001015

For Burt

Contents

Chapter 1 The Torah of the Fetus 1

Chapter 2 Covenantal Fetuses 29

Chapter 3 And the Sons Struggled 47

Chapter 4 Embryology as Theology 65

Chapter 5 Reproductive Theology 89

Epilogue 127

Notes 137

References 207

Name and Subject Index 231

Citation Index 237

Acknowledgments 247

Chapter 1
The Torah of the Fetus

> *How does the fetus rest in its mother's womb? Like a folded writing tablet: its head lies between its knees; its two hands against its two temples;[1] its two heels against its two buttocks; its mouth is closed[2] and its navel is open.*
> —Lev. Rab. 14:8[3]

The appearance of the fetus, be it textually imagined as in antiquity or technologically imaged today, can be quite deceiving.[4] *Leviticus Rabbah*'s "snapshot" of the fetus at rest in its mother's womb conceals as much as it reveals about rabbinic portrayals of the fetus in a variety of narrative textual spaces. Far from embodying a tabula rasa, which the image of a folded writing table might invoke, in rabbinic narratives the fetus inhabits the womb and emerges within it as always already a part of and participant in Israel. And, although *Lev. Rab.* 14:8 imagines the fetus with closed mouth—but open navel—rabbinic narratives about the fetus, and indeed rabbinic fetuses themselves, speak volumes about issues central to rabbinic articulations of Israel. In rabbinic narratives, the fetus is not at rest but consistently called upon to bring to light, enliven, and even personify and internalize certain cultural markers upon which rabbinic Israel centers—if not rests.

Another rabbinic tradition likens the fetus in its mother's womb to a nut floating in a bowl of water.[5] The text explains, "If one puts his finger on it, it sinks from here to there" (*b. Nid.* 31a). Reaching beyond both the superficial image of a here radically deanthropomorphized fetus and the surface reading of a fetus that floats or sinks—as if of little matter—this tradition further bespeaks a fetus that hardly rests, a fetus that cannot be pinned down. In narrative contexts, the rabbinic fetus emerges immersed in a cultural matrix saturated with meanings. When the poked or prodded fetus rises and falls from here to there, it does not simply brush against the borders but speaks to, and strikes at, some very core issues at the heart of rabbinic constructions of Israel.

The earliest rabbinic tradition to imbue fetuses with speech imagines Israelite fetuses singing to God at the crossing of the sea. In the rabbinic imagination, they too would sing, *God is my strength and song and God has become my salvation* (Exod. 15:2) and *Who is like you, God, among the gods?* (Exod. 15:11). They too would celebrate God as their deliverer. A much later tradition creates a dialogue between God and fetuses at Sinai, where after God renders them visible by making windows out of pregnant women's wombs, the Israelite fetuses are called upon to give voice to their parents' acceptance of the Torah—simultaneously articulating their own acceptance.[6] As this tradition would have it, if it were not for its fetuses, Israel would receive no Torah. If not for fetuses, there would be no Israel. In these traditions, fetuses speak along with or on behalf of the people, the "nation,"[7] articulating and bringing into sharp focus Israel's foundational events, its moments of birth: Exodus and Revelation.

Of course, fetuses do not speak for themselves; they are made to speak for others.[8] In the current cultural landscapes within which I write, scientists, cutting-edge photographers, activists, politicians, and scholars are some of the many who use the fetus to articulate their own deeply held convictions. In the rabbinic textual landscape about which I write, fetuses are made to speak for Israel and are used to articulate what the rabbis perceived to be not only central but by virtue of being inscribed onto the fetus in its mother's womb also innate or intrinsic—essential—to Israel. Without collapsing the differences between contemporary cultural and late antique rabbinic discourses about the fetus, this book explores how, for the rabbis of antiquity, in ways akin to—but not identical with—contemporary constituencies, the image of the fetus is made to bear enormous cultural significance.[9]

Rabbinic narratives about the fetus carry both ideological and theological weight. The rabbis summon the fetus to give voice to their vision of Israel, which can neither be envisioned without God nor imagined apart from God's intimate relationship with Israel. If one wishes to know what, according to the rabbis, makes Israel Israel, and who makes Israel Israel, uncover, open up, and look inside their narratives about fetuses, because these traditions play a small but significant part in the larger project of rabbinic self-articulation. When the rabbis fabricate the fetus, they fashion themselves. Conjuring the fetus, the rabbis reproduce themselves writ large—not small—as progenitors conceiving and bringing forth nothing less than Israel itself.

The rabbinic construction of Jacob—*Israel*—in Rebekah's womb in many ways epitomizes the cultural work played out in rabbinic narratives about fetuses.[10] Building upon the scriptural mention of the twins' in utero struggle (Gen. 25:22), midrashic traditions imagine prenatal Jacob performing, embodying, and engendering rabbinic Israel. Already in Rebekah's womb, Jacob is righteous and loved by God, he wishes to study, pray, and observe commandments, and he is circumcised. In contrast, Esau, already in Rebekah's womb, is wicked, uncircumcised, and hated by God, and he desires to worship idols.[11] Indeed, the siblings' biblical prenatal struggle that already foretells "two nations and two peoples" (Gen. 25:23) comes to represent the rabbinic "culture wars" between Israel, who is Jacob, and Rome, who is Esau.[12] Through such portrayals of prenatal Jacob and his other(s), the rabbis establish their pedigree, claim their birthright, and write themselves not only into Rebekah's womb but also into the very beginnings of Israel's genealogy and history.

In the hands of the rabbis, prenatal Jacob represents rabbinic Israel, as if proclaiming, "Peer into Rebekah's womb and behold the origins of Israel." Furthermore, since Jacob *is* Israel, the rabbinic portrayal of prenatal Jacob locates the very beginnings of rabbinic "Israelness" before birth for all Israel.[13] In this way, prenatal Jacob is pregnant with his offspring, both his biblical descendants who, also as fetuses, sing to God as they leave Egypt and accept God's Torah and his later incarnations who manifest Israel—the rabbis.

Rabbinic traditions about prenatal Jacob, while remaining the most expansive and obvious examples of the rabbinic appeal to the fetus as representative of Israel, are part of a broader textual turn to the fetus. Throughout rabbinic narratives, the fetus symbolizes Israel, and that which the rabbis project onto the fetus, what they see when they look inside, is both a reflection of themselves and an embryonic manifestation of Israel. In so doing, the rabbis cast the fetus itself as participant upon their world stage.[14] The rabbinic fetus is to be found, in narrative contexts, not straddling the precarious border between life and not life but centrally enshrined in the no less fraught and even permeable interior spaces from which rabbinic Israel negotiates and inhabits its late antique surroundings.

Articulating Israel

This book places narratives about the fetus at the front lines of rabbinic articulations of Israel. I present rabbinic narratives about the fetus as both ideological and theological records that articulate an idea of, and an ideal, Israel, which cannot, for the rabbis, be thought apart from God. As a corollary to the above assertion that without fetuses there would be no Israel, it goes without saying that, according to the rabbis, there can be no Israel without God.[15] Furthermore, without God there simply could not be any fetuses, a point to which rabbinic discourses about embryology and procreation amply attest. Rabbinic ideology and theology are both overlaid on and interwoven into the very fabric of rabbinic narratives about the fetus because God and Israel are interarticulated and mutually constituted. These narratives consistently concretize the relationship between God and Israel, insisting that Israel is never without God—even from its very beginnings. An inquiry into rabbinic narratives about fetuses thus yields profound insights into rabbinic constructions of both Israel and God.

Building upon the work of previous scholars who have turned to other rabbinic motifs for their insights into rabbinic constructions of Israel, I set forth rabbinic narratives about fetuses as important textual sites where the rabbis not only project themselves onto the fetus but also theorize themselves and Israel through the fetus. Here, the fetus joins the chorus and ranks of, among others, evil empires, heretics, and criminals as a participant in the cacophony of voices and bricolage of images through which rabbinic Israel takes shape. Moshe Herr, Charlotte Fonrobert, and Richard Kalmin have all turned an inward gaze on rabbinic traditions about foreign governmental decrees that ostensibly prohibited definitive Jewish practices.[16] They have shifted attention away from establishing the precise historical contexts of such sources and instead established that this motif presents rabbinic reflections about what it means to be, and what constitutes, Israel. Seen in this way, the motif provides a categorization and classification—which shifts depending on literary contexts—of the "essentials" of rabbinic Israel. Gary Porton has examined the important role traditions about gentiles and converts have played in rabbinic constructions of Israel.[17] Daniel Boyarin has focused on the ways that the early rabbis used the mutually constituting categories of heresy and orthodoxy for self-definition in concert with their Christian counterparts,[18] and Beth Berkowitz has examined how rabbis and Christians invent and authorize themselves through their discourses of capital punishment.[19]

Rabbinic narratives about the fetus both complement the emergent picture of Israel gleaned from these other interpretive angles and provide a different perspective from which to view rabbinic constructions of Israel. Instead of projecting essential aspects of Israel onto external, hostile governments, the fetus allows the rabbis to articulate Israel's essence from an internal—even hyperinternalized—location. The fetus focuses attention on the center of Israel and its (re)production, whereas converts, heretics, and non-Israelites call to mind its borders—however permeable.[20] And the discourse about the fetus is one of creation; it is about the origins and potentials of Israel as a collective body along with those of the individual, and its rhetoric of life stands as a necessary counterpart to the discourse of execution. Finally, the fetus in rabbinic narratives ultimately transgresses chronology and transcends the vicissitudes of history; it provides the rabbis with an image of Israel that illustrates that through past, present, and future, Israel takes shape primarily in relation with God.

To claim a kind of transhistoricity for the rabbinic fetus does not mean that rabbinic traditions about fetuses lack any indication of historical location. Part of the work of this book is to historicize these traditions, to elicit the work that they do in their literary and broader late antique contexts. But part of such contextualization necessitates recognizing that in rabbinic narratives, the fetus—as an image that embodies past, present, and future—allows the rabbis to traverse chronology and construct rabbinic Israel as timeless. Through the fetus, the rabbis cut across time, "anachronistically" reading themselves into the biblical past, reading the biblical past as if it were the rabbinic present, and projecting rabbinic Israel—always already in intimate relationship with God—into a near infinite future.[21]

Similarly, calling attention to the primacy of the relationship between God and Israel in rabbinic narratives about fetuses does not indicate that Israel exists in anywhere near complete isolation. To the contrary, rabbinic narratives about fetuses both reflect and illuminate rabbinic Israel's cultural surroundings. These traditions, both implicitly and explicitly, attest to the shared contexts, concerns, and canons operating through borders of late antique culture. The relationship between rabbinic Israel and its cultural surroundings and evidence of rabbinic embeddedness in late antiquity often come very much into view in narratives about fetuses. For example, *Leviticus Rabbah*'s use of the Greek word *pinaks,* rendered above as "writing tablet," already articulates a common language and thus beckons the exploration of the relationship between Greco-Roman and rabbinic embryology—a relationship that needs to be examined beyond the question of influence.[22] And rabbinic interpretations about prenatal Jacob and Esau present an articulation of Israel in close contact with not-Israel, both pagan and Christian, simultaneously demonstrating the rabbinic adeptness at applying scripture to their own situations and indicating some type of exegetical exchange between these rabbinic traditions and patristic interpretations of Rom. 9:11–13.[23]

But to focus only on how rabbinic traditions enmesh the fetus in the more mundane business of carving out Israel's existence vis-à-vis external others misses the potency of the fetus as an internal image through which the rabbis conceive Israel in extraordinary relation with God and in radical contiguity with their biblical ancestors. Casting a wider view on the entirety of the fourteenth chapter of *Leviticus Rabbah*, where the Greek word *pinaks* appears (14:8), reveals that the primary relationship being articulated through the fetus, and here more specifically through the rabbinic discourse of procreation, is the one between Israel and God, not rabbinic Israel and Greco-Roman culture. At the same time, insisting upon God's central roles in procreation and embryology concretizes the continuity between biblical and rabbinic Israel; just as God is intimately involved in the coming into being of Israel's ancestors, so too God continues to bring forth rabbinic Israel. Similarly, midrashic interpretations about prenatal Jacob and Esau, while most certainly presenting an articulation of Israel in relation to not-Israel, establish that although Israel and Rome struggle with each other, God loves Israel and God knows and sanctifies Israel already from the womb.[24] Furthermore, these passages insist upon the sameness between rabbinic and biblical Israel as they reconceive prenatal Jacob as an ideal embodiment of rabbinic Israel who wishes to pray and study.

Projecting the relationship between God and Israel onto the fetus renders that relationship, which marks the very foundations of "Israelness," not only central but also innate. This innateness provocatively impacts the longstanding question about whether rabbinic Israel constructed itself primarily in either "ethnic" or "religious" terms in ways that I explore below. First, however, it should be noted that focusing on how these traditions construct the rabbinic fetus, and through it Israel, primarily in relation with God also complicates the ease with which the notion of the self is often depicted as bound to that of the "other."[25]

Rabbinic narratives about fetuses touch upon such fundamental questions as whether the rabbis were more focused inward, on some level attempting to bracket off or mitigate current historical locations through exegesis, or whether they were more focused outward, embracing their historical situations and grafting them onto scripture.[26] The related question, what the impact of Christianity was, also presents itself.[27] It might be abundantly clear from outside and in retrospect that rabbinic Israel takes shape within the setting of Greco-Roman antiquity and that rabbinic Israel, to a certain extent, defines itself through its discourses about the "nations" at large and sometimes the "true Israel" in particular. But the question at issue here is whether the rabbis would have seen it that way; would they have seen their own construction of Israel as if it were dependent on and mutually bound up with the simultaneous constructions of their "others"?[28]

The fetus is exceptionally well poised to function as an image through which the rabbis articulate Israel both from an insider perspective and in positive terms. Rabbinic narratives about fetuses are thus uniquely positioned to provide insights into how rabbinic Israel defined itself by what it is, not what it is not. As much as the rabbis used the fetus to traverse chronology, rabbinic narratives about the fetus provide one of the textual sites that allow contemporary readers to hear echoes of how the rabbis would have—and did—conceive Israel. If asked what defines Israel, the rabbis would not have answered negatively, defining Israel by what it is not; if asked what Israel is, the rabbis would not have answered that Israel is not (Christian) Rome, for example. They would have said, "We are Israel," meaning, as Neusner has pointed out, "'we are like that Israel of old' of which the Scriptures speak."[29] The most salient and basic point that midrashic expansions of Jacob and Esau's prenatal struggle make even goes so far as to claim not that "we are *like* that Israel of old," but we *are* that Israel, because Jacob is us. If it is true that, as William Scott Green has put it, "had there been no nations, Israel would have had to invent them,"[30] it does not follow that, according to the rabbis, had the nations not existed, Israel could not exist.

I recognize, as Green does, that "it would be foolish to deny that the extreme distinction between Israel and non-Israel, Jew and non-Jew, the pristine 'us' and the utterly-beyond-the-pale 'them,' is a fundamental component of any Judaic theory of the other."[31] But as Green also points out, "the possession of a fundamental principle of classification does not guarantee its application in a particular circumstance."[32] Rabbinic narratives about prenatal Jacob and Esau seem to present a prime example of such a "fundamental principle of classification" where Israel and not-Israel come into being together rather literally. But the far more prevalent, near omnipresent rabbinic tradition where Israelite fetuses sing to God at the crossing of the sea and thus not only praise God but also proclaim their relationship with God from the womb, which appears to be earlier than traditions about prenatal Jacob and Esau, does not fit this classification scheme—nor do many other rabbinic traditions about fetuses.

Certainly, rabbinic traditions at times call upon "others" while interrogating the collective self, but this might at least sometimes be better considered as the rabbis refining who and what Israel is, not defining Israel by means of what it is not. Although rabbinic traditions about prenatal Jacob and Esau significantly play off the opposition between Israel and not-Israel, even these traditions do not suggest that Israel cannot exist without its others. To the contrary, as Daniel Boyarin has pointed out, one of the interpretations of Gen. 25:23 "effectively erases Esau" at the precise moment that the text manifests the twelve tribes of Israel.[33] Without Esau, Israel does not fall away but proliferates. Without the other, Israel—prenatal and otherwise—still exists in relation with God and its biblical past.

Irad Malkin has noted that, in the wake of the influential work on ethnicity by Frederik Barth, who "claims that there is no 'core ethnicity'—that instead we find conceptual boundaries that an ethnic group creates against others," and due to the influence of Claude Levi-Strauss and other structuralists, "who assume that human beings are mentally predisposed toward binary thinking," a number of scholarly works about "Greeks and Others" have appeared.[34] Malkin voices the possibility and thus the warning "that some of us have been so conditioned by structuralist thinking that bipolar models have come to seem inevitable."[35] Within rabbinics scholarship, Sacha Stern has raised some similar concerns. Stern acknowledges that the opposition between Israel and non-Israel "was an important element in the rabbinic experience of self-identity," but he questions "whether this contrastive dichotomy constitutes indeed the main, *formative* feature of the rabbinic experience of Israel."[36] Ultimately, Stern maintains that a contrastive dichotomy is not formative, writing, "The rabbinic definition of 'Israel' is essentially based on an *introspective* analysis of the rabbis' own features, rather than on an external outlook."[37] Without insisting definitively on either a purely introspective or external outlook prevalent in rabbinic literature as a whole, this book does emphasize what has been called the "aggregative" identity formations along with, and in some ways over and against, "oppositional" forms of collective self-fashioning, highlighting the ways that rabbinic traditions use the fetus to forge a link—and bridge the divide—between biblical and rabbinic Israel.[38]

By constructing the fetus as both an individual Israel and representative of collective Israel, rabbinic narratives about the fetus open themselves up to an extratextual reading that likens Israel itself to a fetus in its mother's womb. Israel emerges as insulated but not impermeable, vulnerable and perhaps precarious but ultimately protected—by God. Israel is nourished by and even flourishes in its larger surroundings—like a fetus in its mother's womb—but Israel can be disembedded from these settings as surely as narratives about fetuses disassociate the fetus from its immediate environs of the womb.[39] The "other" becomes a part of how Israel articulates and refines itself as it, like a fetus, develops and changes, but rabbinic discourse about the other neither encapsulates the whole nor captures the essence of Israel's self-articulation. That essence comes from Israel's enduring relationship with God and its biblical past.

The Fetus as Israel

This book draws attention to the ways that rabbinic narratives use the image of a fetus to "think with"—about the relationships between God and Israel, Israel and its surrounding cultures, biblical and rabbinic Israel, and last but not least, women and men (within Israel). Although some of these traditions, particularly among those on embryology and procreation, might gesture toward a "universal horizon"—where the fetus could serve as representative of humanity more generally—even amid such a potentially universal reach a more localized focus on Israel emerges once the traditions are contextualized.[40] In the broadest terms, I carry over the textual occurrences where the fetus explicitly represents Israel—for example, in the traditions about collective Israelite fetuses at the Exodus and Revelation, prenatal Jacob, individual fetuses being taught, or commanded, Torah—into rabbinic sources about embryology and procreation, assuming that if the fetus illuminates Israel in one context, it does so too in the other.[41] Validation for such an assumption emerges within a number of texts about embryology themselves, which often reveal a specific focus on Israel. For example, in a tradition in *Genesis Rabbah* (72:6) that imagines God changing Dinah from male to female—whether in utero, at, or even after birth—the proof text cited in support of this change is Jer. 18:6, *O house of Israel, cannot I do with you as this potter? said the Lord. Behold, as the clay is in the potter's hand, so are you in my hand, O house of Israel.* A tradition from *Leviticus Rabbah* (23:12) about God fashioning the facial features of the fetus cites Deut. 32:18, *You neglected the Rock that begot you,* which is part of Moses' address to the Israelites before his death.[42] Furthermore, *Lev. Rab.* 23:12 interprets Lev. 18:3, *You shall not copy the practices of the land of Egypt where you dwelt, or of the land of Canaan to which I am taking you,* which is clearly addressed to the Israelites; Lev. 18:1–2 states, *And the Lord spoke to Moses, saying, Speak to the people of Israel and say to them I am the Lord your God.* A close reading of both *Gen. Rab.* 72:6 and *Lev. Rab.* 23:12 demonstrates that their focus is on Israel, and

God's involvement in aspects of fetal development (e.g., sex determination and resemblance) illustrates God's continual involvement in Israel.

Rabbinic traditions that theorize the creation of the embryo perhaps set their sights more toward a "universal horizon" than do those about fetal development. To be sure, the rabbis envision the God of Israel as the God, and creator, of the world, or to use a rabbinic title, "Master of the Universe" (*Ribono shel 'olam*). An extended passage extolling God's roles in (pro)creation recorded in the *Mekhilta of Rabbi Ishmael* consistently contrasts God's powers with those of humanity. Removed from their exegetical context, these traditions might reflect how the rabbis imagined God creating all embryos, but in both their immediate and broader literary context, these traditions are offered as interpretations, elucidations, of Exod. 15:11, *Who is like you, God, among the gods? Who is like you, glorious in holiness, fearful in praises, doing wonders?*—sung by the Israelites in praise of their God, who delivers them from bondage.[43] Likewise, an often cited tradition states, "There are three partners in [the creation of] a person (*'adam*): God, the father, and the mother." Presumably the use of *'adam* signals the universal scope of God's powers in procreation.[44] However, the same *sugya* already marked the fetus as Israel by imagining that it is taught Torah (b. Nid. 30b).[45] Furthermore, the *sugya* itself interprets *m. Nid.* 3:7, which is concerned with a woman's period of birth impurity (Lev. 12:4–6) as commanded specifically to Israel: *And the Lord spoke to Moses, saying, Speak to the people of Israel, saying, If a woman conceives, and bears a male child; then she shall be unclean seven days; as in the days of her menstruation, shall she be unclean. And in the eighth day the flesh of his foreskin shall be circumcised* (Lev. 12:1–3).[46] Finally, the fourteenth chapter of *Leviticus Rabbah*, which plays a pivotal role in my examination of rabbinic theories of procreation, is explicitly attached to, and grounded by, Lev. 12:2.[47] The chapter as a whole juxtaposes, and in many ways conflates, God's roles in creating the world, *'adam,* and each individual embryo. Again, shorn of its exegetical context, *Leviticus Rabbah* 14 might be seen as not only pointing toward a universal horizon but also having actually reached it.[48] Nevertheless, the fact that the chapter presents itself as interpreting Lev. 12:2, clearly addressed to Israel, and is placed in *Leviticus Rabbah*, a compilation hardly exemplary of a rabbinic universalist ideal,[49] has led me to conclude that the chapter uses the fetus not only as an image through which to illustrate God's relationship with humanity but also, and more fundamentally, to render quite concrete God's continued roles in creating, caring for, and sustaining Israel in particular. Rabbinic traditions about embryology and procreation call attention to the ways that the belief in the one God who creates, cares for, delivers, and sustains Israel—from its very beginnings—is essential to being Israel.

My emphasis on the ways that rabbinic traditions cast the fetus as representative of Israel and thus offer insights into rabbinic constructions of Israel specifically is not meant to put forth a decisive statement on, or even engage the question of, whether the rabbis were *either* universalistic *or* particularistic—a dichotomy and taxonomy already exposed as far too simplistic, not to mention political, by other scholars.[50] Nor am I advancing a purely ethnocentric bent, connoting an overarching concern only about Israel and its lineage, pervasive in rabbinic literature in toto. To the contrary, reading the fetus in these traditions as representative of Israel should be seen as undermining a single-minded emphasis on ethnicity understood as synonymous with genealogy or ancestry—not promoting it. Ultimately, reading the fetus *as* Israel reveals that the commonly made distinction between "ethnic" and "religious"—or better, "genealogical" and "covenantal"—constructions of identity is, like that of "particular" and "universal," too simplistic a taxonomy for rabbinic constructions of Israel—as articulated through the fetus.

Genealogy and Covenant

Rabbinic narratives about the fetus consistently point to the overlap, and even interarticulation, of genealogical and covenantal constructions of Israel. Following Joshua Levinson, I use the terms "genealogical" and "covenantal" instead of "religious" and "ethnic" to characterize what he refers to as the two dominant paradigms of fictive ethnicity that contend with each other throughout the rabbinic period.[51] He explains, "According to the former paradigm, inside and outside are established according to biological descent; according to the latter, identity is established by the acceptance of a certain institutionalized belief system."[52]

One of the advantages of Levinson's use of the terms "genealogical" and "covenantal" instead of "ethnic" and "religious" lies in its easier applicability to rabbinic sources; it avoids the possible problems and pitfalls of imposing the categories of "religion" and "ethnicity," both often considered modern classifications and fraught ones at that, onto rabbinic sources.[53] Another advantage of adopting Levinson's terminology stems from its precision, particularly evident in the use of the term "genealogical"; rather than use the broad, elusive term "ethnicity" as a synonym for genealogy or ancestry, which often eclipses or excludes the consideration of other contributing factors to ethnic formations, "genealogical" is simply more exact. At the same time, by including both the genealogical and covenantal paradigms under the rubric of "fictive ethnicity," Levinson allows for the multiple strategies of ethnic formations, which can be constructed through (appeals to) biological descent and systems of beliefs (*and* practices)—among other factors.[54] Furthermore, Levinson astutely notes that the two paradigms overlap and in some texts the difference between them even collapses.[55] As Denise Buell aptly summarizes the preceding two points, "Levinson does not cast the former [genealogical] as 'ethnic' and the latter [covenantal] as 'religious,' instead *both* paradigms help to constitute ethnicity, sometimes in conflict and other times intertwined."[56]

While Levinson points out the potential, and at times realized, overlap between genealogical and covenantal articulations of Israel, his primary interest lies in calling attention to the rabbinic development of a new narrative of identity, the narrative of affiliation, which comes to accommodate the "God-fearers."[57] He writes, "It is against the background of these two converging and conflicting narrations of identity that I want to discuss the emergence of a new type of literary plot and character in the rabbinic literature of this period, whose cultural function, I believe, was precisely to negotiate the faultlines and tensions created by the collocation of these two paradigms of fictive ethnicity."[58] According to Levinson, the God-fearers' ambiguous identity, their having "one foot on each side of the cultural fence,"[59] threatens both of the dominant fictions of ethnic identity.[60] Invoking Kristeva, he describes the God-fearers as "what disturbs identity, system, order, what does not respect borders, positions, rules."[61] They are, for Levinson, "a phenomenon that arises and takes shape on the margins of hegemonic culture, and sometimes against its will."[62]

I suggest that the fetus, both feet being planted firmly within rabbinic cultural borders (themselves somewhat malleable), be seen as, in many ways, the flip side of the God-fearer. The fetus takes shape, and its place, not on the margins of hegemonic culture and not against its will, but at its center.[63] Rabbinic narratives about the fetus work to produce and maintain identity, system, and order; the fetus cannot help but respect the borders, positions, and rules.[64] The fetus, unable to articulate its own thoughts and existing entirely at the will of the rabbis, becomes an ideal vehicle for rabbinic "ventriloquism"—in this case, using the voice of the fetus "as a tactic of self-fashioning."[65] However, I further suggest that rabbinic narratives about the fetus threaten to, and do, undermine the notion that there are two distinct, dominant fictions of ethnicity in rabbinic sources.

My point is not to deny that varied, even conflicting narratives of identity exist in rabbinic documents, which encompass a fairly vast time span and different geographical and cultural locations. My aim, rather, is to call attention to how the fetus, in contrast to the God-fearer and the convert—and it is the latter where the scholarly discourse about the distinction between "religious" and "ethnic" constructions of Israel is most often invoked[66]—provides an image that reflects Israel at its most basic, pristine, and ideal self.

Seeing the fetus as an image through which the rabbis articulate Israel calls into question the very distinction between the covenantal and genealogical paradigms because in these traditions both paradigms take center stage. By imagining the fetus behaving as, embodying, and being Israel already in a covenantal relationship with God, these narratives internalize the covenant—constituted by both practices and beliefs—rendering it and them as innate, intrinsic, and essential to being Israel as genealogy is presumed to be. The fetus emerges as Israel—before birth—not (only) because of its ancestry, but (also) by virtue of the beliefs and practices these traditions imagine it to be expressing.

In rabbinic narratives about the fetus, genealogical and covenantal paradigms not only overlap; they are always already one and the same thing. These narratives, though relatively few in number,[67] might very well articulate the dominant fiction of identity of rabbinic Israel as one that does not entail, does not even recognize, the bifurcation between genealogy and covenant—or for that matter between "ethnicity" and "religion." Only in the case of the anomalous,[68] be it represented by the convert or the God-fearer (and I do not wish to occlude the important differences and degrees of alterity between and among these characters and their plots as played out in rabbinic literature often in conflicting and contradictory ways), do the rabbis make what I see as an ad hoc accommodating move allowing the two deeply intertwined aspects of rabbinic Israelness to be thought of as distinct. Thinking primarily with and through the convert, as others have done, and with and through Levinson on the God-fearer—about Israel—indeed reveals that genealogy and covenant can be construed as distinct; thinking with and through the fetus, however, reveals that they need not be and perhaps were not. Rabbinic narratives about the fetus demonstrate that rabbinic Israel, from its origins and down to its foundations, is steeped in genealogy and saturated with covenant—*and vice versa*.[69]

Part of both the appeal and potency of rabbinic narratives about fetuses is that they function to internalize rabbinic conceptions of Israel, rendering Israel as something innate, literally inborn. These narratives not only entertain but also celebrate the notion of a stable and fixed, core essence of Israel—perhaps in the face of profound instability. As Levinson so eloquently writes, "When cultures feel threatened, they begin to tell tales. Sometimes these are retellings that strengthen the dominant fictions and sometimes they are new or revised narratives. Through these narratives, the imagined community guards its borders and defines for itself who is inside, who is outside, and why." I do not know how threatened the rabbis felt, and if so, exactly what or who caused them to feel it.[70] I suggest, however, that since rabbinic narratives about the fetus define who is inside and who outside from an exceedingly internal position, they encourage us to revise our own understanding of the two dominant rabbinic fictions of identity as one dominant fiction—and to see it in new ways.

Rabbinic narratives about the fetus set forth a radically essentialist and essentializing notion of Israel.[71] The internalization of certain beliefs and practices via the fetus suggests that such beliefs and practices are constitutive of and essential to Israel so much so that they are with Israel from their very beginnings—inscribed on the body as it takes shape. But here too, as Levinson points out, "the rabbis themselves seem to have been aware of the constructed nature of their narratives of identity."[72] Fetuses, clearly, do not sing, pray, or study on their own; they are made to do so for the express purpose of giving voice to the rabbinic visions of Israel. Moreover, despite the essentialism, simultaneously underlying and overt, of these narratives, the fetus itself is not a static entity but a strikingly apt embodiment of both mutability and durability.[73] Thus even the rabbinic appeal to fixity through the image of the fetus, the yearning or grasping for essentials, carries with it a sense of fluidity. In more specific terms, that which the rabbis project onto the fetus develops and expands, like a fetus, over time, reflecting the shifting elements that become constitutive of rabbinic Israel over time. The *Bavli* and post-*Bavli* traditions that imagine the fetus studying or receiving Torah, which are lacking in Palestinian compilations prior to the *Bavli*, provide the clearest evidence of such development.[74]

Finally, I close this section with the undoing of one last dichotomy. As with the distinction between "universal/particular" and "genealogical/covenantal" it should be clear by now that, in my reading, rabbinic narratives about fetuses challenge the distinction between practices and beliefs. While it is hard to surpass such images as the fetus studying Torah, or Israelite fetuses singing to God at Exodus and accepting God's Torah at Sinai, or prenatal Jacob already circumcised and wanting to kick down the doors of synagogues and houses of study to participate in his sons' central practices of being Israel, rabbinic narratives about fetuses do not emphasize practices over beliefs. Instead, rabbinic narratives about fetuses assert the centrality and mutually constituting roles of beliefs and practices to rabbinic Israel.[75] Rabbinic narratives about the fetus once again illustrate the inaccuracy of the already discredited division between rabbinic Israel and the new Israel along the lines of "works righteousness" and "faith."[76] The rabbinic fetus is imagined as doing all that it does in the service of espousing Israel's covenantal relationship with God, ultimately rendering innate Israel's beliefs in a God who created the world and Israel, took Israel out of Egypt, and gave Israel the Torah—and who continues to do so to this very day.

Seeing Fetuses: Terminology, History, and Context

In the early twentieth century, the preferred term for the product of conception was "embryo," but by the end of that century and at the beginning of this one, the term "fetus" had taken over.[77] If, in the span of one century, the terminology and that which it describes could prove so vulnerable to—or adept at—change, then there exists cause for concern about (super)imposing either of these terms onto late antique texts; there is a problem of translation. Despite both the problem of translation and its ever looming danger of anachronism, I have been speaking of fetuses in late antique rabbinic sources as if they are self-evident. However, contemporary feminist scholarship, which has uncovered some of the historical contingencies and uncertainties inherent in fetuses—both real and imaged—and my own desire for precision, which runs somewhat counter to the available sources, necessitate some explanation of my chosen terminology.

Barbara Duden provocatively asserts, "The thing that today also in colloquial speech is called a 'fetus,' the subject that late twentieth-century jurists or theologians call an 'embryo,' the entity that twentieth-century constitutional judges endow with rights, claims, and entitlements, did not exist in pre-modern times. Man's creation in utero was not conceived as the subsequent evolution of fetal, that is, pre-human form."[78] The birth of the fetus, according to Duden, takes place only at the very tail end of the eighteenth century, 1799 to be exact, and thus speaking about fetuses before that moment is to "colonize the past" and to "foreclose the unique historical modern nature of the fetus."⁷⁹ Duden capitalizes on the preponderance of children—not fetuses—depicted in early modern texts and images. She writes, "Illustrations depicting 'how the child sits and rests in the mother's womb' are not rare. 'Nascituri' (children ready for birth) were shown, but never a pre-infantile, pre-human embryonic shape."⁸⁰ Although Duden might astutely bring to light a keen inability to see and therefore reproduce fetuses in both textual and visual representations during the sixteenth through eighteenth centuries, her assertions simply do not hold if one reaches further back into history; while the "false aesthetics" and "willful disregard" of artists, laypeople, and even learned men during these three centuries might have stood in the way of their seeing and representing fetuses in pre-human embryonic form, the rabbis of antiquity did not share this uneasiness.⁸¹

Rabbinic sources exhibit very little hesitation about depicting, in what could be considered *graphic* detail, embryos or fetuses at various stages of development.⁸² The rabbis could not suffer from an inability to see developing fetuses because apparently such "specimens" were examined in the case of a miscarriage in order to determine the "precise" stage of development, which had an impact on halakhic concerns about (im)purities and the determination of firstborns.⁸³ For example, *y. Nid.* 3:3(50d) states, "What is the *shefir merukam* [articulated fetus]⁸⁴ of which they speak? All which begin like a locust.⁸⁵ They do not examine it in water because it is hard and makes it turbid, but in oil because it is soft and makes it clear.⁸⁶ And they only examine it in the sun." In contrast to Duden's eighteenth-century physician, who could not seem to fathom a "relic" from the womb as a developing fetus, seeing instead a mooncalf, mole, or clotted blood, the rabbis worried over determining the presence of a miscarried, but articulated fetus. Furthermore, it seems perfectly natural to them that at the beginning of its formation a fetus looks like an insect—"a pre-human embryonic shape."⁸⁷

The rabbis knew quite well that the contents of the womb are formed over time. They knew this presumably by examination as in the scenario above but most assuredly by exegesis;⁸⁸ scripture teaches them that the fetus is first clothed with skin and flesh and then with sinews and bones⁸⁹ and that its limbs are at first unarticulated and then later articulated.⁹⁰ Directly before *Lev. Rab.* 14:8 describes the fetus resting like a folded writing tablet with head, hands, heels, and buttocks, it states:

It is taught (in a tannaitic teaching): What is the form of the fetus [*tsurat havalad*]?⁹¹ At the beginning of its creation it is like a locust. [Its] two eyes are like two droppings of a fly. Its two ears are like two droppings of a fly. Its two arms are like two cords of crimson silk. Its mouth is drawn like a hair. Its "body" is like a lentil. If it was female, its "body" is like a barley grain in length. It has no developed hands and legs. And the rest of its limbs are attached like an unformed mass [*golem metsumtsamim*]. And concerning it, tradition states, *Your eyes have seen my unformed flesh* [*golmi*]. (Ps. 139:16)

Thus, *Lev. Rab.* 14:8 offers descriptions of a fetus as it develops from its beginning, as an undifferentiated mass and toward its end, as an articulated form. Both the structure and the specifics of the passage indicate that the fetus develops, suggesting that Duden's claim that the developing fetus did not exist in premodern times needs to be nuanced. The prehuman fetal form might not have been rendered in visual arts prior to the very end of the eighteenth century, but it was captured in texts of antiquity. While it may be true that a picture is worth a thousand words, it is no less true that texts can speak volumes. In order to historicize the contemporary fetus, textual images from antiquity need to be considered as well as early modern visual imaging techniques.

My point is not that something new did not occur at the end of the eighteenth century. The systematic collection of different fetuses in order to graphically represent continual gestational development from beginning to end is different than rabbinic sources' more ad hoc examinations, but this does not warrant the claim that prior to such a complete schematic the fetus did not exist. If the birth of the fetus is located in 1799, we foreclose the perhaps equally revelatory finding that although the Hebrew Bible does not have an exact word for fetus, the rabbis have more than one.[92]

The Hebrew words that I translate as "fetus" are *'ubar* and *valad* (*vlad*).[93] In almost all of the texts upon which I focus where either word appears, both words are followed by the phrase "in its mother's womb." To my knowledge, the word *'ubar* is never used to refer to a child that has been born, but the word *valad* sometimes connotes offspring.[94] While one might intuit that the word *valad* would signal a later stage of development, and thus perhaps *'ubar* connotes an earlier one, the sources do not bear this out with any consistency.[95] In most of the midrashic texts with which I am dealing, precision about the age of the fetus remains elusive, and therefore I translate both words as "fetus." If the text or context suggests something prior to eight weeks of development, I sometimes use the term "embryo," in keeping with medical and scholarly tradition,[96] but I do not translate *valad* as child because in rabbinic texts, this word primarily occurs in halakhic contexts about the status of offspring, not children per se, for which the Hebrew words would be *ben*, *bat*, or *tinoq*.[97] Furthermore, rabbinic sources maintain a distinction between fetuses and infants, even those at the moment of birth and newborns of one day, and thus to turn a fetus in its mother's womb into a child occludes such distinctions and does seem to be grossly inaccurate.[98]

The power of rabbinic narratives about the fetus rests in imagining *fetuses* as Israel; their meaning is dependent on the very distinction between fetuses and children, who, according to other rabbinic traditions, also sing at the crossing of the sea and accept the Torah at Revelation.[99] Imagining the developing fetus as both a part of and a symbol for Israel provides the rabbis with an image through which to inscribe Israel at the core of one's being, becoming the very essence through which one takes shape. Seeing fetuses in these traditions, and claiming that the rabbis saw fetuses too, is not an act of "colonization"; to my mind, it is a further historicization of the fetus that Duden and other feminist scholars seek—one that also reveals that to see and speak about fetuses was not, and need not always be, to speak about abortion.[100]

Lynn Morgan opens her article "Embryo Tales" by writing, "Today it is commonplace for human embryos and fetuses to speak to all manner of social issues."[101] She notes the proliferation of fetal images since the 1970s, but her focus is on what embryos were coaxed to say by embryologists in the second and third decades of the twentieth century. Morgan writes, "Although today we tend to associate visual images of human embryos and fetuses with the politics of abortion, I argue that the meanings ascribed to such images vary depending on the context in which they are visualized. I want to denaturalize the human embryo by showing that visual depictions of it were not always considered relevant to abortion or reproductive politics."[102] In the early part of the twentieth century, embryos were mobilized, even produced, to speak about race, nationality, and the relationship between humans and nonhumans—all by virtue of their tails.

The relevance of Morgan's work here lies not in inquiring whether the rabbis knew about embryos' tails[103] but in her distancing of embryos and fetuses from the context of abortion. She writes that "embryo meanings arise out of historically particular social anxieties and controversies,"[104] and she explains in more detail, "Embryos do not themselves pose conundrums or create disputes; rather, social controversies provide the interpretive lenses through which embryos are imbued with meaning."[105] Judging by the paucity of rabbinic materials expressly concerned with abortion, it would seem, perhaps surprisingly, that this was not one of the burning controversies with which they were most concerned.[106] Rabbinic narratives about fetuses, as I have suggested above, are embroiled in formulations of who and what constitutes Israel, and rabbinic fetuses are made to speak about matters central to rabbinic constructions of Israel. One of the most central aspects of Israel that emerges from rabbinic narratives about the fetus and traditions about its creation and care is Israel's relationship with God, which points to a profound difference between early twentieth-century embryologists and late antique rabbis.

In stark contrast to embryological endeavors in the early twentieth century, which according to Morgan worked to make people "understand fetal development as, above all, a biological process,"[107] the rabbis of antiquity worked to imbue embryology with theology. Fetal development, according to rabbinic traditions, is not a biological process but a theological one.[108] And, while "some embryologists and anatomists made a concerted effort to divest the fetal body of its religious and cultural associations in order to convince people that it should be understood as a strictly biological entity,"[109] the rabbis might be seen to have put forth an equally concerted effort to inscribe the fetal body as a cite of religious and cultural associations—and meanings. But there is one significant point of contact: ancient rabbis, like these twentieth-century embryologists, did not have to see embryos and fetuses primarily in the context of abortion.

I have been tempted to suggest that while I do not see seeing fetuses in rabbinic sources as an act of "colonization," I think reading rabbinic narratives about fetuses in light of contemporary abortion debates is a kind of colonization. In the end, although I find such an allegation useful insofar as it encourages closer scrutiny and precision in terms of terminology, history, and context, I find it too limiting for academic endeavors. One could say that writing about the past, translating ancient materials into contemporary, even academic, parlance is always already a colonizing endeavor, or at least one where anachronism must be continually negotiated. Now I prefer to think of it as a question of interpretation, sometimes more constrained by historical context and sometimes less so. I have chosen to highlight the ways in which rabbinic narratives about fetuses give voice to how the rabbis conceived Israel because I think this is the primary meaning—even intent—of the traditions in their contexts. Making these texts speak to contemporary debates explicitly about abortion is simply not the conversation into which I put these texts—these fetuses; it is not the context by which I frame them and not the lens through which I choose to see them here.[110] Instead, I place rabbinic narratives about the fetus and traditions about fetal creation and care within the broader context of feminist scholarship about gender and reproduction, which are, of course, core underlying issues being played out—and fought over—in contemporary abortion debates.

Feminist Readings of Fetal Imaging and Fetal Autonomy

Contemporary feminist scholarship on new reproductive technologies has compellingly illustrated that a significant by-product of increased fetal imaging is the disappearance of the pregnant woman; as the fetus becomes more visible, the pregnant female body becomes increasingly less visible.[111] Although much of this scholarship locates this phenomenon within the past forty years, Karen Newman provides an important historicization demonstrating that today's "free-floating" fetus has its roots in visual representations of the fetus going back long before.[112] Newman acknowledges that "There is no doubt that the media and new visual technologies have endowed the fetus with public persona, a notoriety, even a star status," but she continues, "However much a photograph's power of authentication may seem to exceed its powers of representation and thereby justify such a-historical claims as Petchesky, Sofia, Duden, and others make, in fact the presentation of the fetus as autonomous has a much longer history than these cultural analysts allow."[113] Re-presenting visual renderings from the ninth through twentieth centuries, the bulk of which are from the seventeenth and eighteenth centuries, Newman proposes a "core schema that was reproduced well into the eighteenth century: a uterus separated from the female body and a seemingly autonomous fetal figure," which "suppress completely fetal dependence on the female body by graphically rendering that body as a passive receptacle."[114] I suggest a further historicization of both the "autonomous" fetus and the near-absent female body, as they appear not in the visual arts but in the no less artistic and imaginative literary records of rabbinic literature. Newman opens the door to this more far-reaching historical perspective when she begins her study by voicing her preference for seeing the visual images upon which she focuses not as "visualizations" but, using Bruno Latour's work, as "inscriptions," which would include textual as well as visual representations.

Latour comes to his emphasis on inscriptions and the importance of writing things down in a laboratory setting, explaining, "I was struck, in a study of a biology laboratory, by the way in which many aspects of laboratory practice could be ordered by looking not at scientists' brains (I was forbidden access!), at the cognitive structures (nothing special), nor at the paradigms (the same for thirty years), but at the transformation of rats and chemicals into paper."[115] It is in the "laboratory" of the rabbis, the *beit midrash*, usually rendered "house of study" but for my purposes here reinscribed as the home of interpretation and inscription, that the fetus is both transformed into a writing tablet and imagined as more or less autonomous. Latour continues, "Focusing on the literature, and the way in which anything and everything was transformed into inscriptions was not my bias, as I first thought, but was for what the laboratory was made."[116] So too, the *beit midrash* was made to house rabbinic interpretations.[117] And it is in this space that as the fetus becomes a writing tablet through which the rabbis inscribe Israel onto the body, the woman becomes a house that can be unlocked and opened,[118] almost written away, allowing the rabbis to focus on the fetus as if autonomous and to cast the woman as its receptacle.[119]

The medieval tradition that imagines God turning women's bellies into glass so that God can address Israelite fetuses at Revelation most transparently reveals how rabbinic narratives that foreground fetuses simultaneously background women.[120] In this tradition, the women's bodies—except their wombs, which serve as a type of backlighting—rather literally fade from view as all eyes, including God's, focus on the fetuses. But this *virtual* absence of pregnant women is both already present in and an obvious outgrowth of earlier traditions.[121] The textual focus on the fetus over and against the pregnant woman is evident in the traditions that imagine Israelite fetuses singing to God at the crossing of the sea in order to proclaim *their* praise, along with all Israel's, of God as deliverer and those about prenatal Jacob and Esau wishing to enter their respective houses of worship while Rebekah merely passes them by; it is also apparent in the *Bavli* and post-*Bavli* traditions that imagine the fetus learning or receiving Torah, where the womb itself is transformed into a private *beit midrash*—or Mount Sinai. These traditions, which, as Petchesky writes of contemporary fetal imaging techniques, represent "the fetus as primary and autonomous, the woman as absent or peripheral,"[122] suggest that visual images of the fetus that marginalize or absent pregnant women have a history that can be traced back to textual representations long ago.

By superimposing Petchesky's insights about contemporary fetal images onto rabbinic traditions, I am not suggesting any causal effect between the two; these rabbinic narratives do not in and of themselves contribute directly to contemporary discourses that focus on the fetus at the expense of the pregnant woman.[123] However, the overlap between then and now, between texts about and images of fetuses, has encouraged me to think in terms of, or at least about, historical precedence and similarity—not sameness—across time.

Visual renderings of the autonomous fetus, be they of the seventeenth and eighteenth centuries or twentieth and twenty-first centuries, are heirs to a long-standing tradition of laying bare and writing off the woman in order to draw out the fetus. Rabbinic narratives about the fetus *and* traditions about its creation and care are part of this history, but these sources themselves rehearse and recast far older portrayals of women as passive in the process of generation already apparent in ancient Greek sources.[124] Contemporary images that present "the fetus as primary and autonomous, the woman as absent or peripheral,"[125] are but the most recent manifestations of textual imprints left long ago and still holding sway. As Nathan Stormer has written, "The womb and the public have been linked to one another since antiquity through understandings of conception that absent women from the process of genesis."[126] Today's images of free-floating fetuses are mirrored and underscored by the contemporary rhetoric of conception that tenaciously portrays women as passive.[127] And theories of procreation, as Carol Delaney has demonstrated, are linked not only to ideologies of gender but also often to ideas about God.[128] Rabbinic narratives about fetuses are likewise linked to rabbinic theories of procreation, which are in turn indelibly linked to rabbinic notions of God, and all, working in tandem, marginalize women. By turning a spotlight on one literary historical example of the ways in which cultural conceptions of God, gender, and reproduction are mutually constituted, further light will be shed on how these concepts are still deeply intertwined. Minimally, this book offers a further historicization of contemporary fetal imag(in)ing and fetal subjectivity, or "autonomy," than is often presented.

Structure, Parameters, and Chapter Outline

Structure

The body of this book consists of four chapters. The first two chapters focus on rabbinic narratives about fetuses, the latter two on rabbinic traditions about embryology and theories of procreation. Although the book might appear structurally divided, the two parts ultimately produce an organic whole.

The approach foregrounded in the earlier chapters, which reads rabbinic narratives about fetuses as important textual sites where the rabbis articulate that which is central—even innate—to Israel, informs and permeates my readings of rabbinic embryology in the latter chapters. I have chosen to begin with rabbinic narratives about fetuses read in such a way precisely because this type of framing illustrates that rabbinic embryology, in addition to demonstrating rabbinic embeddedness in late antiquity, also provides insights into rabbinic constructions of both God and Israel.[129] Moreover, this seems to me to be the main point and primary function of these traditions. The rabbis are not asking how much Greek in Jewish Palestine, to use Lieberman's phrase;[130] they are demonstrating God's active participation in the continual creation of Israel. Rabbinic traditions about embryology and procreation render manifest and material—literally inscribing in flesh and blood—the centrality of the belief in a God who creates and cares for Israel. Rabbinic embryology thus emerges as a largely theological endeavor, which further demonstrates how the rabbis turned to the fetus, here specifically its creation and care, to articulate that which is essential to Israel—an immanent and intimate God. If the first two chapters are seen as highlighting the ways in which Exodus and Revelation become continual events enacted in every generation by fetuses, the latter chapters demonstrate how Creation itself continues, since the creation of the embryo is likened to the creation of the world; embryogeny recapitulates cosmogeny.[131]

The other connecting thread through the chapters is the displacement, at times partial and at times complete, and the overall passivity of women. Although one might think that seeing fetuses means seeing pregnant women and that to write about fetuses is also to write about pregnant women as actively present, rabbinic traditions consistently demonstrate that this is not always the case. The rabbis show themselves as adept as their counterparts, throughout late antiquity and unto today, at calling on fetuses and embryology not only to articulate the collective self but also to represent, reify, and write hierarchical constructions of gendered selves into the very nature of things.

Rabbinic embryology as presented here proceeds along much the same lines that Eve Keller has noted regarding early modern embryology. She writes, "The story of embryology in the seventeenth century looks therefore in two directions: toward concerns about the self and the manner of its construction and toward the ways in which gender functions in the process."[132] Although I deal much more explicitly with how gender functions in the last two chapters of the book, the construction of Israel as normatively gendered male is ever present in the first two chapters. When the rabbis reflect upon what constitutes Israel, maleness serves as both the norm and model as well as the ideal. The two parts of this book should be seen as mutually illuminating to the extent that constructions of the collective rabbinic self (Israel) are interarticulated with constructions of gender.

Hierarchical constructions of gender are evident both in rabbinic theories of procreation and rabbinic embryology, as well as in the presumed, and often explicit, gender of the rabbinic fetus. Rabbinic theories about procreation are overwhelmingly far more aligned, though by no means identical, with what has come to be known as a "one-seed" theory of generation, where primacy is given to the male contribution over the female's in the creation of the embryo. Furthermore, rabbinic embryology, as a theological endeavor, attributes the development and care of the fetus to God, thereby erasing women's active roles even in nurturing and protecting the fetus.[133] One might reasonably assume that female, as well as male, fetuses sing to God after crossing the sea and that female fetuses are included among those who accept the Torah at Revelation—surely they are among those who are created and cared for by God. However, when the rabbis imagine individual fetuses, they imagine them as male—to the point that the one female fetus that makes it into rabbinic literature, Dinah, is "made male."[134]

Topical Parameters

This book follows the rabbinic gaze and looks at the rabbis looking at fetuses, often at the expense of pregnant women themselves. The claims made throughout this book about the absenting or obscuring of pregnant women should not be taken as suggesting that rabbinic narratives have nothing to say about pregnant women in other contexts; it simply reflects my findings in this specific context. Similarly, this book does not attempt an exposition of "the womb" in rabbinic literature. Furthermore, I have chosen not to highlight the womb as the place from which rabbinic Israel is constituted and within which it takes root, instead preferring to focus on the incorporation of fetuses into the discursive "field" through which rabbinic Israel articulates itself. Although the language of the texts consistently locates the fetus "in its mother's womb," rendering the womb rhetorically present, I think that the womb ultimately slips from view and the focus in these traditions is fixed upon the fetus. Especially when the word *valad* is used, the phrase "in its mother's womb" appears to function as a linguistic distinction between miscarriages or offspring that have been born and those yet to be born, not as indicating any profound significance to the womb itself.[135]

Rabbinic traditions about embryology and theories of procreation, which by and large figure the womb as passive (but sometimes deadly), seem to undercut reading too much significance into the womb itself in this context. Certainly, a "Jewish" womb is presumed by these traditions, as is a "Jewish" father (or seed), and perhaps a "Jewish" womb is an implicit prerequisite. However, what marks the fetus as Israel is not its passive dwelling in a passive vessel but its imagined beliefs and actions that espouse a relationship with God.

Textual Parameters

Most of the chapters focus on rabbinic traditions from tannaitic (ca. third century CE) and amoraic (fourth to sixth century CE) compilations of Palestinian provenance, the latter always figuring more prominently because rabbinic narratives about the fetus and midrashic traditions about embryology are more abundant there.[136] Parallels from the Babylonian Talmud (*Bavli*) are considered when significant, and traditions unique to the *Bavli* are included when they are so well known that to leave them unexamined would significantly impact a sense of the completeness of this project, for example, the fetus studying Torah and the "two-seed" procreation theory. Both of these traditions, moreover, resonate with those found in Palestinian compilations prior to the *Bavli* and inform post-*Bavli* medieval sources, so their consideration is crucial—not in order to present rabbinic materials as a seamless whole but to provide a sense of how the motif of the fetus develops over time. Some traditions from *Midrash Tanhuma* (ca. eighth century) are incorporated for similar reasons. Such development is central to Chapter 2, which covers rabbinic narratives about fetuses from the tannaitic through medieval periods. It is in that chapter especially that I have opted for flexible parameters when traditions exist outside of Palestinian compilations that are relevant to the specific motif under consideration, but all attempts have been made to note when I am citing from a tannaitic, amoraic, or medieval compilation.

The primary objective of this project is to set forth rabbinic narratives about the fetus and rabbinic embryology in midrashic traditions;[137] an in-depth exploration of early Christian and patristic sources about the fetus and embryology is beyond the scope of this study.[138] Where rabbinic traditions themselves seem to be in dialogue with early Christian or patristic sources, I explore the possible relationship between them. I also make note of some broad-based commonalities between patristic and rabbinic theories of procreation, which demonstrate both groups' adaptation of ancient Greek theories of generation to fit their theological purposes. More detailed comparison between rabbinic and early Christian and patristic sources about the fetus and embryology awaits further study, and I hope that this book, with all its limitations vis-à-vis comparative exploration, will contribute to realizing such potentially fruitful work.[139]

Chapter Outline

Chapter 2, "Covenantal Fetuses," begins with what I consider to be the earliest extant rabbinic tradition about fetuses, where Israelite fetuses sing to God at the crossing of the sea. It stretches forward to include the latest tradition considered in this study, where Israelite fetuses serve as guarantors for their parents so that Israel can receive the Torah. I also juxtapose these traditions with others about individual fetuses that experience their own exoduses and revelations. By locating Israelite fetuses, as a collective, at Exodus and Revelation and by imagining individual rabbinic fetuses partaking in their own privatized versions of these two most fundamental events of Israel's formation, the rabbis internalize the covenantal relationship between God and Israel. What emerges from these traditions is that the construction of rabbinic Israel depends on the covenant, which I understand to be encapsulated in the acknowledgment of God as deliverer from "Egypt" and the deliverer of Torah—here projected onto fetuses. A mutual covenantal relationship emerges explicitly when the tannaitic tradition about singing fetuses is joined with the medieval one about fetuses serving as guarantors so that Israel can receive the Torah. In the earlier tradition, Israelite fetuses sing, *Who is like you, God, among the gods?* (Exod. 15:11), and in the latter one, God reciprocates, *Happy are you, O Israel, Who is like you?* (Deut. 33:29).

Chapter 2 covers the broadest chronological range of traditions presented in this study, and it serves well to chart out some of the territory. Furthermore, casting such a wide view, which encompasses tannaitic to medieval sources, allows one to see both the continuity of the motif of using fetuses to articulate essential aspects of Israel and how the construction of rabbinic Israel develops over time. Finally, this chapter focuses on the use of the fetus for positive, internal constructions of Israel; Israel is defined by what it is—in a covenantal relationship with God—not by what it is not, and the texts do not explicitly invoke rabbinic Israel's "others," in order to articulate the collective self.

Chapter 3, "And the Sons Struggled," focuses on traditions about Jacob and Esau's struggle in Rebekah's womb, demonstrating that the rabbinic typology of Jacob as Israel and Esau as (Christian) Rome, long noted by scholars, is projected onto both Jacob and Esau as fetuses. Already in utero, Jacob represents rabbinic Israel as a collective; here rabbinic Israel takes shape in relation to its others, in relation to biblical Israel, and in relation with God. I consider the possibility of an exegetical exchange between rabbinic and patristic interpretations of prenatal Jacob and Esau, particularly Origen's interpretations of Romans 9, which represents a diametrically opposing typology in patristic sources, where Jacob represents the New Israel, and Esau, the Jews. This chapter also examines the much broader question of the impact of Christianity on rabbinic Judaism through the narrow prism of rabbinic and patristic interpretations of prenatal Jacob and Esau.

Chapter 4, "Embryology as Theology," demonstrates that despite the overall consonance between rabbinic and Greco-Roman embryology, rabbinic embryology adapts ancient embryology to suit its theological purposes. Since many of the specific details about pregnancy and fetal development are consistent with those evident in Greco-Roman sources and lacking in biblical sources, rabbinic embryology provides an important trope through which to examine the situatedness of the rabbis in their larger late antique setting. While rabbinic embryology contributes significantly to contemporary concerns about how the rabbis negotiated their relationship with their broader geocultural surroundings, the sources themselves more profoundly testify to how the rabbis used embryology as a vehicle through which to expound upon Israel's relationship with God. Rabbinic embryology serves theology, and it functions primarily to give shape and texture to the relationship between God and Israel.

Chapter 5, "Reproductive Theology," focuses on rabbinic theories of procreation. Much of this chapter revolves around an in-depth exploration of the fourteenth chapter of *Leviticus Rabbah*, which interprets Lev. 12:2, *When a woman* tazria' *and gives birth to a male*. I explore how and why this verse, which could have been mobilized in support of women's active contribution to the creation of the embryo by interpreting it to mean "when a woman *emits seed*," was instead consistently read as "when a woman *conceives*"—receives seed. Although the fourteenth chapter of *Leviticus Rabbah* as a whole provides both the most extended rabbinic engagement with this verse and the most extensive Palestinian discourse about procreation, it remains largely overlooked in scholarship about rabbinic theories of procreation, which often focus on one (counter) tradition from the *Bavli*. Here, *Leviticus Rabbah* 14 provides the lens through which to explore rabbinic theories of procreation not only because it hinges upon interpreting Lev. 12:2 but also because it reveals the extent to which the rabbinic discourse about procreation is once again thoroughly imbued with theology. Instead of asking whether the rabbis adopted a "one-seed" or "two-seed" theory of generation, which is the common question put to rabbinic sources, the chapter demonstrates that the question itself is an imposition that ultimately obscures the primary message of these traditions. The rabbis are not asking how men and women contribute to procreation, but how God, men, and women—in that order—create the embryo.

The Torah of the Fetus

I began this chapter with a text that likens the image of the fetus to a *pinaks*, a folded writing tablet. A parable in *Genesis Rabbah* uses the same Greek word to describe the Torah into which God looked and created the world.[140] If fetuses "take their meanings from the scripts that they are asked to read,"[141] the overlapping imagery between the "original" Text and origin stories—perhaps only coincidental—becomes quite consequential. Instead of seeing the fetus in rabbinic narratives as a blank slate, an empty image devoid of meaning and cultural significance, this book explores the ways in which the rabbis of antiquity called forth the fetus to help articulate, essentialize, and embody that which is central to Israel—without which, Israel would not be. Rabbinic narratives about the fetus and midrashic traditions about embryology not only serve as important textual sites in which the rabbis imagine Israel; they also inscribe Israel onto the body as it takes shape. As God looked into the Torah to create the world, the rabbis looked to the fetus to conceive Israel.

Chapter 2
Covenantal Fetuses

From the womb of my mother, you are my God.
—Psalm 22:11

Two times the Babylonian Talmud states, "Nation can mean only fetuses."[1] Although in its contexts, this statement appears connected to particular midrashic interpretations of specific verses, I use it here to call attention to the ways that rabbinic traditions, from the third through tenth centuries CE, use fetuses to articulate and internalize what is most central to rabbinic Israel's collective identity, its national character: the covenant between God and Israel.[2] At Israel's moments of birth, the Exodus from Egypt and the Revelation of Torah at Mount Sinai, the rabbis imagine Israelite fetuses singing along with, and then speaking on behalf of, Israel, ultimately giving voice to their acceptance of its national charter—the Torah. As one tradition states, "The Torah was founded upon fetuses."

Almost a century ago, Julius Preuss wrote, "The not infrequent expressions found in the sermonizing sections of the *Midrash* such as 'the children began to sing hymns in their mother's wombs, and they praised the Lord, etc.' are naturally not to be taken literally."[3] Without suggesting that these traditions be taken literally, I do take them quite seriously. Rabbinic narratives about fetuses are important textual sites where the rabbis reveal that which is most foundational to rabbinic Israel—its covenantal relationship with God—by projecting it onto the fetus, a symbol for Israel as it takes shape.

Collective Israelite Fetuses

One of the most pervasive rabbinic traditions about the fetus recorded already in tannaitic compilations teaches that after Israel crosses the Red Sea, the fetuses join in singing their God's praises.⁴ At a moment of national birth, when Israel ceases to be just Jacob as an individual and becomes a collective people, the rabbis consistently assert that the fetuses in their mother's wombs praised God. The *Mekhilta of Rabbi Ishmael* (*Shirata* 1) states:⁵

> *I will sing unto God* . . . [*God is my strength and song*] (Exod. 15:1–2). R. Yosi the Galilean says: "Behold scripture says, *Out of the mouths of babes* [*'olalim*] *and sucklings you have founded strength* (Ps. 8:3). *Out of the mouths of babes*: these are the fetuses that are in their mother's womb. As it is said, *Or as a hidden untimely birth I had not been;* [*as fetuses*⁶ (*'olalim*) *that never saw light*] (Job 3:16). *And sucklings*: these are those who suck from their mother's breast. As it is said, *Gather the children and those that suck the breasts* (Joel 2:16)." . . . R. Meir says, "Even the fetuses that are in their mother's womb opened their mouths and sang before God, as it is said, *Bless God in the congregations, the Lord from the womb* [*mimakor*]⁷ *of Israel* (Ps. 68:27)."⁸

The *Mekhilta* first juxtaposes Exod. 15:1–2 and Ps. 8:3, because both verses use the word strength (*'oz*). R. Yosi the Galilean interprets the word "babes" (*'olalim*) mentioned in Ps. 8:3 to refer to fetuses in their mothers' wombs, based upon his interpretation of Job 3:16, *fetuses* [*'olalim*] *that never saw the light*.⁹ According to the interpretation attributed to R. Yosi the Galilean, the word "babes" in Ps. 8:3 teaches that the fetuses in their mothers' wombs sang to God at the sea. Soon after, the *Mekhilta* cites a tradition attributed to R. Meir, which also asserts that fetuses sang to God. The statement attributed to R. Meir uses Ps. 68:27, midrashically read so that *mimakor Israel* is understood as "from the womb, or source, of Israel." Thus fetuses, Israel at its source, opened up in song to praise God after the crossing of the sea. These collective Israelite fetuses recognize God as the God who delivered them out of Egypt, and thus they praise God for their deliverance.¹⁰

This tradition magnifies the scope and importance of the Exodus, which climaxes with the miracle of the crossing of the sea. It was so grand that even fetuses and nursing babes experienced the event and sang God's praises. Likewise, just three months, or one trimester, later, fetuses will witness, and partake in, the Revelation of Torah at Mount Sinai, as the following tradition makes clear.

I cite the tradition as it appears in the medieval compilation *Midrash on the Ten Commandments,* but after presenting the text, I discuss some of its textual precursors. In all its variations, the tradition consistently imagines that before God gives the Torah to Israel, God asks for guarantors that they will fulfill it. Here, after God rejects Abraham, Isaac, and Jacob as suitable guarantors, Israel offers its children, specifically its fetuses and sucklings:

They said before God, "Behold, our children [*baneinu*]." Immediately the Holy Blessed One said, "Give me these guarantors and I will accept them." Immediately the children of Israel brought their women with sucklings and their pregnant women and the Holy Blessed One made their bellies like glass and they [the fetuses] speak with God. God said to them, "Do you see that I want to give the Torah to your parents, and you are the guarantors for them, that they will fulfill it?" They said to God, "Yes." God said to them, "I am the Lord your God who brought you out [of Egypt]?" They said to God, "Yes." "There will be no other gods before you?" They said to God, "No [there will be no other gods . . .]." God said to them, "You will not swear falsely by the name of the Lord your God?" They said to God, "No, [we will not swear falsely . . .]." And so it was that they answered God yes to all the yes questions and no to all the no questions/commandments. And from where do we know that the Torah was founded upon fetuses in their mothers' womb and sucklings? As it is said, *Out of the mouths of babes and sucklings You have founded strength* (Ps. 8:3). And there is no strength except for Torah. As it is said, *God will give strength (= Torah) to his people* (Ps. 29:11). And when the Holy Blessed One saw Israel, that with all of their hearts they were intending and from so much love they were hurrying to receive the Torah, God praised them and exalted them, as it is said, *Happy are you, Israel: Who is like you?* (Deut. 33:29).[11]

This text magnifies the scope and miraculousness of Revelation at Sinai such that even fetuses in their mother's wombs, again coupled with suckling babes, participated in this foundational event. Just as the fetuses sang to God, who took them out of Egypt and parted the sea for them, here the fetuses accept God's Torah on behalf of their parents and upon themselves, attesting that they will have no other Gods but God and, once again, that God is the God who brought them out [of Egypt], and so forth.

The miracle of the crossing of the sea is matched, and surpassed, at Revelation, where God peers into women's wombs and converses with the fetuses, asking, not commanding, in this rabbinic refashioning of Revelation, if they will serve as guarantors—as collateral—for their parents and accept the covenant upon themselves.[12] The fetuses agree, thus ensuring and insuring that God's covenant with Israel will be fulfilled on into the future. What better image upon which to project continuity, a very future, than the fetus?

The future orientation of this text is central. Revelation not only takes place in the present, as the fetuses accept the covenant upon themselves but it stretches forth endlessly into the future, through the fetuses of coming generations. Like Ps. 29:11, with its future tense assertion that, midrashically read, God will give Torah to God's people, this midrash insists on the future promise of Israel, embodied by its fetuses. If Abraham, Isaac, and Jacob cannot serve as Israel's guarantors, then clearly no past generation can serve as Israel's guarantor.

Although the fetuses' participation grasps the reader's attention, it should not occlude from view that the tradition reconceives Revelation itself. Gone is the Israel who fears God, who fears that God's voice will bring death, preferring to remain ignorant of the details or hide behind Moses (Exod. 20:16). In this reimagined Revelation, Israel presents its women, neither separating from them nor the mountain, as Exod. 19:15 and 19:12 require.[13] In fact, excised from the text is any reason Israel might fear God, who now so benevolently speaks with fetuses. The thunder and lightning, the chaos and fear, so present in the biblical account of Revelation have been removed. The awesomeness of the event, however, has not so much been left behind or forgotten as internalized, witnessed by fetuses in their wombs, now alight, in the place of the sky and mountain.[14] And yet, also gone is the God who requires no collateral, no guarantee, that God's gift will be fulfilled in future generations. What emerges from this text, through the image of the hidden fetus now revealed and a softer, kinder God who asks for assurance and converses with fetuses, is a renewed, eternally renewable, covenant, emphasizing the willingness of Israel—from within, at its core, and into the future.

Although I have cited this tradition from one of its medieval versions, parallel traditions appear in earlier compilations. The *Mekhilta of Rabbi Shimeon* on Exod. 19:17 previously suggested that God asked Israel for guarantors before God gave Israel the Torah:[15] "The Holy Blessed One said, 'Behold, I need guarantors [*arevim*].' [Israel said], 'Behold, heaven and earth will be our guarantors.' God said to them, 'They are busy.' They said, 'Our children [*baneinu*] will be our guarantors.' God said, 'Behold they are good guarantors,' as scripture says, *Out of the mouths of babes and sucklings, You have founded strength* (Ps. 8:3)."[16] This midrash, like the one about singing fetuses discussed above, cites Ps. 8:3, *Out of the mouths of babes and sucklings, You have founded strength*. Perhaps here too, "babes" should be understood as referring to fetuses. *Song of Songs Rabbah* (1:4), attributes an expanded version of this tradition, which also cites Ps. 8:3, to R. Meir, the tanna who ostensibly claims that the fetuses sing after crossing the sea.[17] Despite the fact that both traditions fail to explicitly mention fetuses, this might have been obvious through the common verse, Ps. 8:3, or the shared attribution to R. Meir. Regardless, later traditions do not hesitate to explicitly mention the fetuses' participation at Revelation, thereby either making manifest that which already seemed implied, or, by further fabricating the tradition, to enhance the miraculousness of the event.

I have followed the tradition about fetuses at Revelation backward, possibly establishing that already in earlier sources, the rabbis imagined fetuses partaking in this event. It is, however, quite certain that the tradition about fetuses at the crossing of the sea travels forward, from tannaitic compilations through amoraic sources and into medieval ones, where, in the *Midrash on Psalms*, the two traditions appear in close proximity, as interpretations of Ps. 8:3, *Out of the mouths of babes and sucklings, You have founded strength*.[18] God has laid the foundations of strength, of Torah, in Israelite fetuses. By making the fetuses not only the guarantors for their parents but also the direct recipients of Sinaitic Revelation, and by including fetuses at the Red Sea as those who also experience the Exodus, the rabbis internalize the covenantal relationship between God and Israel.

Although the tradition about fetuses singing at the crossing of the sea and the one about fetuses at Revelation exist chronologically separated, the two traditions form a textual unit, a dialogue of sorts, traversing any historical gap. When brought together, they give voice to the covenantal relationship between God and Israelite fetuses suggested by both traditions. According to the tannaitic tradition, the singing fetuses at the crossing of the sea would have sung, *Who is like you, God among the gods?* (Exod. 15:11), and in reciprocal fashion, at the end of the medieval tradition about the fetuses receiving God's Torah, God states, *Happy are you, Israel: Who is like you?* (Deut. 33:29).[19]

Rabbinic Fetuses

Like the rabbinic portrayal of Israelite fetuses who praise God for their deliverance from Egypt and through the sea, another rabbinic tradition imagines that each and every fetus praises God. And, like the Israelite fetuses who receive Torah at Mount Sinai, the rabbis imagine that every fetus receives Torah.[20] In what follows, I examine the recurrence of praise and study attributed to the individual fetus in rabbinic sources. Further, I juxtapose God's deliverance of Israel out of Egypt with God's continual deliverance of each fetus from the womb, and I also juxtapose God's revelation of Torah to the Israelites at Mount Sinai with God's teaching or delivering Torah to the fetus, thereby making both Exodus and Revelation events not only located in the past, but continually enacted in the rabbinic present.

Beyond the often repeated tradition about the collective Israelite fetuses of the generation of the Exodus praising God as their deliverer, *Leviticus Rabbah*, a fifth-century Palestinian midrash on the book of Leviticus, imagines that all fetuses sing God's praises. *Lev. Rab.* 4:7 interprets Psalms 103 and 104, which mention the word soul five times: "R. Yehoshua ben Levi said: 'Five times the word soul is written here. Five times stands for the five worlds that a person sees. *Bless the Lord, O my soul: and all that is within me* (Ps. 103:1). [This is said] at the time that one dwells in its mother's womb."[21] Here, Ps. 103:1 is interpreted as "Bless the Lord, O my soul, from within the womb, the first world one sees." *Lev. Rab.* 4:7 does not specify for what the fetus praises God, but Psalms 103 and 104 provide ample statements affirming God as the creator of everything. Furthermore, Ps. 103:4 states, [*Bless the Lord, O my soul . . .*] *Who redeems your life from the pit, who encircles you with loving kindness and compassion.*[22] Although *Lev. Rab.* 4:7 does not explicitly state that the fetus utters this specific verse while in its mother's womb, the biblical context and proximity of these verses suggest that, once again, God redeems or delivers all Israel from the womb, just as God delivered the Israelites—even those in the womb—from Egypt.

That God delivers the fetus from the womb is further apparent in the fourteenth chapter of *Leviticus Rabbah*, which provides a series of traditions about the creation and care of the fetus. Although this chapter will be discussed at length in the latter portion of this book, here I mention two traditions, which credit God with delivering the fetus from the womb. *Lev. Rab.* 14:2 likens the womb to a prison, in which God cares for the fetus and from which God releases and "brings forth" the fetus. *Lev. Rab.* 14:4 interprets Job 38:8, *Who shut up the sea with doors, when it broke forth and came out of the womb*, to describe the gestation and birth, or delivery, of the fetus from its mother's womb, suggesting that just as God let the sea issue out of the womb, God brings forth the fetus from the womb.

The crossing of the sea itself has been interpreted as nothing short of a miraculous birth story on a national level.[23] Ilana Pardes characterizes the parting of the Red Sea as the preeminent wonder God performs for the Israelites, explaining that the passage "marks the nation's first breath—out in the open air—and serves as a distinct reminder of the miraculous character of birth. Where there was nothing, a living creature emerges all of a sudden." She continues, "It is an intensified miracle: a wonder on a great scale. The two enormous walls of water, the ultimate breaking of the waters, and the exciting appearance of dry land all seem to represent a gigantic birth, a birth that is analogous to the creation of the world."[24] Thus, God "births" the Israelites out of Egypt, and, in like fashion, God brings forth every fetus from the womb.

Before God delivers the fetus from the womb, however, according to rabbinic traditions from the *Bavli* and post-*Bavli* compilations, God delivers the Torah to the fetus. The *Bavli* (*Nid.* 30b), in the context of an extended discourse about the fetus attributed to R. Simlai,[25] states, "And they teach it [the fetus] all the Torah in its entirety."[26] In order to substantiate this claim, the text first cites Prov. 4:4, applying it to the fetus, *He taught me also, and said to me, Let your heart hold fast to my words: keep my commandments and live*. Presumably this is a fitting proof text for the fetus because it teaches that if the fetus keeps the commandments, the fetus will live, that is, be born, and/or it is fitting because the previous verses state, *Hear, <u>you children</u>, the instruction of a father. . . . For I give you good doctrine, do not forsake <u>my torah</u>* (Prov. 4:1–2). The *Bavli* then brings another proof text, "And scripture says, [*As I was in the days of my youth*] *when the teaching sod of God was upon my tent* (Job 29:4)." This verse is also applied to the fetus in its "tent," or dwelling, which is to say, in its mother's womb.[27] But the *Bavli* then pauses to consider why this second verse was cited, because presumably one proof text would be enough to prove that the fetus learns Torah. The text answers, "You might have said that a prophet was the one who stated it; Come and learn, *When the teaching of God was upon my tent* (Job 29:4)." This answer is somewhat ambiguous, because according to rabbinic traditions, both Solomon, traditionally thought to be the author of Proverbs, and Job were prophets.[28] In either case, the concern is that one might think that only Solomon or Job knew Torah in the womb.[29] Thus the *Bavli* repeats Job 29:4, asserting that each fetus learns Torah, not just Solomon or Job.[30] Finally, although the text does not explicitly mention who teaches the fetus Torah, both proof texts suggest that the fetus learns Torah from God.

Although neither tannaitic nor Palestinian amoraic compilations record a parallel to the tradition about the fetus learning Torah, post-Talmudic sources record a similar, though slightly modified tradition. *Midrash Tanhuma* (*Tazria'*) explicitly maintains that God teaches the fetus Torah: "So this fetus, before he comes forth from his mother's womb, the Holy Blessed One commands him, 'From this you shall eat and from this you shall not eat and this is unclean to you.' And when he accepts upon himself in his mother's womb all of the commandments that are in the Torah, after that he is born. As scripture states, *When a woman conceives and gives birth to a male* (Lev. 12:2)."[31] According to this tradition, God first teaches, or commands, the fetus the instructions of *kashrut*, echoing the language of Deuteronomy 14. Furthermore, the fetus is born only after it has accepted all of the commandments in the Torah, and in contrast to *b. Nid.* 30b, where at birth the newborn is struck by an angel causing him to forget what he has learned,[32] here the fetus apparently does not forget what it has learned upon birth. Here the fetus is born only once it has accepted the Torah and its commandments, and in doing so, internalized the covenant, ensuring both the fetus's future and that of the covenant.

The medieval tradition about the collective Israelite fetuses at Revelation discussed above combines elements of these *Bavli* and post-*Bavli* rabbinic traditions that imagine that the individual fetus learns or receives Torah and the tannaitic tradition about the collective Israelite fetuses singing to God at the crossing of the Red Sea as well as amoraic traditions, which already imagined that Israel offered its children as guarantors that the Torah will be kept throughout the generations. The individual fetus that learns or receives Torah, thus internalizing the covenant, is, in the medieval tradition, writ large and projected upon the collective Israelite fetuses such that Revelation itself becomes internalized.

Contexts

Rabbinic traditions about fetuses participating, on both collective and individual levels, in Exodus and Revelation should be seen as part of the larger rabbinic project of magnifying the significance—and establishing the timelessness—of these events for rabbinic Israel. According to rabbinic traditions, Exodus and Revelation did not simply take place in the past, as the nation was coming into being; these two foundational events continue to be experienced in their own day and presumably into the future. For example, the Mishnah states, "In every generation Israel is obligated to see itself as if it went forth from Egypt. . . . Therefore, we are obligated to thank, praise, laud, glorify, exalt, honor, bless, extol and adore the one who did, for our fathers *and for us,* all these miracles" (*m. Pes.* 10:5).[33] This mishnah, made famous through its incorporation into the Passover Haggadah, links rabbinic Israel, and all future generations, with the generation of the Exodus because all of them experience the Exodus. A lesser-known tradition, from the *Mekhilta of Rabbi Ishmael*, which is roughly contemporary with the Mishnah, also links Israel, past, present, and future. Here, however, the connection is even placed in the mouths of the Israelites as they come forth from Egypt, singing to God at the Red Sea. Interpreting the mention of "my father's God" in Exod. 15:2, *The Lord is my strength and song, and he has become my salvation; he is my God, and I will praise him; my father's God, and I will exalt him,* the *Mekhilta* (*Shirata*3) states, "The congregation of Israel said before the Holy

Blessed One, 'Master of the Universe, not only on account of the miracles that you have done for me do I sing songs and hymns before you, but also for the miracles that you did for my fathers and for me, and for those that you will do for me in every generation.'"[34]

In these two traditions, the rabbis and the Israelites meet, as the rabbis look back to the Exodus and place themselves in it, and the Israelites themselves, according to the rabbis, look both back to their predecessors and forward to their future. At the splitting of the sea, time collides, bringing generations of Israel together.

In addition to the rabbinic insistence that every generation experience the Exodus, so too every generation experiences Revelation. A tradition recorded in *Midrash Tanhuma* interprets Exod. 19:1, which states "this day" to teach that whenever one engages in the study of Torah, it is as if that person has experienced Revelation at Sinai: "Ben Zoma states, 'Why is it written *In the third month* [*when the people of Israel were gone forth out of the land of Egypt, this day came they into the wilderness of Sinai*] (Exod. 19:1)? That day is not written, but *this day* [in order to teach] that it is as if on this day they came into the wilderness of Sinai. Every day that you study Torah it is as if *this day* you received Torah from Sinai."[35] Like the "as if" clause above, which places rabbinic Israel alongside the Israelites as if they too experienced the Exodus from Egypt, this tradition places rabbinic Israel alongside Israelites at Revelation.

Another tradition from *Midrash Tanhuma* goes further, proclaiming that all souls actually received Torah at Mount Sinai.[36] In the context of a lengthy exposition about the creation of the embryo, *Midrash Tanhuma* (*Pekudei* 3) states, "R. Yohanan said, 'What is the meaning of the verse, *Who does great things past finding out; and wonders without number* (Job 9:10)? Know this: all the souls from *'adam* until the end of the world were all created in the six days of creation, and all of them were in Gan Eden and all of them were at the giving of the Torah, as scripture states, [*And not with you alone do I make this covenant and this oath;*] *but with the one who stands here with us today before the Lord our God and with the one who is not with us this day* (Deut. 29:14).'"[37]

These rabbinic traditions construct Exodus and Revelation as both historical and transhistorical events, not only foundational to Israelite collective identity during the biblical period, but also foundational to rabbinic Israel.[38] The rabbis situate these events in time; they read them as having actually occurred to the specific generation of the Exodus—including the fetuses—and make these events timeless or eternal, for in every generation

Israel partakes in them. Moreover, as the traditions examined in the previous sections demonstrate, Israel experiences these events as fetuses, suggesting that beyond seeing themselves *as if* they were at the beginning, the birth, of Israel, Israel itself is conceived and born again and again through its fetuses.

The fetus links the biblical past, where the Exodus and Revelation occurred to Israel as a collective, and the rabbinic present, where Exodus and Revelation continue to occur to individuals, as the rabbis use the fetus to articulate what constitutes collective Israel. By projecting Exodus and Revelation onto the fetus in its mother's womb, the rabbis emphasize the continuity between the biblical past and the rabbinic present, even suggesting parity between the two. By appealing to the fetus, moreover, the rabbis internalize Exodus and Revelation, thereby internalizing the covenantal relationship between God and Israel. The internalization of the covenantal relationship between God and Israel through the fetus—past, present, and future—is what makes these traditions unique vis-à-vis rabbinic articulations of Israel.

Essentializing Israel

My reading of rabbinic narratives about fetuses for the ways they illuminate rabbinic constructions of Israel has much in common with the approach taken by some scholars to another recurring rabbinic motif. Moshe Herr, Charlotte Fonrobert, and Richard Kalmin have all examined rabbinic traditions about Roman governmental decrees that ostensibly prohibit certain practices, such as Sabbath observance, circumcision, and, according to *Bavli* traditions, Torah study, for the insights they provide into rabbinic constructions of Israel.[39] Fonrobert suggests that these traditions should be read "as rabbinic self-reflections, as indicators of what the rabbis considered to be the 'essence' of Judaism."[40] She further points out, "By projecting the prohibition of these practices onto a hostile government, a government that self-evidently had stigmatized the practices in order to destroy the Jewish community, the rabbis emphasized how essential they were. Therefore, in their literary (as opposed to historical) context, these lists of prohibited practices direct the reader's attention to what the rabbis considered to be the heart of Jewish life."[41] Moshe Herr, also writing about such traditions, points out, "Apparently, the Romans deliberately aimed their enactments at the most important and crucial of the commandments, the non-observance of which would render Judaism a soulless body."[42]

Rabbinic traditions about the fetus present another means by which to examine what lay at the "heart of Jewish life" for the rabbis, which complements—and supplements—the traditions about governmental decrees. Through the image of the fetus, the rabbis turn inward, projecting the very "heart" and "soul" of rabbinic identity onto Israel as it takes shape, not outside onto hostile governments. Furthermore, while a turn to the motif of prohibitive decrees inevitably highlights specific aspects, or practices, precisely because those external markers of Israel might be vulnerable to outside prohibition, rabbinic traditions about the fetus bring into view central elements of being Israel that cannot be so easily seen and thus prohibited: the belief in God as the God who brought Israel forth—from Egypt and the womb—and who revealed, and continues to reveal, the Torah to Israel.[43]

Rabbinic traditions about the fetus reveal that the covenantal relationship between God and Israel is foundational to, and constitutive of, rabbinic Israel's collective identity. This is precisely what cannot be addressed, or prohibited, by foreign governments. Rabbinic accounts of specific practices the Roman government is said to have prohibited might imply that what is being undermined is Israel's covenant with God, but they do not explicitly articulate this. Focusing only on the construction of rabbinic Israel evident in traditions about governmental decrees against certain practices might unwittingly reify the notion that that which is essential to rabbinic Israel is (only) its practices, or "laws," thus allowing presumably hostile outsiders to define Israel, perhaps on their terms. But a focus on the fetus, on all that the rabbis project onto the fetus, opens up an interior space for an internal articulation of that which the rabbis deem essential, and foundational, to Israel. Rabbinic narratives about the fetus serve as poignant reminders that quintessential practices are performed in order to express, indeed to fulfill, that which is essential to Israel, its covenant with God—even from its very beginnings.

In addition to, and perhaps even more than, any specific act, be it study, communal prayer, or circumcision, all of which may be precarious because vulnerable to outside prohibitions, rabbinic Israel is built upon the belief in a covenantal relationship between God and Israel, which can most likely endure, even in the face of external prohibitions, at least for a time.[44] Furthermore, in the traditions upon which I focus in this chapter, it is the covenant itself, which is traced back to the Exodus from Egypt and Revelation at Sinai in the collective memory of rabbinic Israel, that the rabbis project onto the fetus.[45]

Rabbinic traditions about the fetus enhance contemporary scholarly endeavors to reconstruct what lay at the heart of rabbinic Israel because they not only reveal certain practices, or external manifestations, of being Israel as essential but they also internalize the foundations of rabbinic Israel: Israel's covenantal relationship with God established through the Exodus from Egypt and the Revelation of Torah.

Developing Israel

My claim that through the fetus the rabbis internalize being Israel in no way indicates that what is projected onto the fetus, which reflects the rabbinic concept of Israel, remains static. To the contrary, as the fetus develops over time, so too the rabbinic conception of Israel and that which the rabbis conceive as central to it. Most notably, as I have consistently mentioned, only the *Bavli* and post-*Bavli* compilations project the study or acceptance of Torah into the womb.

In and of themselves, rabbinic traditions about the fetus, since relatively few in number, might not be able to support any grand claims about the construction of rabbinic Israel as a dynamic process. However, since these traditions support other studies that have established the preeminence of Torah study as a unique contribution of the *Bavli*, it seems appropriate to contextualize rabbinic traditions about the fetus among such larger scholarly projects.

The *Bavli's* portrayal of the fetus studying Torah, which highlights the centrality of Torah study for the rabbis, is consistent with recent research about the heightened or "exaggerated" centrality of Torah study in the *Bavli*, as recently elucidated by both Richard Kalmin and Jeffrey Rubenstein.[46] Kalmin, in his article comparing Palestinian and Babylonian traditions about Roman decrees, which was discussed above, concludes, "the most significant difference is Torah study, mentioned more frequently in the Bavli than any other *mitzvah*, with the possible exception of circumcision, while in Palestinian compilations it is mentioned perhaps not at all."[47] Rabbinic traditions about the fetus, though on a much smaller scale, yield similar results, since it is not until the *Bavli* that the fetus is imagined as learning Torah.

I am not suggesting that Torah study was not important to rabbinic Israel before the *Bavli*. Indeed, according to a Palestinian amoraic tradition,

Gen. Rab. 63:6, Jacob as a fetus wished to enter the study house, but the text falls short of explicitly maintaining that Jacob actually learned Torah as a fetus. Again Kalmin's remarks are applicable here when he writes, "For Palestinian rabbis, Torah study is only one among many important religious observances and practices; significant yes, but not to the extent that it overshadows other religious activities as it does for their Babylonian counterparts."[48] So too in *Gen. Rab.* 63:6–8, Jacob's prenatal embodiment of rabbinic Israel is not constructed through (the desire for) Torah study alone, but accompanied by other practices and attributes, such as prayer, circumcision, righteousness, and observance of mitzvot more generally.[49] Moreover, in the *Bavli* the fetus does not desire to enter the study house, rather it is already there, as the rabbis reconfigure the womb as a "private" house of study where the fetus learns Torah from, and/or with, God.

Perhaps in the *Bavli*, in contrast to other rabbinic compilations, the rabbis imagine the fetus as themselves, as representatives of Israel, instead of using the fetus to represent Israel as a whole.[50] In the *Bavli*, beyond maintaining that the fetus learns Torah, the rabbis further rabbinize the fetus when they imagine that fetuses curse those who do not transmit halakhah to a student. *B. Sanh.* 91b states, "R. Hanah b. Bisna said in the name of R. Shimeon the Just: whoever withholds a halakhah from a student, even fetuses in their mothers' wombs curse him."[51] Even if the rhetoric is understood as hyperbolic, it is evident that the rabbis do not hesitate to project their own views, even their own practices, onto the fetus. These fetuses know *halakhah*, at least enough to know when it is being withheld from a student, suggesting that the Torah the fetuses learn in the womb includes rabbinic teachings, or oral Torah, as well as written. Certainly this tradition functions to highlight the rabbis' own critique of one who withholds a teaching from his student, but nevertheless, by invoking the fetuses in this context, the rabbis bring them into their house of study.

The *Bavli*, when it comes to rabbinic traditions about the fetus, seems more interested in modeling the fetus after the rabbinic elite, not all Israel, again confirming Kalmin's findings in another context, where he concludes that Babylonian rabbis are less engaged with non-rabbis than are Palestinian rabbis.[52] It is interesting to note that the *Bavli* lacks any parallels to the Palestinian traditions about Jacob (*Israel*) as a fetus, and in its parallel to *Lev. Rab.* 4:7 where all fetuses praise God, according to the *Bavli*, only David sings to God from the womb (*b. Ber.* 10a).[53] Furthermore, the *Bavli's* version of a tradition about the fetus observing the fast of Yom Kippur, in contrast to that of the *Yerushalmi* version, attaches the lesson to a well-known rabbi.[54]

After the *Bavli*, medieval traditions carry forth the motif of the fetus learning Torah, modifying it and making it clear that, according to *Midrash Tanhuma (Tazria')*, the individual fetus receives Torah directly from God, apparently as a condition of its birth. The *Tanhuma* text does not state that the fetus studies Torah, rather that God commands the fetus Torah, perhaps indicating a shift away from the *Bavli's* more particular rabbinization of the fetus who studies Torah, and returning to the use of the fetus as representative of all Israel, who accept God's Torah. And then, *Midrash on the Ten Commandments* quite literally renders Israelite fetuses, and with them all fetuses to come, the only acceptable representatives of Israel, eternalizing the revelation of Torah—through the fetuses.

The significance of pausing to consider the later development concerning the fetus learning or receiving Torah lies in revealing that what becomes internalized in the rabbinic imagination, what becomes depicted as the primary expression of the covenantal relationship between God and Israel, here exemplified by that which the rabbis project onto their fetuses, changes over time. As seen above, tannaitic and amoraic sources internalize and eternalize the Exodus from Egypt by way of the fetus, and, as I will demonstrate in the latter part of this book they also emphasize God's roles in (pro)Creation, but only the *Bavli* and post-*Bavli* sources magnify the revelation or reception of Torah by projecting it onto the fetus as well.

Covenant and Contact

Rabbinic traditions are not alone in making the Exodus a transhistorical event; patristic sources also make the Israelite Exodus from Egypt, and Revelation (albeit a much more limited view of it, which focuses on the giving of the Decalogue alone) events that still occur in the present.[55] Origen, for example, commenting on Exod. 20:2, states,[56] "These words, therefore, are addressed not only to those who departed from Egypt, but much more to you, who now hear them. If only you depart from Egypt and do not further serve the Egyptians, God says, 'I am the Lord your God who brought you out of the land of Egypt, out of the house of bondage.'"[57] Here Origen suggests that departing from Egypt and receiving the Ten Commandments are present possibilities, as Origen, according to Marc Hirshman, aims "to create a bridge between the textual source and the listener."[58] Later in the same homily, Origen continues, "But do not think that these words [Exod. 20:3] are spoken only to that 'Israel' which is 'according to the flesh.' These words are addressed much more to you who were made Israel spiritually by living for God and were circumcised in heart, not in the flesh."[59]

Origen's interpretations construct the Exodus and the beginning of the Decalogue as continually relevant, even more real and pertinent for the present than they were for the past as he seeks to demonstrate how "Israel according to the flesh" has been superseded by "Israel of the spirit."[60] Origen does not invoke fetuses in these interpretations, nor, as yet, has he made a generational or genealogical connection, which an invocation of fetuses suggests. However, according to Origen, following Paul in a statement replete with genealogical concerns, the parting of the sea represents ancestral baptism, or rebirth. In Origen's homily on the departure of Israel from Egypt (*Exod. Hom.* 5), interpreting 1 Cor. 10:1–2, *For I do not want you to be ignorant of the fact, brothers and sisters, that our ancestors were all under the cloud and that they all passed through the sea. They were all baptized into Moses in the cloud and in the sea*, Origen states, "Do you see how much Paul's teaching differs from the literal meaning? What the Jews supposed to be a crossing of the sea, Paul calls a baptism; what they supposed to be a cloud, Paul asserts is the Holy Spirit. He wishes that to be understood in a similar manner to this which the Lord taught in the Gospels, 'Unless a man be born again of water and the Holy Spirit, he cannot enter the kingdom of heaven' [John 3:5]."[61] And later in the same homily Origen links the past "baptism in Moses" with the present baptism in Christ: "He [Paul] calls this 'baptism in Moses consummated in the cloud and in the sea,' that you also who are baptized in Christ, in water and the Holy Spirit, might know that the Egyptians are following you and wish to recall you to their service."[62]

Origen's accusation that the "Jews" see the crossing of the sea simply or only as a literal crossing of the sea is erroneous. The rabbis, as I have suggested above, also deviate from the literal meaning of the text,[63] seeing the crossing of the sea as the birth of the people Israel, which continues through the birth of each fetus. Although rabbinic sources do not explicitly interpret Exodus as God birthing Israel, though they imagine God birthing the world at Creation,[64] locating the fetuses at the crossing of the sea implies that they see this story as one of birth as well. Recall that in Pardes's reading the crossing of the sea evokes Creation itself, the birth of the world, not re-creation or rebirth. For the rabbis, an operative metaphor and even allegorization of the splitting of the sea is birth; for Paul and Origen, it is baptism. Despite the difference, both readings succeed in achieving continuity between the biblical past and the present, making the Exodus live on in perpetuity. I am not suggesting any type of direct exegetical or polemical exchange between these two readings, merely noting that in the third century CE, rabbinic and patristic sources both continue to lay claim to the biblical Exodus, interpreting it as their own.[65]

The timelessness of the Revelation of Torah is a bit more fraught when considered in patristic and rabbinic contexts. In the broadest terms, the "Law" is insufficient for Christianness. While the Decalogue remains, the other mitzvot have been considered nullified and superseded.[66] If placed in this context, the *Bavli's* image of the fetus studying Torah, perhaps inclusive of rabbinic interpretations, along with *Midrash Tanhuma's* portrayal of God commanding the fetus the laws of kashrut and *all of the commandments of the Torah*, asserts that the Revelation of Torah, and the covenant it represents, which encompasses much more than the Decalogue, has not been superseded or replaced, nor is it insufficient. Revelation as it was, which for the rabbis includes rabbinic interpretations, continues to occur to Israel as fetuses. Locating the Israelite fetuses at Sinai as guarantors for the Torah, in addition to bringing Sinai to each individual fetus, projects Revelation into the future, for all time. Although in the tradition from the *Midrash on the Ten Commandments* the Israelite fetuses explicitly agree to the Ten Commandments, in its medieval Jewish context there would be no misunderstanding this as affirming the future of the Decalogue alone. Again, I am not suggesting direct polemics surfacing in these traditions, but I am noting that these rabbinic traditions assert the timelessness of the Revelation of the Torah, in and of itself and all inclusive as it were, in the face of competing interpretations of the covenant.[67]

Finally, although I have continually stressed the future-reaching aspect of the tradition from the *Midrash on the Ten Commandments,* where the fetuses embody the future of Israel and its covenant, it is worth pausing to consider, albeit briefly and however conjecturally, this medieval textual move from offering "our children" as in earlier traditions, to more specifically offering "our fetuses."[68] Why do these later versions insist that the best, the only, guarantors for Israel are its fetuses? While this might be an internal development, a logical fruition of the combination of preceding rabbinic traditions as I have suggested above, taking elements from the tannaitic tradition about the Israelite fetuses singing at the crossing of the sea and later traditions about the individual fetus learning or receiving Torah and then projecting them back onto Revelation at Sinai, might this tradition not only assert the ongoing nature of Revelation, but also suggest the purity of infants, their lack of any (original) sin? Whether or not such a point was intended, it should be noted that according to this tradition, prior to birth, baptism, or circumcision,[69] the fetuses guarantee the covenant and accept it upon themselves. Moreover, in this text God rejects Abraham, Isaac, and Jacob not only because they represent the past, which cannot here guarantee the future, but because God has found fault with each of them.[70] In contrast, the fetuses are blameless, innocent, and pure.[71]

Even a brief juxtaposition of rabbinic traditions and Origen's interpretations on the Exodus demonstrates that both construct Exodus as continually relevant—experienced by those in the present no less, and for Origen even more, than the past. Whereas rabbinic traditions are concerned with making Revelation—in its broadest sense—continual, Origen focuses on the ongoing relevance of the Decalogue alone, the rest of the "Law" having been superseded.[72] Origen consistently appears to look over his shoulder and see Jews' claims to biblical Israel and its covenant with God; rabbinic interpretations, in contrast, turn inward, seeing fetuses as their link to their own biblical past. The polemical, supersessionist readings in Origen have no obvious counterpart in the rabbinic traditions; nor should such polemics, on the part of the rabbis be presupposed—the rabbinic emphasis on the covenantal relationship between God and Israel more likely being an outgrowth of biblical sources than a response to Christian claims to the covenant.

Despite the fact that both rabbinic and patristic authors lay claim to the covenantal relationship between God and Israel, I find no evidence of contact between the two in rabbinic traditions about fetuses, or other rabbinic traditions about the Exodus and Revelation, examined here. As the rabbis look to an internal image, the fetus, to articulate the foundations and fundamentals of Israel, they need no "other," no contrasting image, through which to define, let alone conceive, Israel. All that is needed is the Torah, which is with Israel from its very beginnings and continually given to Israel as it takes shape.

Conclusion

In the traditions presented above, the rabbis repeatedly locate the beginnings of the covenantal relationship between God and Israel with the fetus. However, to read these traditions for the insights they provide into rabbinic constructions of the fetus in and of itself[73] would be to miss the point; the rabbis invoke the fetus in order to internalize the covenant between God and (rabbinic) Israel, collapse the distinction between biblical and rabbinic Israel, and project the covenant infinitely into the future. In these traditions, which reach into the womb and attach themselves to the fetus, the rabbis conceive and articulate nothing less than Israel itself. The fetus in these traditions represents Israel, and it provides a fitting symbol and an apt image with which to theorize the foundations of rabbinic Israel. Through the fetus, the rabbis lay claim to biblical Israel and internalize its foundations, establishing the covenant between God and Israel as eternal and Exodus and Revelation as ongoing events. In the chapters in the second part of this book, I demonstrate that rabbinic traditions about procreation establish that Creation itself is reenacted through each embryo. In the following chapter, however, I examine rabbinic traditions about prenatal Jacob (Israel), again reading these traditions for their insights into rabbinic constructions of Israel and further exploring the question of Jewish-Christian exchange, briefly broached above, in much more depth and detail.

Chapter 3
And the Sons Struggled

And the sons struggled inside her;
and she said, If it be so, why am I thus?
And she went to inquire of God.
And God said to her,
Two nations are in your womb,
and two peoples shall be separated from your womb;
and the one people shall be stronger than the other people;
and the elder shall serve the younger.

—Gen. 25:22–23

In stark contrast to the poignant reconciliation between Jacob and Esau recounted in the book of Genesis, a tradition in *Genesis Rabbah* denies any such reconciliation. Interpreting Gen. 33:4, *And Esau ran to meet him [Jacob], and embraced him, and fell on his neck, and kissed him; and they wept*, R. Yannai maintains that Esau did not come to kiss Jacob at all, but instead he came to bite him; they weep not out of the emotion of coming together after their long separation but over their respective injuries: Jacob's neck and Esau's teeth (*Gen. Rab.* 78:9). As much as this rabbinic interpretation betrays the biblical text,[1] it reveals that in many instances "rabbinic exegesis of the Biblical account of Esau and Jacob constitutes a web of veiled references to Rome and Israel."[2] And if rabbinic traditions insist upon reading irreconcilable differences between Israel and Rome into Jacob and Esau's epic moment of reconciliation, it should come as no surprise that they read the twins' prenatal struggle in this same light.

It has long been noted that in many rabbinic texts, Esau is symbolic of (Christian) Rome and Jacob symbolizes (rabbinic) Israel, and that conversely, in patristic sources, Jacob is symbolic of the true Israel—the Church—and Esau symbolizes the Jews—the "Synagogue."[3] Marc Hirshman has characterized the core of contention between early Christian and rabbinic interpreters as a "battle over biblical exegesis," where both interpretive communities lay claim to the title Israel.[4] In the midst of such competing claims for the title Israel, is it any wonder that one rabbinic passage tries to fix the identities of Jacob as Israel and Esau as not-Israel rather definitively—even as fetuses?

Gen. Rab. 63:6–8, while engaging in the broader concern about demonstrating just *who* is Israel, moves on to articulate more precisely *what* Israel is—or what it means, according to the rabbis, to be Israel. Moreover, this passage inscribes the very beginnings of being Israel onto Jacob's fetal body; since Jacob *is* Israel, this passage further suggests the prenatal beginnings of all Israel.[5]

This chapter begins by highlighting the ways in which *Gen. Rab.* 63:6–8 applies the typological reading of Jacob as (rabbinic) Israel and Esau as (Christian) Rome to Jacob and Esau already as fetuses, thus casting these biblical—and subsequent—fetuses as participants in the rabbinic effort to delineate who and what constitutes Israel. I further examine *Gen. Rab.* 63:6–8 in light of patristic interpretations of Romans 9, exploring the possible relationship between rabbinic and patristic readings of *prenatal* Jacob and Esau. Finally, I consider the ways in which creating a narrative dialogue between these sources might help determine whether Esau, in *Gen. Rab.* 63:6–8, is best considered metonymic of Christian Rome in particular or pagan Rome more generally and how *Gen. Rab.* 63:6–8 illuminates the extent of the impact Christianity had on rabbinic Judaism.

Genesis Rabbah 63:6–8

Throughout *Gen. Rab.* 63:6–8, the rabbis claim their inheritance of Jacob, their birthright as Israel. They do so by reconceiving their father Jacob in their own image, such that *prenatal* Jacob already embodies and engenders *rabbinic* Israel. Although neither as blatantly deceptive as Jacob's theft of his own father's blessing (Genesis 27) nor as outright conniving as Jacob's purchase of his own (brother's) birthright (Genesis 25), the rabbis cunningly establish that Israel is always already rabbinic Israel—even before Israel is born.

At the same time that *Genesis Rabbah 63* makes prenatal Jacob into the embodiment of rabbinic Israel, it casts prenatal Esau as the current manifestation of not-Israel, Rome. *Genesis Rabbah*'s consistent portrayal of Jacob and Esau as oppositive (id)entities, from their very beginnings and throughout their lives,[6] suggests that these traditions have much to do with the construction of collective rabbinic Israel's identity in the rabbis' own political-cultural setting, when no reconciliation between Israel and Rome seems imminent. *Gen. Rab.* 63:6–8 accounts for the irreconcilable differences between rabbinic Israel and Rome by writing them back into the biblical story of Israel's origins and in so doing making them congenital, part of the very makeup of being—or not being—Israel.

Gen. Rab. 63:6 begins by interpreting Gen. 25:22, *And the sons struggled within her,* in light of the rabbinic understanding of Gen. 25:23, *Two nations are in your womb and two peoples shall be separated from your womb*: "And the sons struggled together [*vayitrotsatsu*] *within her.* R. Yohanan and Reish Lakish [interpreted the word *vayitrotsatsu*]. R. Yohanan said, 'this one ran [*rats*] to kill this one and this one ran to kill this one.' R. Shimeon ben Lakish said, 'this one permitted[7] the [forbidden] commands of this one, and this one permitted the [forbidden] commands of this one.'"[8] The midrash asks what Jacob and Esau struggle over, and it offers multiple answers, often invoking the differences between Israel and Rome. According to a statement attributed to R. Yohanan, the two are locked in mortal combat—each trying to kill the other.[9] Although R. Yohanan's interpretation does not indicate what the two are fighting over, the next interpretation, attributed to R. Shimeon ben Lakish, imagines each one trying to do that which the other forbids, and presumably the struggle comes from their mutual attempts to stop each other from performing such deeds.[10] R. Shimeon ben Lakish thus imagines a religious or cultural motivation behind their struggle, where each *fetus* is attempting to follow its own laws—perhaps even if it kills them.

A third interpretation of Gen. 25:22, attributed to R. Berekiah, states, "Do not say that [only after] Esau went forth from his mother's womb did he attack him (Jacob). But [even] while he was in his mother's womb, his fist *zoro*] was stretched out against him. As it is written, *The wicked are estranged [zoru (make fists)] from the womb [they go astray from the womb]* (Ps. 58:4)."[11] In contrast to the previous two interpretations, which envision a mutual struggle between Jacob and Esau, this last tradition highlights Esau's culpability, imagining the already wicked Esau attacking the presumably already righteous, perhaps innocent and defenseless, Jacob.

One final interpretation of Gen. 25:22 again applies Ps. 58:4 to Esau:[12] "*And the sons struggled together within her.* The sons hastened within her. She passes by houses of idolatry and Esau kicks to go out.[13] As it is written, *The wicked are estranged from the womb* (Ps. 58:4). She passes by synagogues and houses of study and Jacob kicks to go out. As it is written, *Before I formed you in the womb, I knew you* (Jer. 1:5)."[14] Already, prenatal Jacob, who is known (and elected)[15] by God, and who follows God's laws and wishes to study those laws and pray to his God, emerges looking like rabbinic Israel. In contrast, Esau, who is wicked and estranged from God, and who follows other laws and wishes to worship other gods, resembles pagan Rome. If any doubt exists that these interpretations operate on a national as well as an individual level, *Gen. Rab.* 63:7 makes the connections between the individual and the collective, or the personal and the political, quite clear:[16] "*Two nations are in your womb* (Gen. 25:23): Two proud nations are in your womb. This one is proud in his world and this one is proud in his world.[17] This one is proud in his kingdom and this one is proud in his kingdom. Two proud nations are in your womb: Hadrian of the nations [of the world] and Solomon of Israel. Two hated nations are in your womb: All the nations hate Esau and all the nations hate Israel. Those who hate your children are in your womb, as it is written, *But Esau I hated*[18] (Mal. 1:3)." Here the midrash explicitly connects Esau with Rome and Jacob with Israel; Rebekah is pregnant with Jacob and Esau, and they, in turn have within them their future offspring:[19] Solomon and Hadrian, Israel and Rome.[20] The passage portrays both nations as proud and hated by others.[21] The last line, as rendered above, also notes the hatred between Rome and Israel.[22] However, commentators have suggested an alternative reading, which states, "Those hated by your Creator are in your womb."[23] This reading has the disadvantage of emending the text, but it has the advantage of being both closer to the biblical proof text, which has God express God's hatred for Esau,[24] and more in line with the overall message of this passage, which highlights Esau's wickedness and estrangement from God. Furthermore, Mal. 1:2, states, *Yet I loved Jacob* and then continues to point out that God hated Esau (Mal. 1:3). Thus the text simultaneously asserts God's love of Jacob/Israel and God's hatred of Esau/Rome already in the womb.[25]

Gen. Rab. 63:7 then interprets the continuation of Gen. 25:23: "*Two peoples shall be separated from your womb.* R. Berekiah said, 'From here we learn that he (Jacob) was born circumcised.'"[26] Jacob, already in Rebekah's womb, bears the physical mark of Israel; Esau, already in the womb, signifies otherness.[27] But the separation between Israel and not-Israel does not hinge only upon circumcision, as *Gen. Rab.* 63:6–8, taken as a whole, makes clear; Israel and not-Israel are distinguished by virtue of God's love and, both stemming from and contributing to this, their practices.

To the extent that there exists an overarching difference between Jacob and Esau—Israel and Rome—that emerges from this passage, it is the distinction between wickedness and righteousness. Heretofore *Gen.*

Rab. 63:6–7 alludes to the centrality of righteousness to rabbinic Israel only through implication: Esau's wickedness implies, and through opposition even substantiates, Jacob's righteousness. *Gen. Rab.* 63:8 brings righteousness front and center: "*And when her days to be delivered were fulfilled behold, there were twins in her womb* (Gen. 25:24). Later [the word for twins is written] plene and here it is deficient. [Here it does not say], 'Behold there were twins [*te'omim*] in her womb' but twins [*tomim*] is written. There [where it is written full[28] it refers to] Peretz and Zerah, both of them righteous. Here [it refers to] Jacob and Esau, one righteous and the other wicked."[29]

According to *Gen. Rab.* 63:6–8, Jacob and Esau, already as fetuses, exemplify, even typify, the separation between Israel and Rome bodily, theologically, and "through works." The difference between Jacob and Esau, Israel and Rome, is illustrated through different theological beliefs (monotheism or idolatry), and concomitant practices (observance of commandments, which includes circumcision, worship through study and prayer or observance of other laws and "strange" worship). Running through these traditions is the construction of Jacob/Israel as righteous, and thus loved by God, and the representation of Esau/Rome as wicked, and thus estranged from and hated by God—even *before they are born.*

Gen. Rab. 63:6–8, with its focus on Jacob and Esau in utero, is unique among extant rabbinic compilations.[30] In fact, Gen. 25:22–23 receives remarkably little attention in the rabbinic corpus as a whole.[31] The rabbis in *Genesis Rabbah,* however, were not the first to use prenatal Jacob and Esau to reflect upon their own circumstances; a first-century preacher of the people Israel, Paul, used Gen. 25:23 for his own purposes centuries prior to the rabbis.[32]

Genesis Rabbah 63, Romans 9, and Origen

One of the earliest midrashic readings of Gen. 25:23 appears in Paul's letter to the Romans (9:6–13):[33]

For not all who are descended from Israel belong to Israel, and not all are children of Abraham because they are his descendants; but "Through Isaac shall your descendants be named" [Gen. 21:12]. This means that it is not the children of the flesh who are the children of God, but the children of the promise are reckoned as descendants. For this is what the promise said, "About this time I will return and Sarah shall have a son." And not only so, but also when Rebecca had conceived children by one man, our forefather Isaac, though they were not yet born and had done nothing either good or bad, in order that God's purpose of election might continue, not because of works but because of his call, she was told, "The elder will serve the younger." As it is written, "Jacob I loved, but Esau I hated."[34]

A cursory reading of Romans 9 already presents some compelling reasons for putting this passage in dialogue with the traditions from *Gen. Rab.* 63:6–8 set forth above—even without immediate concern over any precise avenue of transmission.[35] Others have already noted how *subsequent* patristic interpretations of Gen. 25:23, which assert that "the younger" signifies the true Israel, might have impacted—or not impacted—the rabbinic interpretation of Jacob as signifying *rabbinic* Israel. However, little attention has been given to the points of contact and contrast between materials specific to both *Genesis Rabbah* 63 and Romans 9 that exceed the mention of this verse.[36]

To begin with, both Rom. 9:10–13 and *Gen. Rab.* 63:6–8 reflect specifically upon Jacob and Esau before they are born. Such rabbinic interest in Gen. 25:22–23 qua Gen. 25:22–23, with a focus on prenatal Jacob and Esau, is astonishingly localized in the rabbinic corpus—appearing only in *Genesis Rabbah* 63.[37] Moreover, both passages cite Mal. 1:3, *But Esau I hated*. Even though *Genesis Rabbah* does not cite Mal. 1:2, *Yet Jacob I loved,* God's love of Jacob over and against Esau is implied throughout the passage—not in the least by way of the rabbinic application of Jer. 1:5, which in the context of *Genesis Rabbah* 63 bespeaks God's sanctification ("election") of Jacob/Israel. And finally, given the concern over righteousness I see as an overarching element in *Gen. Rab.* 63:6–8, the latter part of Romans 9 should also be considered: "What then are we to say? Gentiles, who did not strive for righteousness, have attained it, that is, righteousness through faith; but Israel, who did strive for the righteousness that is based on the law, did not succeed in fulfilling that law. Why not? Because they did not strive for it on the basis of faith, but as if it were based on works. They have stumbled over the stumbling stone" (Rom. 9:30–33).[38] Righteousness—and how to attain it, as well as precisely who has attained it—not only serves as a possible additional point of contact between *Gen. Rab.* 63:6–8 and Romans 9 but also illustrates their strongest point of departure:[39] According to Paul, Jacob and Esau, while not yet born, had done nothing either good or bad; the point is that neither, before they were born, were righteous (or wicked). However, according to *Genesis Rabbah* 63, already prenatally, Jacob had done everything good, and Esau, everything bad—illustrating that one (Israel) is entirely righteous and the other (Rome), entirely wicked.

The dialogue between *Gen. Rab.* 63:6–9 and Romans 9 that I have created necessitates speculation about how these two disparate—by all counts—sources could present such striking overlap: focus on prenatal Jacob and Esau; citation of Mal. 1:(2–)3; and a concern about righteousness. Due to the improbability that the rabbis knew Paul's letter unmediated, subsequent early Christian and patristic sources need to be considered as a likely route of exchange.[40] Gerson Cohen and Israel Yuval have previously explored the relationship between patristic interpretations of Romans 9 and rabbinic traditions, but neither focused specifically on *Gen. Rab.* 63:6–8; Cohen does not mention these traditions, and Yuval, even though he cites *Gen. Rab.* 63:7, does not put the passage fully in dialogue with Romans 9 or its later interpretations.[41] Instead, both scholars cite a number of patristic sources, drawn from Western and Eastern authors,[42] which interpret Gen. 25:23 such that Jacob stands for Christians, and Esau represents the Jews.[43] The various patristic passages cited do provide compelling evidence, as both scholars claim, for an overall environment, or *Zeitgeist,* within which rabbis and church fathers continue their biblical namesake's struggle with their own Esau. Cohen asserts, "Indeed, the claim must have reached at least some Jewish ears, for it was being shouted far and wide, and in virtually identical terms."[44] Yuval goes quite a bit further when he characterizes the Jewish position as "reactive and defensive"[45] and writes that on the topic of election, "Pauline thought seems to have preceded that of the Sages and even to have caused the latter to defend itself."[46] Neither scholar, however, locates what Visotzky has recently dubbed "the smoking gun"[47]—in this instance *Gen. Rab.* 63:6–8—although both make passing mention of the most likely impetus for such rabbinic (f)ire: Origen.[48]

Determining a likely path of transmission between patristic and rabbinic sources is at best a difficult undertaking. However, Origen, who lived in Palestine during the third century CE, where he wrote both his *Homilies on Genesis* and his *Commentary on the Epistle to the Romans,* provides a logical place from which to explore the possibility of an exegetical exchange surfacing in *Gen. Rab.* 63:6–8 and Romans 9.[49]

In *Hom. Gen.* 12:1, Origen does not expand upon Paul's interpretation of Jacob and Esau. He clearly cites Rom. 9:11–13, almost verbatim, and claims that it would be tedious to examine Paul's "enigmas" and "mysteries." At the risk of such tedium, I recite the relevant section of his homily because establishing at least the possible proximity of Romans 9 to rabbis in Palestine during the third century—and therefore later—is precisely the issue here:

It would be tedious if we wished now to examine the leaping of the children while they still remained in the womb. It would be tedious if we should mention the interpretations and enigmas which the Apostle wrote about these matters, what mysteries, what reasons they contain; why it is said of them, "before the children are born or do anything good or evil in this world": "One people shall overcome the other and the elder shall serve the younger"; why, before they proceeded from their mother's womb, it is said by the prophet: "I have loved Jacob, but have hated Esau." These matters surpass both my ability to speak and your ability to hear.[50]

Paul's comments about prenatal Jacob and Esau having done neither evil nor good, the use of the latter part of Gen. 25:23, and the application of Mal. 1:2–3 are all here, ostensibly presented live in a public sermon in third-century Palestine.[51] Origen also mentions Gen. 25:22, which does not appear in Romans 9 but does appear in *Gen. Rab.* 63:6.

Later in the same homily (12:3), Origen comments on Gen. 25:23, now much more expansively interpreting Paul's invocation of that verse to explicitly teach that the Church has risen over the Synagogue. He writes, "How 'one people has risen over the other,' that is, the Church over the Synagogue, and how 'the elder serves the younger' *is known even to the Jews themselves* although they do not believe. I think it is superfluous, therefore, to speak about these things *which are well known and very commonplace to everyone.*"[52] He continues, "I think that this can be said *also* of us as individuals, that 'two nations and two peoples are within you.' For there is both a people of virtues within us and there is no less a people of vices within us."[53] Although at this point Origen has applied God's response to Rebekah to each of his listeners,[54] the internalized distinction between virtues and vices so quick on the heels of his previous interpretation would seem to indicate that the virtues and vices also reflect back to his distinction between "Church" and "Synagogue," respectively. By Origen's testimony, the Jews know that Christians interpret (virtuous) Jacob as "the Church" and (wicked) Esau as "the Synagogue."

All that is lacking in the *Homilies on Genesis* is Paul's assertion that Jacob's "election" is based on "promise"—not "works." Origen broaches this part of Romans 9 in his *Commentary*, also written in Caesarea, during the same period that he wrote his *Homilies*.[55] He writes, "before the birth occurred, and before the boys had any good or evil deeds among men, the divine election was reckoned toward Jacob, as it is said, 'The elder will serve the younger,' and 'Jacob I loved, but Esau I hated.'"[56] He continues, now connecting Rom. 9:12 and 9:8, "But he teaches why these things are said in this way, 'in order that according to election the purpose of God might abide not by works, but by the one who calls'; that is in order that it might not be those who are sons of the flesh, but those who are sons of God who are reckoned as descendants."[57] Later in the commentary, Origen turns to Rom. 9:30, writing, "He says, 'What then are we to say? That Gentiles, who were not seeking righteousness, have attained righteousness, but a righteousness that is from faith.' This perhaps appears to contradict what we said above, either that each person must cleanse and purify himself in order to become a useful vessel and a vessel of mercy. . . .[58] How then is he saying here, 'Gentiles, who were not seeking righteousness, have attained righteousness'? Consider then whether we can reply in this way. It is one thing to seek, another to have it *inborn*."[59]

Taken together, Origen's *Homilies on Genesis* and his *Commentary* place Romans 9 in Palestine during the third century, within earshot of the rabbis—as Gerson Cohen suggested. Of course, this does not provide an airtight case proving that the rabbis knew Origen's interpretations of Romans, but it does suggest the plausibility of an "exegetical encounter,"[60] one that is strengthened not only by geographical and (relative) chronological proximity[61] but also by the general interest in *prenatal* Jacob and Esau— heretofore unexplored in extant rabbinic compilations—the concern about righteousness, and the explicit mention of Mal. 1:(2–)3 in both Origen and *Genesis Rabbah* 63.[62]

With a plausible explanation as to how at least some rabbis living in Palestine between the third and fifth centuries might have become acquainted with Romans 9, it is now possible to probe beneath some of the surface-level similarities between Romans 9 and *Gen. Rab.* 63:6–8 set forth above and explore the underlying differences between *Gen. Rab.* 63:6–8 and Romans 9. In stark contrast to the image of Jacob and Esau having done neither good nor evil before they are born, the rabbis assert precisely the opposite.[63] In its elaboration of the prenatal struggle between Jacob and Esau, *Gen. Rab.* 63:6–8 moves well beyond asserting that Jacob is Israel, which means rabbinic Israel, and Esau is Rome, both pagan and Christian. The passage goes on to articulate what being Israel means—both by seeing *prenatal* Jacob as the manifestation of rabbinic Israel and casting *prenatal* Esau as rabbinic Israel's "other(s)." Israel—from its very beginnings— means worship of, and thus belief in, one God, observance of God's commandments—that is, study, prayer, and circumcision—and righteousness, all of which bring about God's love (Mal. 1:2)[64] and God's "election" (Jer. 1:5): *Before I formed you* [= Israel] *in the womb I knew you, and before you came forth from the womb I set you apart/made you holy, and I set you as a prophet to the nations.* The application of Jer. 1:5 in *Gen. Rab.* 63:6 suggests that Jacob, here all Israel not just one lone prophet, is called by God and set apart and made holy "from the womb" through mitzvot. At the same time, *Gen. Rab.* 63:6–8 explains that being not-Israel means worshipping idols, following other laws, being uncircumcised and wicked, all of which bring about estrangement from God (Ps. 58:4) and ultimately justify God's—and Israel's—hatred (Mal. 1:3). *Gen. Rab.* 63:6–8 does not recognize any bifurcation between "works" and "call"—even for fetuses—because both are mutually implicated, not mutually exclusive.[65] Esau and the nations he engenders are spurned as a result of their wicked ways, but Jacob is called Israel and rabbinic Israel merits God's call by virtue of its righteous ways.

Much of *Gen. Rab.* 63:6–8 stands in sharp contrast to Origen's claim that Jacob represents the Church. The interpretations upon which I have focused from *Gen. Rab.* 63:6–8, taken as a whole, *re*-affirm that Jacob represents rabbinic Israel and insist that he has always done so—even as a fetus.[66] Furthermore, in contrast to Origen's explicit assertion that Esau is the Synagogue, Israel according to the flesh, as it were, *Gen. Rab.* 63:6–8 consistently marks prenatal Esau as (Christian) Rome *in the flesh*.

But what of Origen's concomitant claim, shared by a number of other patristic authors, that Gen. 25:23, *the elder will serve the younger,* means that the Synagogue serves the Church? Origen's assertion that already in the third century this commonplace reading is known even to the Jews themselves is largely unsupported by any direct rabbinic evidence.[67] Even in *Genesis Rabbah* 63 that biblical phrase receives little direct attention and seems to present little difficulty for the rabbinic claim to Jacob as Israel. Nevertheless, both Daniel Boyarin and Israel Yuval have asserted that patristic uses of Gen. 25:23 had a direct impact on the rabbis. Yuval asserts that "the Jewish identification with Jacob emerged from internalizing the Christian position and confronting it,"[68] and Boyarin claims that the ways that Christian writers could exploit the sequence of the elder and younger influenced rabbinic interpretations.[69] Boyarin, in turn, "exploit[s] the temporal paradoxes of the midrashic equation of Esau with Christianity," which suggest that "rabbinic Judaism was born on the heels, indeed, holding the heel, of its elder brother, the Church."[70] In order to more fully engage what Boyarin cleverly submits as his "midrash that never was," it is helpful to return once again to the midrash that was—*Genesis Rabbah* 63—and examine some of the temporal paradoxes that the passage itself sets forth.[71]

The one direct interpretation of the latter part of Gen. 25:23 in *Genesis Rabbah* 63—or elsewhere in rabbinic literature—states, "*And the elder shall serve the younger.* R Huna said, 'If [the younger] is worthy, [the elder] will serve [the younger]; and if not, [the elder] will enslave [the younger].'"[72]

This interpretation, attributed to a fourth-century rabbi,[73] asserts that the fulfillment of Gen. 25:23 will come in the future—not much of a stretch given the grammar of the verse. In other words, "the elder *will* serve the younger." As direct as R. Huna's reading is, it is anything but explicit. This reading could be applied to any subjugation and any oppressor throughout time with no alteration; the emphasis is on Israel's worthiness, not on Esau.[74] The future-oriented reading appears more explicitly in *Gen. Rab.* 63:8, commenting not on Gen. 25:23 but on Gen. 25:26: "A [Roman] prefect asked one from the house of Silna,[75] who will seize [power] after us? He brought a piece of paper and took a quill and wrote on it, *And after that his brother came forth, and his hand seized Esau's heel* (Gen. 25:26)."[76] Both traditions offer Israel comfort by acknowledging that although presently the younger, second-born son serves, such reality is temporary since Israel will be served in the future, just as Gen. 25:23 promises.[77] The final statement in *Gen. Rab.* 63:8 uses Jacob's/Israel's current servitude and suffering to further identify the younger son [*tsa'ir*] as rabbinic Israel: "This teaches how much suffering (*tsa'ar*) this righteous one suffered [*mitsta'er*]."[78] *Gen. Rab.* 63:8 ends right where it begins, with *the younger* Jacob's/Israel's righteousness.

The contrast between the rabbinic identification of the younger Jacob as rabbinic Israel and Origen's, among other patristic authors, identification of the younger Jacob as the Church could not be more apparent; both claim Jacob as their own, and both spurn Esau the elder. However, in addition to identifying the elder Esau as Rome—be it pagan or Christian[79]—as in the interpretations from *Genesis Rabbah* 63 presented thus far, *Gen. Rab.* 63:8 also makes Jacob—not Esau—the elder[80] and at times even the only son.[81] It does this, however, not when interpreting Gen. 25:23 but when interpreting Gen. 25:25, *And the first came out red, all over like a hairy garment; and they called his name Esau.*

One of the interpretations of Gen. 25:25, *And the first came forth red,* states, "Why did Esau come forth first? So that he would come forth and take his foul matter with him. R. Abbahu said, 'Like a bath attendant who washes the bath house and afterwards bathes the king's son, so too why did Esau come forth first? So that he would come forth and [take] his foulness with him.'"[82] At first the midrash suggests that Esau came forth first with all his foul matter so that Jacob can be born without such filth—perhaps pure. R. Abbahu's *mashal*, however, does not quite match up with the interpretation in any straightforward manner; either Esau is now simply the filth that is cleaned away by the bath attendant and thus not considered a son at all, or perhaps Esau is the servant after all, who bathes the king's—or is it "the King's"—(only) son. Regardless, any familial relationship, any likeness or resemblance, between Jacob and Esau, as well as Israel and (Christian) Rome, is washed right out of the text.

Gen. Rab. 63:8 later brings a likely subtext of the very question of why Esau is born first, *Israel is my son, my firstborn son* (Exod. 4:22), to the surface.[83] Interpreting the latter part of Gen. 25:25, *And they called his name Esau*, the text states, "[God said] 'What a waste that I created you in my world.' R. Yitzhak said [that God said] 'You call your swine by name [Esau], I call my firstborn son [Jacob] by name, *Israel is my firstborn son* (Exod. 4:22).'" Here God names Jacob as the firstborn, the elder, and God disowns Esau, wishing that he had never been born—again ultimately making Israel not only the firstborn but also the only son.

That Jacob/Israel is God's "firstborn" son is also at issue in one of the other interpretations of the earlier part of Gen. 25:25: "*And the first came forth red*. A *matrona* asked R. Yosi bar Halfota, 'Why did Esau issue forth first?' He said to her, 'The first drop [of semen] was Jacob's.' He made a comparison for her, 'If you put two pearls in a tube, does not the one that you put in first come out last? So too, the first drop was Jacob's.'"[84] According to this tradition, Jacob is the elder since he was conceived first. Although this interpretation acknowledges that Jacob/Israel and Esau/Rome are brothers, it still finds a way to make them essentially different.[85] Esau is clearly the "bad seed," and Jacob the good.[86] This distinction, somewhat muted here because they both still originate in Isaac, is not as slight as it seems if one recalls the very beginning of *Gen. Rab.* 63:8, which portrays the one as entirely wicked, the other wholly righteous.

According to *Gen. Rab.* 63:6–8, from conception through gestation and birth, Jacob and Esau are truly separated. Indeed, there are two nations in Rebekah's womb, and they are two divided and disparate peoples. Jacob and Esau might have inhabited the same womb, but they were already worlds apart in that very womb. The question that remains, given that Jacob is always already rabbinic Israel, is who is Israel's other? With whom does rabbinic Israel contend?

Who Is Esau in *Genesis Rabbah* 63?

Jacob Neusner, in an article sharply critiquing his own prior work that failed to recognize the impact of Christianity upon Judaism, writes, "What went wrong? The answer is simple. I began my research with perfect faith in a dogma of Judaism and therefore also of scholars of Judaism. It is that Christianity never made any difference to Judaism. So I took for granted, without knowing it, that I too would find that Christianity never made any difference. My original results then conformed to the premise with which I had commenced work."[87] Neusner goes on, in this article and numerous other works to postulate the tremendous and unsettling impact that Christianity, beginning in the fourth century,[88] indeed had on Judaism. Two decades after Neusner's article, having come to expect that Christianity made just such a difference and even more judging from statements like "The confrontation with Christianity lies at the very heart of Midrashic and Talmudic Judaism,"[89] "quite a lot of the distinctive Jewish culture was, to be vulgar about it, repackaged Christianity,"[90] and the far more evenhanded "In order to understand properly Jewish or Christian exegesis in late antiquity it is essential to understand each other's interpretations and the influence of one upon the other,"[91] I have begun to wonder if the time has come at least to consider if something might be going wrong again.

Obviously, the overall point that rabbinic and patristic interpretations are mutually illuminating is worth exploring, even proclaiming; comparative work can very well lead to more nuanced understandings of the many exegetical twists and turns made by both rabbinic and patristic sources in certain textual spaces and possibly lead to "thicker" description of rabbinic and Christian late antiquities. However, to assume that there is an exegetical encounter, or worse, anti-Christian polemic, or worse still, the internalization of Christian positions throughout rabbinic sources, especially already beginning in the third century, runs the risk of significantly misrepresenting rabbinic literature or at least presents a picture of, as Carol Bakhos puts it, "rabbinic engagement with Christianity that may be a bit distorted."[92] Such broader discussions about the impact of Christianity on rabbinic sources have a direct impact on the much more specific question at hand here: just who is Esau in *Genesis Rabbah* 63.

I came to *Genesis Rabbah* 63 with the assumption that Esau in this passage clearly represents Christian Rome. There is ample evidence to support this claim, beginning simply with its fifth-century redaction date. Add to that its clear, to use Neusner's especially apt term in this context, "*genealogization* of Rome," the making of Rome a sibling, a twin, it appeared obvious to me that such a relationship fits better with Christian than pagan Rome.[93] I also shared the reasonable assumption that not only would the rabbis have been aware of the potential for Christian exploitation of Gen. 25:23, but they were, in fact, aware that such potential had been realized. Did not Origen assert precisely this—in Caesarea—making it "gospel"?

The juxtaposition of *Gen. Rab.* 63:6–8 and Origen's writings on Romans 9, moreover, adds substantial evidence to seeing Esau as representative of specifically Christian Rome in *Genesis Rabbah* 63. Heretofore, scholars have depended on far less proximate sources, both rabbinic and patristic, to posit Jewish-Christian contact through and rabbinic defensiveness concerning Gen. 25:23—even in the absence of the direct citation of the verse itself.[94] Reading Esau as Christian in *Genesis Rabbah* 63 makes for a nice neat symmetry lying underneath the interpretive and historical asymmetry posited by both sides. Origen reads Jacob as the new Israel and Esau as the Jews, and the rabbis counter that Jacob is rabbinic Israel and Esau the Christians. I have little doubt that *Gen. Rab.* 63:6–8, with its incessant claim that Jacob embodies rabbinic Israel, through mitzvot, righteousness, and divine election, engages such Christian readings and even surpasses them by making Jacob rabbinic Israel already as a fetus. At the same time, it is striking, and I think significant, that this first appears in a fifth-century compilation and that throughout *Gen. Rab.* 63:6–8, Esau still looks far more pagan than Christian. However much an "Esau who wishes to sit with a prayer shawl and study Torah with the righteous in heaven is almost obviously a Christian,"[95] is the same obviously true about an Esau who wishes to worship idols and whose descendants can attain a royal mantle like Diocletian, who ruled Rome between 285 and 305 CE and is explicitly invoked in *Gen. Rab.* 63:8?[96] If Christian worship resembled idol worship enough for the rabbis not to distinguish between the two, how much of an impact did Christianity, or the Christianization of Rome, make, and how close were these two "siblings"?[97]

I remain bothered by the lack of direct engagement with Gen. 25:23 in rabbinic literature as a whole. Assuming that the rabbis, knowing Christian interpretations of this phrase, simply felt it better to leave well enough alone and thus willfully refused to directly engage this text until they could hardly ignore it in *Genesis Rabbah* 63 is an argument from silence, one that not only presumes that Origen can speak for the rabbis but also that the rabbis would have read Gen. 25:23 as Christians did. The "counter"-interpretation in *Gen. Rab.* 63:7, which amounts to "If Jacob/Israel merits he will be served" with its radical turn inward, appears to lack any gusto given the weight patristic uses of "the elder will serve the younger" presumably holds over the rabbis. It is possible that the rabbis, knowing the Christian interpretation, deflected and diffused it so that it surfaced in their interpretations on surrounding verses, Gen. 25:22; 24–26.[98] *Gen. Rab.* 63:8, interpreting *And the first came forth red*, might be an example of such a strategy, where the "elder" and "younger" distinction is superimposed upon and suffused through the interpretations of the birth order of Esau and Jacob. And here, where cumulatively, Jacob becomes both elder and younger, first and last—in other words the only legitimate son—it is possible that this is both a response to Christian readings of *the elder will serve the younger* and an attempt to ward off the temporal paradoxes that inhere in making Christianity, through Esau, the older brother.

It is worth considering, however, whether the rabbis might not have focused on Gen. 25:23 for reasons of their own. Instead of grafting patristic interpretations onto rabbinic sources, thus allowing patristic exegesis to set the terms of a debate under which rabbinic exegesis can only be "reactive and defensive,"[99] and instead of relying only on an argument from rabbinic silence concerning this verse, I suggest an alternative reason for why the rabbis did not dwell upon Gen. 25:23. Gen. 25:23, *and the elder shall serve the younger*, becomes undone already in Gen. 25:29–34, when Jacob becomes the firstborn, the elder by birthright, and in Gen. 27:36, where Jacob's birthright is again mentioned along with his receiving his father's blessing.[100] Perhaps Gen. 25:23, then, posed no special problem to rabbinic interpretations that understand Jacob as Israel. Taking the rabbis at their word, the more prominent subtext of *Gen. Rab.* 63:8 might very well be their knowledge that *Israel is God's firstborn son*, as Exod. 4:22 states. The identification of Jacob as Israel need not be evidence that "the Jewish identification with Jacob emerged from internalizing the Christian position and confronting it." The identification of Israel with Jacob is biblical, not "Jewish"; the rabbis could hardly have seen Jacob any other way—even as a fetus.[101] That the rabbis chose to portray prenatal Jacob struggling with prenatal pagan Esau, or at least Esau as much idol-worshipper as Jesus-worshipper, should caution against the notion of Christianity as an all-encompassing or all-consuming force throughout rabbinic literature.

My point is not, of course, that there was no contact between Jews and Christians but to question the degree of impact that such contact can meaningfully be made to bear and still leave rabbinic literature intact enough so that it does not become, at its essence or heart, a response to Christianity. Even if, despite the pagan cloaking, Esau is best read as Christian Rome in *Gen. Rab.* 63:6–8 and *Gen. Rab.* 63:6–8 is best read as reacting to patristic interpretations of Gen. 25:23, such reaction is exceedingly localized—hardly supporting that Christianity looms that large over or in front of rabbinic interpretation. And even if one amasses all the instances of anti-Christian polemic or exegetical encounters in rabbinic sources, we are far off from establishing that the confrontation with Christianity is at the center of rabbinic literature and not at its margins.

In the end, the answer to "Who is Esau in *Genesis Rabbah* 63?" is that he is both pagan and Christian because for the rabbis, at least here, they appear to be one and the same thing. The conflation of the two constructs Christian and pagan in the figure of prenatal Esau suggests two additional points. First, the emphasis in this text, as in rabbinic exegesis more generally, is on creating and articulating Israel; Esau, as pagan and Christian, helps insofar as he is not-Israel. However, Israel does not depend on not-Israel, as the passages in *Genesis Rabbah* 63 that effectively erase Esau make clear. For the rabbis, Israel is first, last, elder, and younger, who takes shape known and loved by—and in relation with—God. Israel, through mitzvot and righteousness, merits that love and *that* relationship. Second, I find Neusner's emphasis on the genealogization of Rome, the transition "from enemy to sibling," compelling, although as surely and as soon as *Gen. Rab.* 63:6–8 places (Christian) Rome along with rabbinic Israel in one womb, the point seems to be to undermine any relation and any kinship whatsoever between them, thus complicating the ease with which contemporary scholars have come to read the two primarily as brothers—and sons.

Rebekah's Sons

As a corrective to a previous generation's faulty familial portrait of Judaism as the "mother" of Christianity, more recent scholarship has moved on to present late antique Judaism and Christianity as siblings, often invoking the image of Jacob and Esau in Rebekah's womb.[102] Alan Segal draws on this image in order to emphasize both the "overwhelming similarities" and "great areas of difference" between Judaism and Christianity.[103] Daniel Boyarin writes, "Like many twins, Judaism and Christianity never quite formed separate identities. Like closely related siblings, they rivaled each other, learned from each other fought with each other, perhaps even sometimes loved each other."[104] Meanwhile, the rabbinic depictions of prenatal Jacob and Esau from *Genesis Rabbah* make these same twins *essentially* different and project their difference into that mythic womb of a mythic time long ago, which is the very beginning.[105] As much as current scholarship pushes the "parting of the ways" later, the rabbinic traditions in *Genesis*

Rabbah 63 cannot seem to push it back early enough; as we explore the ways they never parted, in *Genesis Rabbah* 63 they explore never being related at all, despite being in the same womb.

The transition from "enemy to sibling" and the "genealogization of Rome" that Jacob Neusner documents is simultaneously ever present and eclipsed in *Gen. Rab.* 63:6–8.[106] On the one hand, Rome is thoroughly genealogized insofar as Esau comes to be in Rebekah's womb. On the other hand, Rebekah is not Israel, only Jacob is Israel. From the very beginning of Israel, which is Jacob, Esau is already entirely separated, excised. The point of *Gen. Rab.* 63:6–8 is not that they share a womb; the point is that even in that womb—at their very beginnings—they are wholly different. The shared womb that evokes a common space for contemporary readers is figured by the rabbis as a battleground highlighting the ways that Esau and Jacob never had anything (else) in common. More than simply portraying these fetuses as brothers and sons, the rabbis are ever aware that they are conceiving their very father and the father of their enemies. The focus in *Genesis Rabbah* 63 is not only on the fetuses as Rebekah's sons, but on prenatal Jacob and Esau already being and fathering their respective offspring: (rabbinic) Israel and (Christian) Rome.

Conclusion

Gen. Rab. 63:6–8 constructs prenatal Jacob and Esau as wholly separate peoples who simultaneously already embody and engender two totally different nations. It is true that this rabbinic passage is fruitfully compared and contrasted with Origen's interpretations of Romans 9 insofar as both rabbinic and patristic interpreters lay claim to Jacob/Israel as their own inheritance. However, focusing only on how *Gen. Rab.* 63:6–8 engages others' interpretations and constructs Esau as rabbinic "others" passes too quickly over how this passage uses *prenatal* Jacob as a vehicle through which to articulate what it means to be (rabbinic) Israel and to make a statement about when being (rabbinic) Israel begins. By conceiving Jacob as rabbinic Israel, *Genesis Rabbah* 63, like many rabbinic traditions, erases the difference between biblical and rabbinic Israel; they are one and the same thing because Jacob was always rabbinic Israel. Unique to *Gen. Rab.* 63:6–8, however, is that not only does rabbinic Israel begin with Jacob, but it begins with *prenatal* Jacob.

Focusing on Origen (and Paul) and other patristic interpretations, with their attention to "the elder will serve the younger," ultimately leaves uninterpreted the fact that in *Genesis Rabbah* 63 Jacob—as a fetus—represents rabbinic Israel. Allowing early Christian and patristic sources to set the terms through which rabbinic sources are examined, coupled with what is perhaps an overestimation of the impact Christianity had on the rabbis, has contributed to the occlusion of one of the central lessons *Gen. Rab.* 63:6–8 makes; being Israel—for Jacob and the nation he engenders—begins with fetuses.[107]

This chapter has focused on the differences between Jacob and Esau already as fetuses rather than on their coming into being in a shared womb because *Genesis Rabbah* 63 internalizes being Israel through prenatal "pregnant" Jacob, not pregnant Rebekah. Although Rebekah's womb might provide an inviting image from which to emphasize the similarities between Jacob and Esau, *Genesis Rabbah* 63 is far more interested in their irreconcilable differences. Furthermore, putting any particular emphasis on Rebekah's womb would be at odds with the lack of significance the rabbis attribute to pregnant women and wombs in their traditions about embryology and procreation, which are explored at length in the chapters that follow.

Chapter 4
Embryology as Theology

According to a rabbinic tradition, the Roman emperor Antoninus asks Rabbi Yehudah haNasi, "When is the soul placed in humans?" Rabbi initially answers at the moment of birth, but Antoninus counters, asserting that ensoulment occurs at conception. Ultimately Rabbi agrees—*because scripture supports Antoninus.* In another tradition, R. Abbahu converses with Greek speakers, teaching *them* about the nonviability of a child born after eight months of gestation, something widely attested to in Greco-Roman sources. What's more, he teaches it to them *in Greek,* but he has presumably learned this lesson from scripture.

Both of these traditions explicitly articulate the interchange, and here even the interchangeability, of Greco-Roman and rabbinic embryology. Yet they also demonstrate how the rabbis buttress such common notions through appeals to scripture. In doing so, the rabbis achieve two things. First, they make it appear as if their embryology comes from the Bible rather than from Greco-Roman culture. And second, both traditions demonstrate that rabbinic embryology is steeped in theology because the proof texts cited to support that the soul is given at conception and to prove the nonviability of the "eight-month child" make it clear that God places the soul in the embryo at that time and that God decides who shall live and who shall die, even among fetuses. Since rabbinic traditions about embryology weave together ancient notions culled from the rabbis' cultural surroundings and theological aspects of biblical materials, rabbinic embryology offers significant insights into both how the rabbis situated themselves within their Greco-Roman context and how they conceived their God.

In *Imperialism and Jewish Society,* Seth Schwartz asks how the rabbis could not have been influenced by their environment.[1] He begins his book by asserting that "It is intuitively obvious that the ancient Jews (assuming that they behaved like a recognizably human group) were profoundly affected by the imperial powers under which they were constrained to live."[2] The exploration of rabbinic traditions about pregnancy and embryology undertaken throughout this chapter confirms that Greco-Roman notions about these topics have profound effects on rabbinic sources—and in ways far more productive than constraining.

Despite the fact that birth stories and genealogies appear often in the Hebrew Bible, biblical sources are almost completely silent when it comes to the details of pregnancy and the topic of embryology.[3] Rabbinic traditions on embryology fill such enormous gaps left by biblical materials that they indicate an almost revolutionary shift in the development of this discourse, providing substantial evidence for situating Palestinian rabbinic sources within their larger geocultural milieu. Writing on a related topic, the physiology of menstruation in talmudic sources, Charlotte Fonrobert has suggested "the possibility of a rabbinic engagement of such debates in their cultural environment, by means of which they absorbed notions circulating in late antique culture." She continues, "Taking such a possibility into account adds to our understanding as to how the rabbis located themselves in relationship to the larger cultural context of late antiquity."[4] I suggest that not only do rabbinic sources on the topic of embryology point to the possibility of rabbinic engagement with and absorption of notions circulating in late antique culture, but they also establish the likelihood of such engagement. Put simply, Greco-Roman embryology is, by and large, the context within which rabbinic discourse about the fetus, and the rabbinic fetus itself, takes shape.[5]

And yet, such contextualization, even situatedness, does not mean sameness; rabbinic traditions do not by any means merely adopt Greco-Roman notions of embryology verbatim. Nor should rabbinic embryology be seen in terms of simple reaction to, or against, Greco-Roman embryology. As Schwartz also points out, "It is equally obvious that the effects of imperialism were not limited to reaction—to the impulse to 'circle the wagons' that has so often been attributed to the Jews by historians and others."[6] In the specific case of embryology, rabbinic sources adapt Greco-Roman ideas, ultimately producing a unique blend[7] of traditions that demonstrates the rabbinic embeddedness in both their Greco-Roman and biblical "worlds."[8]

Numerous scholars have already posited a certain degree of rabbinic knowledge of Greco-Roman notions about pregnancy and fetal development.[9] There is, broadly speaking, consonance between rabbinic and Greco-Roman sources on these topics. Similar questions are posed, and to almost any given question, the various answers exist within largely overlapping possibilities or parameters.[10] Assuming broad consonance between Greco-

Roman and rabbinic embryology, which situates the rabbis well within Greco-Roman culture, I highlight how the rabbis adapt such embryology, persistently asserting God's roles in pregnancy and fetal development. In the midrashic texts presented throughout this chapter, I suggest that rabbinic embryology is largely a theological endeavor, and I read these texts specifically for the insights they offer into how the rabbis conceived their God and constructed the relationship between God and Israel.[11]

The presentation of texts roughly adheres to the process of fetal development as depicted in the sources excluding traditions about conception, which I discuss in the following chapter. I begin with rabbinic sources on ensoulment, move on to traditions about fetal formation and development, then turn to traditions about the duration of pregnancy and the production of breast milk, and finally, I consider traditions about sex determination and resemblance, thus working through the process of fetal development from start to finish—as the rabbis imagine God does—with various stops along the way.

Ensoulment

Opinions about the moment at which one acquires a soul vary in Greco-Roman writings of antiquity, ranging from conception, formation, which may or may not be the same as movement, or birth.[12] Although the Hebrew Bible does not consider at which precise point ensoulment occurs, the same options suggested in Greco-Roman sources make an appearance in rabbinic literature.[13] However, in comparison with the significant amount of debate surrounding this issue in Greco-Roman writings, rabbinic traditions on the soul of the fetus are relatively clear—and relatively few. All rabbinic traditions that explicitly address the topic maintain that the fetus has a soul, and moreover, that the soul is given by God.[14]

The *Yerushalmi* (*Kel.* 8:3[31c]), *Ecclesiastes Rabbah* (5:10.2), and the *Bavli* (*Nid.* 31a)[15] all record a tradition that states there are three partners in the creation of humans:[16] God, the father, and the mother. God contributes the soul, presumably prenatally in both talmudic versions, and explicitly to the fetus in *Ecclesiastes Rabbah*[17] The tradition does not mention when God provides the soul, just that God does.[18]

Only one tradition in Palestinian sources explicitly addresses the moment at which ensoulment occurs. *Gen. Rab.* 34:10 states:

> [Antoninus] asked [our Rabbi] further,[19] "From when is the soul placed in humans?"
> [Rabbi] said to him, "From when one issues forth from his mother's womb."
> [Antoninus] said to him, "If meat sits without salt for three days, does it not spoil?,[20] rather [say that the soul enters] from the time of conception."[21]
> And Rabbi agreed with him because scripture supports him, [*All the while my soul is in me*] *and the spirit of God is in my nostrils* (Job 27:3). *You have granted me life and favor and your providence* [*has preserved my spirit*] (Job 10:12). From when did you place the soul in me? From when you conceived me.

Whether or not such a conversation between Rabbi and Antoninus took place, the text gives voice to the exchange of ideas between rabbis and "Greeks" on the topic of ensoulment specifically, and embryology more generally.[22] Furthermore, this text explicitly articulates the path of such an exchange—from Greeks to rabbis. At the very least, this tradition suggests that the rabbis were not averse to Greco-Roman notions about embryology, and it plausibly indicates that they were aware, perhaps even self-consciously, of such "borrowing" and here sought to set forth some sort of methodology, a kind of checks and balances. Therefore, the text demonstrates that such "foreign" notions need to be located within scripture, and, in the process, they become not foreign at all but intrinsic—rooted in the Bible. Furthermore, Rabbi is not the only convert in the text insofar as he adopts the opinion of Antoninus, but the Bible is also converted into a vehicle of support, almost a "rubber stamp" for one of the late antique opinions about ensoulment. However, simultaneously, Greco-Roman notions about embryology are themselves converted, or adapted, and a seemingly more abstract discussion about ensoulment becomes a way to concretely render God manifest, immanent—in a word, involved—in embryology and, through it, in Israel. Both of the proof texts that support Antoninus's view make it clear that not only is the soul in the fetus "all the while" (Job 27:3), but moreover, God has placed the soul there, when God conceived this individual Israel.

The parallel tradition in the *Bavli* (*Sanh.* 91b) works the same way, but this version presents the options for ensoulment as either conception or formation, which according to other rabbinic traditions occurs after forty days of gestation.[23] Here again, because of scriptural support Rabbi ultimately agrees with Antoninus that ensoulment occurs at conception.[24] However, elsewhere the *Bavli* seems to suggest that the soul is formed (or given) after forty days of gestation, an opinion also set forth in some Greco-Roman and patristic sources.[25]

B. *Men.* 99b states, "R. Yohanan and R. Eleazar[26] both said, 'The Torah was given in forty days and the soul is formed [or given][27] in forty days.' All who keep the Torah, his soul is kept, and all who do not keep the Torah, his soul is not kept." The rhetoric of the text functions to link the giving of the soul and its preservation with the giving of the Torah and its preservation, and it implies that God, who gave the Torah to Israel, also gives Israel its souls. The text does not cite a specific proof text that establishes that ensoulment occurs at forty days; it is taken for granted.[28] Nevertheless embryology is imbued with theological significance: just as God gave the Torah to Israel after forty days (e.g., Exod. 24:18 and 34:28–29), God gives the soul to Israel forty days after conception.[29]

Regardless of when rabbinic sources place the exact time at which the soul is given to the embryo, the discourse about ensoulment situates rabbinic sources within Greco-Roman culture. The Rabbi and Antoninus text renders the exchange between Greco-Roman and rabbinic embryology explicit, and it also demonstrates both the rabbinic attempt to locate such notions within scripture and the rabbinic predilection for imbuing embryology with theological significance. The question about ensoulment provides the rabbis with a way to imagine God actively involved in Israel—its formation and preservation.

Fetal Formation and Development

In midrashic traditions, fetal formation, no less than ensoulment, becomes a platform from which to assert and explore God's relationship with Israel. According to these traditions, formation occurs at forty days, which although unsubstantiated in biblical sources, is roughly consonant with some Greco-Roman opinions about the time of formation.[30]

Lev. Rab. 23:12 elaborately implicates God in the formation of the embryo when it fabricates a conversation between Job and God, which explores the dilemma God faces if a pregnant woman commits adultery. Interpreting Job 10:3, *Is it good that you despise the work of your hands?* the text imagines that Job says to God, "After you have worked all forty days [to establish the embryo's likeness to its father], you go back and spoil it [and form the embryo in the likeness of the adulterer]."[31] The text later likens God to a sculptor, chiseling the embryo's facial features like one who sculpts the image of a king.[32] But when a new king arises, the artist worries over whose image his work should reflect. So too, God's hands grow weak from adultery, and the text cites Deut. 32:18, *Of the rock [tsur] that begot you, you are unmindful (teshi)*, interpreted to teach the adulterers that "you have weakened [*hitshatem*] the strength of the creator [*yotser*]." The formation of the embryo is the work of the God's hands, right down to its facial features.³³

These two brief excerpts cannot do justice to the entirety of *Lev. Rab.* 23:12, a tradition itself almost entirely concerned with issues of divine justice and providence. Although this tradition demonstrates that midrashic sources attest to fetal formation at forty days, it much more potently illustrates that rabbinic embryology is deeply entwined with theology, such that in midrashic sources when there is a fetus, there is God, and Israel—and the relationship between them. Here the rabbis do not even attempt to prove the specifics of fetal formation from scripture. The reckoning of forty days for the completion of formation is simply asserted, reflecting an utter lack of concern that this may well come from Greco-Roman culture—with no basis in the Bible.³⁴ What does come from the Bible, however, is that Israel is the work of God's hands. And here the text mobilizes the image of the formation of the embryo to powerfully depict, even mold, fashion, and sculpt an image of the God of Israel.

The wider textual context within which these passages appear interprets Job 24:15, *The eye also of an adulterer waits for the twilight, saying, No eye shall see me,* and the point of this tradition is to illustrate that God sees Israel. God does not simply watch over Israel at a distance as an impartial observer, even one who sees all, but God actively oversees and shapes Israel. The tradition renders this remarkably concrete through its image of the embryo in formation.

At the same time that the image of the embryo is here used to inform rabbinic constructions of God, it further serves to construct Israel. Taking into consideration the yet wider context of this tradition in *Leviticus Rabbah* 23, which interprets Lev. 18:3, *After the doings of the land of Egypt, where you dwelt, you shall not do, and after the doings of the land of Canaan, where I bring you, shall you not do; nor shall you walk in their ordinances,* the text not only concerns itself with distinctive facial markings that signal anxieties about paternity and lineage, but also with ethnonational markers that demarcate Israel's uniqueness among other peoples and in relation with God. Using the image of the embryo and the (potential)³⁵ consequences adultery has on it individually and Israel collectively, this midrash defines Israel against the other nations: they commit adultery, but Israel should not do as they do. Of course, the text imagines well that Israel does commit adultery, and it warns that in so doing, the embryo, Israel, and God, insofar as Israel's adultery weakens God and presumably the relationship between God and Israel, all pay a price.

The embryo in this text is thus used to articulate messages of theological and national, as well as religious or moral import. Israel should not follow in the other nations' ways or "walk in their laws."[36] Israel has its own ways, laws, and God, and all of this distinction is illustrated through and even thrust upon the forty-day-old embryo. This becomes all the more complex if such articulations of Israel's uniqueness vis-à-vis its relationship with God and notions of Israel's difference vis-à-vis other nations, while grafted onto the embryo, reflect incorporation of Greco-Roman embryology.

Even if the specific claim of fetal formation at forty days does not come from Greco-Roman sources, the concern over when formation occurs locates the rabbis as participants in late antique cultural investigations about embryology. In midrashic sources, however, the rabbis are not concerned with embryology in and of itself, but what it reflects about the nature of the relationship between Israel, even in utero, and God.[37] In *Lev. Rab.* 23:12, the assertion that the embryo is formed at forty days requires no proof text, nor can one be easily found, but God's work in creating Israel (Job 10:3), or "birthing Israel" (Deut. 32:18), is biblically well founded. In bringing both assertions together, one possibly relaid from surrounding culture and the other from the Bible, the rabbis imbue embryology with theological significance and meaning, making it their own.

If there is no obvious biblical basis for the formation of the embryo at forty days, this does not mean that the rabbis do not attempt to ground this lesson in scripture. Although such an attempt is absent in *Lev. Rab.* 23:12, *Gen. Rab.* 32:5, a tradition also concerned with divine justice, provides biblical support for the formation of the embryo at forty days, or at least seems to do so. Explaining why God floods the earth for forty days and nights instead of another length of time, *Gen. Rab.* 32:5 states, "R. Yohanan said, 'They spoiled the form that was given in forty days, therefore [*I will cause it to rain upon the earth*] *forty days and forty nights* (Gen. 7:4).'"[38] According to this tradition, the generation of the flood merited destruction presumably because of its adulterous unions, which as seen above, spoil the form of the embryo.[39] Although scripture does not explicitly attest to the formation of the embryo at forty days, the text makes it appear as if it does by interpreting Gen. 7:4 in a way that juxtaposes God's causing the rain to come down for forty days and forty nights with the formation of the embryo at forty days. At the same time, the text establishes that just as God caused the rain, God forms the embryo, again overlaying embryology with a theological point.[40]

Beyond asserting that God forms the embryo at forty days, midrashic sources further implicate God in the very process of fetal formation. Greco-

Roman sources also consider the order of fetal development, and they assert that the fetus develops from the "outside to inside," meaning skin and flesh are formed first, followed by bones and sinews.[41] *Gen. Rab.* 14:5 and *Lev. Rab.* 14:9 interpret Job 10:11, *You have clothed me with skin and flesh, and knit me together with bones and sinews.* Since the verse says skin and flesh first, and afterward bones and sinews, it is quite easily read as describing the order of fetal formation. That God forms the embryo in such a fashion, as already evident in Job 10, is made even more explicit in the continuation of *Lev. Rab.* 14:9: "R. Abbahu[42] states, 'the Holy Blessed One does a great good with women in this world, in that He does not begin forming the embryo with sinews and bones, because if He began in such a way, it would split her belly and go forth.'"[43]

Even rabbinic traditions that describe the appearance of the developing embryo are supported by scripture and demonstrate God's involvement in Israel. *Lev. Rab.* 14:8 describes the shape of the embryo[44] in its mother's womb as an unformed mass, citing Ps. 139:16, *Your eyes have seen my unformed shape.* The description of the embryo simultaneously signals, once again, that God sees Israel and, moreover, bringing in the broader context of Psalm 139, that God fashions Israel: *For you have formed my insides; you knit me together in my mother's womb* (Ps. 139:13).

Lev. Rab. 14:8 provides one final image, in answer to the question "how does the fetus lay in its mother's womb?" Using a Greek loanword, the text answers, "it lay like a folded *pinaks* [writing tablet]; its head lies between its knees, its two hands on its two sides [or temples], and its two heels on its buttocks."[45] Coincidentally, but nevertheless perspicaciously, the word *pinaks* also appears in a tradition that likens the Torah, with which God created the world, to writing tablets used by an architect in building a palace (*Gen. Rab.* 1:1). The use of the Greek loanword in both contexts, to describe the Torah and the fetus, leads me to suggest in conclusion to this section, but pertinent for this entire project, that the fetus offers the rabbis its own unique instruction, like the Torah, about God and Israel, and the relationship between them.

Pregnancy and the Production of Breast Milk

The Hebrew Bible almost always neglects to remark on the time between the beginning of pregnancy and birth, as if the woman becomes pregnant and immediately delivers the child.[46] When Gen. 25:24 mentions that Rebekah's days were fulfilled, it does not specify how many days have passed, nor does the Bible reckon pregnancy by months or divide those months into "trimesters," much less consider the advantages or disadvantages of sexual intercourse to the fetus and the woman during such trimesters. The Bible also lacks any explanation for the production of breast milk. Rabbinic sources, in contrast, consider nine months, or roughly 270 days, of pregnancy normative, divide those nine months into "trimesters,"[47] discuss during which trimester sexual intercourse with a pregnant woman is harmful or beneficial,[48] proclaim the nonviability of "eight-month children," and explain how breast milk is produced, once again demonstrating at least broad consonance with the discourse about pregnancy in Greco-Roman culture. Many of the midrashic traditions that fill in such details about pregnancy further illustrate that rabbinic embryology is suffused with theological, as well as physiological, speculation, and I focus on these passages, highlighting such theological overtones.

Mention of nine months of pregnancy appears in a number of rabbinic sources, but two traditions from *Leviticus Rabbah* combine this "fact of life" with a theological message.[49] The first has to do with God's transforming the pregnant woman's menstrual blood into breast milk during the nine months of pregnancy (*Lev. Rab.* 14:3), and I return to this below. The second tradition teaches that throughout the nine months of pregnancy, God gives light to the fetus (*Lev. Rab.* 31:8).[50] The text's mention of nine months represents a casual statement about the duration of pregnancy, about which there is no scriptural basis offered—or transparently available. The midrash's primary concern is with the theological implications of Lev. 24:2, where Moses commands the Israelites to bring oil to make a continual light in the Tent of Meeting.[51] The midrash asks, putting the rhetorical question into God's mouth, "All nine months that you were in your mother's womb, I gave light to you. Do I need your light?" The text makes clear that Israel needs God, but not the other way around.

This tradition depicts God as more impenetrable than *Lev. Rab.* 23:12, where God is imagined as deeply affected by Israel's actions. The discrepancy between the constructions of God in both traditions serves as a reminder that despite the overall theological bent that I see present in midrashic traditions about embryology, rabbinic theology is not consistent or systematic but far more nuanced, complex, and multivalent. Nevertheless, *Lev. Rab.* 31:8 still portrays God as deeply involved in caring for and sustaining Israel, already in utero; it just also asserts God's self-sufficiency, as if to protect God from any weakness so powerfully depicted in *Lev. Rab.* 23:12.

Gen. Rab. 20:6, interpreting *I will greatly multiply [harbah 'arbeh] your pain and your pregnancy* (Gen. 3:16), uses this verse to discuss both the shortest and normative number of days of pregnancy, and it also suggests that God determines both, again making a theological claim through embryology. The text first sets the shortest gestation time for viable birth at 212 days: "R. Aba bar Zutra in the name of Shmuel: All who are *harbah* [which has the numerical value of 212], *I will multiply ['arbeh]*. All who are 212 days, live."[52] The text not only maintains that the shortest gestation for a viable birth is seven months,[53] consonant with Greco-Roman sources,[54] but it also explicitly asserts that God is responsible for preserving one born at this time: God multiplies them. Still interpreting Gen. 3:16, the text later states, "R. Berekiah and R. Biba in the name of Shmuel: 'A woman only gives birth on the 271st, or 272nd, or 273rd day. [This is] nine months plus the days of conception."[55] In the context of *Gen. Rab.* 20:6, this statement is again a midrashic reading of how God multiplies pregnancy, that is, by making it a particular length. In other words, God has established the duration of "full-term" pregnancy at roughly 270 days.[56]

Interpreting Gen. 3:16 to teach that God establishes the duration of pregnancy, *Gen. Rab.* 20:6 here ignores and possibly subverts the biblical context and content of the verse, which appears as a curse to Eve, and presumably all women. In the place of a curse, the text takes this opportunity to make it clear that God blesses pregnancy and birth.[57] Although not recorded in Palestinian sources, a statement in the *Bavli*, using *gematria*, accounts for the 271 days of pregnancy by citing Ruth 4:13, *And the Lord gave her pregnancy* (= 271), reinforcing that the duration of pregnancy is God's gift, no less than pregnancy itself.

Gen. Rab. 20:6, right in the middle of the two traditions about the durations of pregnancy and still interpreting Gen. 3:16 in a way that emphasizes God's roles in procreation, records a tradition about the nonviability of the child born during its eighth month of gestation, a belief well documented in Greco-Roman sources.[58] The same tradition appears in *Gen. Rab.* 14:2, where the theological message that God determines who shall live and who shall die, even among fetuses, is arguably stronger, since here the passage is offered as an interpretation of Gen. 2:7, *And the Lord God formed ha'adam*:[59] "*And God formed [vayyitser]* . . . [there is a] formation for nine [months] and formation for seven [months]. R. Huna said: '[if] it [the fetus] is formed for seven [months] and born at seven or nine, it lives. [If it is formed for seven and born at] eight, it doesn't live. If it is formed for nine and it is born at seven, it does not live, how much more so [it does not live if it was formed for nine and born] at eight.'" R. Huna presents the belief in the nonviability of the eight-month child as if it appears in scripture.[60] The lexical oddity of the doubling of the *yod* in the word for "formed" (*vayyitser*)[61] in Gen. 2:7 teaches that there are two formations or, more specifically, God creates fetuses that will be born after seven months and nine months of gestation. By implication at first, and then spelled out, no one born during the eighth month will survive. The tradition seems logical, but the assertion that one created to be born at seven months does not survive if it is born at eight months is not logical unless one presupposes the nonviability of the eight-month child. The logic of the second example, that if one created to be born at nine months and is born at seven months does not live, all the more so it does not live if it is born at eight months, is similarly questionable; it too requires the a priori belief in the nonviability of the eight-month child. Nevertheless, the tradition presents the interpretation as scripturally motivated, leaving no hint that the rabbis are grafting a widely held late antique notion about embryology onto the Bible.

All of this changes with the continuation of the tradition, which appears in all of the parallels:[62] "They came before R. Abbahu: From where [do we know] that the one who is formed for seven [months] lives? He said to them, from your own [language] I will prove it to you: [infants of] seven months [are more likely to survive than those] of eight."[63] This is no casual acknowledgment of rabbinic cultural embeddedness; *Gen. Rab.* 14:2 and parallels employ the Greek alphabet and language, not to mention Greek exegetical methods,[64] rendering quite manifest, even baldly proclaiming, the connection between rabbinic and Greek embryology. Not since the Rabbi and Antoninus tradition about ensoulment discussed at the beginning of this chapter has there been a clearer indication of the intersection among ancient notions of embryology. But this tradition, in stark contrast to the Rabbi and Antoninus one, does not locate the rabbis on the receiving end. The belief in the nonviability of eight-month children is not presented as something learned from Greeks; the nonviability of eight-month children is first learned from scripture, and then this "scripture" *and* embryology are translated into Greek and transmitted to Greeks.[65]

I do not know why this tradition goes to such great lengths to deny the rabbinic assimilation of Greco-Roman notions about the nonviability of eight-month children only to disclose it so blatantly in its very rhetoric and even language. The attribution of the Greek lesson to R. Abbahu is of course apt, since his acculturation to things Greek is well documented. But the tradition signals the acculturation of R. Huna, and I think as well the rabbis more generally, not only about the nonviability of eight-month children, but also more broadly in the case of embryology.[66] Perhaps again, as in the Rabbi and Antoninus tradition, the rabbis are all too aware of their own indebtedness to ancient embryology. And here, instead of openly proclaiming that the path of transmission goes from Greeks to rabbis, they attempt to deny it, and the use of Greek in the text is a crack in the edifice of their own making. They may try to hide that rabbinic embryology is, to a large extent, Greco-Roman embryology, but this just cannot be hidden. But the rabbis are not trying to hide their acculturation, at least as it pertains to embryology. They are, instead, adapting embryology and, in so doing, illustrating their acculturation—and their difference.

At the same time this text signals the similarity of rabbinic and Greco-Roman embryology on the fate of eight-month children, it articulates a contrast. Helen King writes, "We do not know how Greek religion accounted for the death of a child ... we do know how Hippocratic medicine coped with the death of a newborn child. The Hippocratic solution to the problem *refers not to gods or spirits,* but to an unavoidable law of nature related to numbers."[67] In contrast, rabbinic literature, in one of its explanations for the death of a newborn, indeed refers to laws of nature, but those that God sets.[68] Eight-month children do not survive because, according to this motif, God does not create them to survive: there are two formations, one for seven and one for nine.[69] The rabbis theologize the nonviability of the eight-month child, explaining why some fetuses do not survive (God has God's reasons), but also implicating God in the process of forming and sustaining most of Israel.

One more midrashic tradition that mentions nine months of pregnancy further illustrates how rabbinic traditions theologize the discourse about pregnancy and embryology in order to construct God as intimately involved in Israel's formation and here, quite specifically, Israel's sustenance. *Lev. Rab.* 14:3 states, "R. Meir said, 'All nine months [of pregnancy] that a woman does not see blood, it is logical that she should see [it].[70] What does the Holy Blessed One do? He raises it up to her breasts and makes it milk so that when the child goes forth their will be food for it to eat.'"[71]

The transformation of (menstrual) blood into milk appears in Greco-Roman writings as one of the leading theories for the production of breast milk.[72] *Lev. Rab.* 14:3, although here without any apparent acknowledgment or hesitation, works from, and with, this theory, transforming it into a theological lesson:[73] God transforms the blood and produces the milk.[74] In the context of *Lev. Rab.* 14:3, which most immediately interprets Job 10:12, *You have granted me life and favor and your providence has preserved my spirit,* the physiology of the production of milk is one of the examples of divine favor, or "life and mercy," that God performs for Israel. This tradition links God's care of the fetus, set forth repeatedly in *Lev. Rab.* 14:2–4, with God's continued care for the child. Again, God watches over—and sustains—Israel.

The bridge that this tradition makes between God's—prenatal and postnatal—care of this individual Israel also carries with it another connection that deepens and expands the theological message of all of the traditions about embryology examined thus far. Rabbinic assertions that God cares for, sustains, and nurtures the fetus are themselves pregnant with the notion that God does the same for all Israel.[75] The fetus in these texts, over which God watches, protects, and indeed forms, represents Israel. And that God is this intimately tied up with the individual fetus represents how God is so occupied with Israel.

Rabbinic discourse about embryology uses the fetus in the pregnant woman's body, and pregnancy itself, to illustrate, even probe, the depths of God's care for Israel. These traditions might appear to focus on the formation of the fetus and on pregnancy, but they no less, and possibly more profoundly, reflect rabbinic constructions of God.[76]

Sex-ing the Fetus and Face-ing the Fetus: Inherited Traits

A tradition recorded in the *Yerushalmi, Genesis Rabbah,* and the *Bavli* suggests that God changed Dinah, the daughter of Jacob and Leah, from male to female either at the moment of birth or even after Dinah was born.[77] Along similar lines, *b. Bab. Metz.* 87a maintains that God changed Isaac's facial features well after he was born in order to render Abraham's paternity certain.

Not all rabbinic traditions about sex determination and resemblance set such "miracles" after birth; some of them suggest that the embryo's facial features and its sex are completed at forty days, and yet others leave the time of such prenatal markings unspecified. Nevertheless, I consider these traditions at the end of this chapter for two reasons. First, since some sources do suggest that these changes might occur at or just after birth I discuss them here, in keeping with the order of fetal formation as presented in rabbinic traditions to which I have roughly adhered. Furthermore, the miraculousness of these traditions, which place sex determination and resemblance so late in development, serves to highlight God's involvement in these matters even when they occur prenatally. In other words, these rather extreme examples represent a difference of degree, not of kind.

The second reason that I discuss sex determination and resemblance here is because theories about such inherited traits are fundamental to Greco-Roman theories about generation, and therefore they set the scene for my examination of rabbinic theories of procreation in the next chapter.[78] Once it becomes clear that rabbinic sources often invoke God in order to explain a person's physical characteristics, and in doing so they differ from Greco-Roman sources but are consistent with rabbinic conceptions of embryology seen throughout this chapter, the failure inherent in any attempt to explain rabbinic theories of procreation solely by asking whether the rabbis adopted either a "one-seed" or "two-seed" theory of generation becomes obvious. Part of the work of this chapter has been to challenge the notion that rabbinic sources, despite their embeddedness in Greco-Roman culture, simply adopt anything, without further adapting late antique cultural notions about embryology to serve their theological purposes, and needs. Beyond looking for similarity among rabbinic and Greco-Roman embryology, which at least in broad strokes is readily apparent and has been well documented, I have been interested in exploring some of the differences by highlighting theological motivations and meanings that I see as central but have been left underinterpreted.

The *Mekhilta of Rabbi Ishmael,* in the context of a sustained presentation about the differences between God and humanity's powers of (pro) creation, states, "It is the rule among people that one goes to an image maker and says to him, 'Make for me an image of my father.' And does he [the image maker] not say to him, 'Let your father come and stand before me or bring me a likeness of him and I will make his image?' But this is not so for the Holy Blessed One. [God] gives to man a son from a drop of liquid and he resembles the image of his father."[79] As far as I have been able to determine, this passage from the *Mekhilta,* a tannaitic midrashic compilation on part of the book of Exodus, is the earliest midrashic tradition to set forth a theory of inherited traits in children.[80] And according to this tradition, God determines both that the child will be male and that he will resemble his father.[81] This tradition also implies a concern specifically over paternal influence, or even anxiety over paternity, and this is in keeping with most traditions about facial resemblance set forth below.

Despite the *Mekhilta* tradition's suggestion of God's involvement in determining the sex of the child, or fetus,[82] and the clear assertion of God's decisive role in this found in the traditions about Dinah, much of the scholarship about sex determination in rabbinic sources centers on a tradition recorded in *b. Nid.* 31a.[83] This passage attributes the child's sex to the partner who "emits seed" first[84] *and* assumes that each partner reproduces not itself but its "other," perhaps here its opposite:[85] "If a woman emits seed first she gives birth to a male; if a man emits seed first she gives birth to a female."

In the context of this study, it should be noted that extant Palestinian sources do not record this teaching.[86] Furthermore, in contrast to the *Mekhilta* tradition cited above and other Palestinian traditions set forth below, the *Bavli* tradition makes no mention of God in determining the sex of the offspring; sex determination is decided by the human partners, irrespective of God, who in other traditions is depicted as the other "partner" in procreation.[87] The very lack of any mention of God might contribute to the scholarly interest in this version of the tradition specifically; it simply sounds more "scientific."[88] My interests, of course, lie precisely in the interarticulation of such science and theology that I see permeating many rabbinic sources—especially of Palestinian provenance—ostensibly about embryology, and therefore I focus on Palestinian traditions about sex determination that implicate God in the process.[89]

Lev. Rab. 14:7 states, "*Give a portion to seven and also to eight* (Eccles.11:2). *Give a portion to seven*: these are the seven days of *niddah*. *And a portion to eight:* These are the eight days of circumcision. The Holy Blessed One said, 'If you keep the days of *niddah*, I will give you a son and you will circumcise him on the eighth [day].' [As it is said], *And on the eighth day the flesh of his foreskin shall be circumcised* (Lev. 12:3)."[90] Without any appeal to the emission of seed, and instead invoking behavioral and ritual actions, this tradition nevertheless both accounts for why some offspring are girls and some boys and attributes the ultimate decision to God.[91] Furthermore, God's control over this matter is attached to scripture (Eccles. 11:2), which might be more apt than at first apparent because Ecclesiastes 11 meditates on the lack of human understanding of the world and of God's workings in it, and a few verses later than the verse cited in this midrash, states, *Just as you do not know how the life-breath gets into the fetus in the womb of a pregnant woman, so you cannot know the work of God who makes everything* (11:5).[92] Sex determination, among other matters, is not for humans to understand, but there exist some ways for people to act that influence the divine process.

A tradition in *Gen. Rab.* 72:6 illustrates God's role in sex determination much more dramatically, and it too suggests some role for human influence.[93]

Overturning *m. Ber.* 9:3, which characterizes a man's prayer that his wife give birth to a son as ineffective, this tradition imagines the effect that human prayer has on God's sex-ing the fetus rather concretely:[94]

And afterwards she gave birth to a daughter [and called her name Dinah] (Gen. 30:21). We have learned in a mishnah: If a man's wife is pregnant and he said may it be Your will that she give birth to a male, behold this prayer [takes God's name] in vain.[95] The House of R. Yannai said this is taught concerning a woman who is giving birth[96] [but before this time such prayer is not wasted]. R. Yehudah bar Pazi said, "Even when the woman is giving birth He can change [the sex of the fetus] as scripture states, *Cannot I do with you as this potter.* . . . [*Behold, like the clay in the potter's hand, so are you in My hands, O House of Israel*] (Jer. 18:6).[97]

Although R. Yannai's assertion that God can change the sex of the fetus until birth has begun seems acceptable, R. Yehudah's further claim, that God can change the sex even during birth is challenged: "An objection was raised: Scripture states, *And afterwards [ve'ahar], she bore a daughter* (Gen. 30:21)." Since scripture says "afterwards," then the sex change must have occurred *before* birth. R. Yehudah responds, even rises, to the challenge: "He said to them, 'the essence of Dinah's creation[98] was male but from Rachel's prayer that said, *May the Lord add to me another ['aher] son* (Gen. 30:24), it was made female."[99] R. Yehudah appeals to a verse that appears in the biblical text after Dinah has been born, suggesting that God can change the sex of the child even after birth.[100]

Whether or not the specific example of God changing Dinah's sex from male to female occurs right before Leah begins to give birth, sometime earlier during gestation, or even after birth, God determines Dinah's sex. Although the *Bavli* parallel first relegates Dinah's example to a miraculous event and then suggests that it occurs before forty days of gestation, the Palestinian sources do not show any anxiety about God's role in determining, and then changing, Dinah's sex, even at the onset of labor. Nor do the Palestinian sources indicate that God's role in sex determination is limited to this specific example of Dinah. Both the *Yerushalmi* and *Genesis Rabbah* frame this tradition by the Mishnah's general statement about the sex of the fetus being beyond the realm of human influence, and both sources reject that sex determination is completely removed from human influence. However, the parental influence is through prayer—not through their seed. Furthermore, both traditions also assert that God determines the sex of the fetus, and only God can change that in response to human prayer. One can indeed pray and these prayers are in fact heeded, and thus even a rabbinic inquiry into sex determination articulates the theological message that God both hears Israel and, like a potter with clay, shapes Israel.[101]

In addition to attributing sex determination primarily to God, midrashic traditions also imagine that God further fashions Israel by shaping the embryo's appearance. *Gen. Rab.* 72:6 bears some resemblance to *Lev. Rab.* 23:12, which I discussed above: just as God determines and then changes the sex of the fetus, so too God shapes the facial features and can change them. Other Palestinian traditions attribute parental, or more accurately paternal, influence to God as well.

The "three partners" tradition at *y. Kel.* 8:3, maintains that the man contributes the marrow, bones, and tendons, and the woman contributes the skin and flesh and blood.[102] God contributes the *ruah, nefesh,* and *neshamah,* that which animates the body. This tradition, which attributes the dark parts of the body to women and the light parts of the body to men, represents a general rabbinic explanation of heredity, but it does not provide any information about rabbinic understanding of specific inherited traits or how and why the child resembles the parent.[103] The *Bavli*'s version and *Eccles. Rab.* 5:10, which follows it, add that God provides the facial features of the fetus, perhaps drawing from the Palestinian sources discussed above.[104]

Although the *Bavli* seems to leave open the possibility that God might shape the facial features to resemble either parent, both the *Mekhilta* (*B'shalakh* 8) and *Lev. Rab.* 23:12 only consider that the fetus, which is presumably male, will resemble the male partner.[105] Neither tradition entertains the possibility that a child, male or female, might resemble the woman, suggesting that the concern about resemblance is a concern about paternity, leaving maternal influence untheorized either because it is of less interest or because it is more obvious.[106] If the latter, the obviousness of maternal resemblance is left implicit in Palestinian sources, never explained by an appeal to a theory of woman's seed, like Hippocratic sources, since in Palestinian sources, the woman has no seed.[107] Nor is there ever any explicit mention that the environment of the womb or the woman's blood would contribute to any likeness between the woman and child, as others, including some patristic authors arguing for the both the divinity and humanity, or flesh and bloodness, of Jesus suggest.[108] If maternal resemblance is ignored in rabbinic traditions because it is obvious, paternal influence emerges as nothing short of miraculous.[109] And if *Lev. Rab.* 23:12 and the *Mekhilta* (*B'shalakh* 8) implicitly demonstrate rabbinic concerns about paternity, paternal anxiety becomes explicit in the following traditions.

Gen. Rab. 53:6 interprets Gen. 21:2, rendered rather literally as *And*

Sarah became pregnant and bore to Abraham [l'Avraham] a son for his old age:[110] "*To Abraham a son in his old age*—this teaches that she did not steal seed from another.[111] *For his old age*—this teaches that his [Isaac's] facial features were like his [Abraham's]."[112] Since Gen. 20 places Sarah in Avimelech's house, and Gen. 21:1 begins with *And God visited Sarah*, followed by Gen. 21:2, which announces Isaac's birth, this tradition worries about Abraham's paternity. The textual peculiarity of *l'Avraham* puts such concerns at rest as it comes to signify that Sarah gives birth to Abraham's son, from his seed, who reflects or mirrors his face, but of course the repeated assertion of Abraham's paternity also gives voice to an underlying anxiety.

Presumably, God makes Isaac resemble Abraham, along the same lines as the *Mekhilta* (*B'shalakh*),[113] and as attested to in *b. Bab. Metz.* 87a and in a later tradition from *Midrash Tanhuma* (*Toldot* 1), where paternal concerns more obviously take on national proportions:[114] "At the time that Sarah was passed from the hand of Pharaoh to the hand of Avimelech and she became pregnant with Isaac, the nations of the world were saying, 'Can a man one hundred years old beget? Rather, she became pregnant from Avimelech or from Pharaoh.' And there was doubt in Abraham's heart about these things. What did the Holy Blessed One do? God said to the angel appointed over the creation of the embryo, make all his features like the image of his father so that they will all testify that he is the son of Abraham."[115] This tradition projects the rabbinic concern about Abraham's paternity evident in *Gen. Rab.* 53:6 directly onto Abraham, as he now worries if Isaac is his son. In direct response to Abraham's anxiety, God fashions Isaac in his image.

Although *Midrash Tanhuma*'s redaction date is the eighth century CE, amoraic compilations similarly link concerns about paternal resemblance and ethnonational identity. Just as Abraham, the father of (the father of) Israel, is taunted by the nations, so too Israel is taunted. *Song of Songs Rab.* 4:12, states:

The nations were taunting Israel and saying, "*And the Egyptians made the sons of Israel serve with rigor* (Exod. 1:13). If they forced them [to serve] with labor, all the more so with their bodies and their wives!" At this moment the Holy Blessed One said, *A garden closed up is my sister, my bride* (Song 4:12). What does *a garden closed up* mean? The Holy Blessed One said, "My garden is closed up, but she is disgraced." R. Pinhas said, "At this moment the Holy Blessed One called to the angel appointed over pregnancy and said, 'Go and shape their facial features like their fathers.'" . . . God testified on their behalf that they are the sons/children of their fathers.[116]

The parallel in *Pesikta de Rav Kahana* (11:6) makes the nations' accusation more explicit, "*You are the sons of Egyptians*. If the Egyptians were ruling over the souls [*benafshoteihem*] of Israel, were they not also ruling over their wives [*benashoteihen*]?" But the point is clear enough in the *Song of Songs Rabbah* version: Israel's paternity is being questioned, and I think on both fronts. Certainly the specific claim is that the sons of Israel are not the fathers of their children, which is answered by the now familiar proof of paternity, which involves God face-ing their fetuses to resemble them. But also in play is the *possibility* that Israel are no longer God's children. The *mashal* (parable) that precedes the passage I have cited tells of a king who has left his two daughters unmarried only to return and ask for proof of the paternity of his now pregnant daughters' fetuses—seeking testimony to the offsprings' legitimacy and lineage.[117] This sets the scene for the *nimshal* cited above, where God, who has left his sons in Egyptian bondage, now provides divine proof for Israel's paternity, testifies on Israel's behalf that they are the fathers of their sons, and in doing all this, affirms that despite God's apparent abandonment of Israel, God is still their father. Just as in the *mashal*, Song of Songs 4:12, *A garden locked is my sister, my bride*, is attached to the daughters of the king, in the *nimshal*, God's sons, Israel, are the "locked garden" ever faithful to God, who in turn, is faithful to them. The difference between the *mashal* and *nimshal*, which articulates the difference between a king of flesh and blood and God, is that God never questions Israel's fidelity and pure lineage, instead asserting at the outset that Israel is a locked garden who has been disgraced—defaced and unmanned—by the nations' false accusations. God, as Israel's king/father, responds by (re)face-ing Israelite children so that they testify to their fathers' potency and paternity, thus putting the nations in their place and settingGod in God's place as the one who "fathers" all Israel, a trope I explore in the following chapter.

Conclusion

Midrashic traditions about fetal development and pregnancy are exemplary products of rabbinic imagination born out of the creative integration of Greco-Roman embryology and biblical (and rabbinic) theology. The overall consonance among late antique cultural notions about embryology—rabbinic sources included—presents itself through the similar questions posed, for example, when does ensoulment occur? when is the embryo formed? how does the fetus develop? how is breast milk produced? and it is further evident in some of the overlapping answers to these questions. For most of these inquiries, rabbinic absorption of contemporaneous cultural ideas about fetal development and pregnancy serves to fill the biblical silences on these topics. Nevertheless, rabbinic traditions often attach these notions to available biblical passages, some more likely and others less, making it appear as if the Hebrew Bible contains rabbinic, which is to say, Greco-Roman, embryology. It does not. In the process of infusing biblical sources with details about embryology, superimposing current ideas onto biblical precedents, rabbinic sources adapt late antique cultural notions about the fetus, theologizing and "rabbinizing" them.[118]

I have intentionally used the terms consonance and adaptation instead of influence and accommodation for most of this chapter. Consonance seems more apt than influence because if the rabbis were part of and participants in late antique culture, not an isolated group with clearly defined boundaries, they cannot be said to be subject to *outside* influence. In addition, on the specific topic of embryology, adaptation is more accurate than accommodation. Seth Schwartz discusses rabbinic accommodation in the context of the rabbis and idolatry.[119] However, whereas there are multiple passages that prohibit idolatry in the Hebrew Bible that could be construed as biblical constraints on the rabbis' endeavor to successfully live among pagans, thus causing or compelling the rabbis to make accommodations (intentional or not), the Hebrew Bible has no prohibition on embryology. Furthermore, accommodation might carry with it a sense of reluctance; it might be something that one is "forced" to do. Again, the Bible says remarkably little about the details of pregnancy—from conception through birth. There were, then, few biblical constraints, and the rabbis were not "forced" to make any accommodations by anybody other than themselves. What the rabbis did in most cases was adapt Greco-Roman theories of embryology, which they shared, to the one clear biblical theory of embryology that they inherited and held fast to, namely that God is the master of all things concerning pregnancy *and* the creator of the embryo, as the next chapter will demonstrate.

The rabbinized fetus, at issue in the first part of this book, here emerges entangled in a rabbinized discourse always already interwoven with Greco-Roman notions about fetal development and pregnancy. In most instances, the consonance between rabbinic and Greco-Roman embryology remains implicit in the texts and therefore naturalized. Most sources do not pause to reflect upon where the discourse about embryology originates, making the rabbinic embeddedness in its larger geocultural surroundings seem self-evident—and unproblematically so. In these cases, the rabbinic contribution to the already variegated, complex cultural discourse about embryology does not signal a rabbinic need for constraint or even accommodation but instead provides yet further evidence of rabbinic participation in late antique culture insofar as the rabbis adapt, and/or mimic, notions about fetal development and pregnancy in order to *produce* their own discourse about these topics, which is consistently (re)framed by or refracted through a rhetoric of theology.

However, two traditions, no less imbued with theological import than all others in this chapter, do explicitly acknowledge the interconnectedness of Greco-Roman and rabbinic embryology. Moreover, these two traditions—in varying and even opposing ways—proclaim Greco-Roman *influence* on rabbinic embryology. The purported exchange between Rabbi and Antoninus about ensoulment suggests that rabbinic embryology develops—like the fetus, according to ancient sources—from outside in: a late antique concern about the time of ensoulment is grafted onto biblical verses that attribute ensoulment to God. In contrast, the tradition that incorporates the Greco-Roman belief about the nonviability of eight-month children inverts the relationship between late antique and rabbinic embryology, turning it inside out so that the Greco-Roman notion about the nonviability of the eight-month child comes from scripture and originates in God. Here the rabbis have quite fully internalized, even swallowed, this outside knowledge, and through R. Abbahu, they spit it back, derisively, thinly veiling but not totally suppressing the derivativeness *and* the difference of rabbinic embryology. R. Abbahu both mocks and mimics the Greek speakers with his response, and this tête-à-tête exchange not only turns the relationship between rabbinic and Greco-Roman embryology on its head in this particular textual context but also invites speculation as to whether, beyond exhibiting consonance and adaptation, rabbinic traditions about fetal development and pregnancy suggest *resistance* to a more or less hegemonic discourse of embryology in late antiquity. Certainly, this text's double translation, or forked tongue—simultaneously Greek and Hebrew, "medical" and "theological," and its ultimately transliterated and transformed, rabbinized Greek—encourages at least some gesture toward postcolonial theory and its investigations into the complex relationship between dominant and minority cultures.

Beth Berkowitz has profitably applied postcolonial theory about resistance and mimicry to rabbinic traditions about capital punishment.[120] Despite the difference in topics, one of which could be cast rather starkly as my concern with a "life-giving" and hers with a "death-meting" discourse, there are some striking similarities in addition to considerable divergences, which I briefly address here.

After first contending that Roman discourse about capital punishment shaped the rabbis' own discourse and then highlighting one text that renders manifest the connection between Roman and rabbinic methods of decapitation, Berkowitz, using the work of James Scott and Homi Bhabha on strategies of power reversals and mimicry, suggests that rabbinic traditions about capital punishment authorize the rabbis, over and against the Romans, as the proper arbiters of execution. But in the midst of such triumphalism, she questions whether the rabbis might have worried that they have become too much like Romans. Here also, might there be a concern that rabbinic embryology is too Greco-Roman? Berkowitz answers, "The Mishnah creates an executioner that looks like the Roman one but with a rabbinic face. Rather than understanding rabbinic decapitation either as an unexamined borrowing from Rome or as totally unrelated to it . . . we can understand it as something more, as an appropriation of power."[121]

Similarly, rabbinic traditions about fetal development and pregnancy should not be seen only as representative of rabbinic borrowing in a simplistic sense; these traditions create a fetus—and construct a God—with a rabbinic "countenance." But here the rabbis do not appropriate power in such a way as to authorize themselves regarding questions about the beginnings of life as they might be undertaking in their discourse about one of the ways in which life could end; their consistent point is that only God has this authority.[122] In rabbinic traditions about embryology the rabbis don't so much appropriate power for themselves, but by imbuing embryology with theology they establish that this power is only appropriately allocated to God.[123]

Rabbi, "our Rabbi," here serving as the paradigmatic rabbi indicative of all rabbis, apparently reverses his opinion about ensoulment in express agreement with the Roman emperor Antoninus, who in this context stands in for (Greco-)Romans.[124] But there is reason to believe that if scripture offered no possible support, and perhaps it is significant that the text calls upon two proof texts, Rabbi would not have agreed with Antoninus.[125] What looks like a reversal on the part of Rabbi, ends up being, or being passed off as, a return, and a reclaiming, of something originally expressed in scripture—by, and about, God.[126] While it does not seem like Rabbi here either simply placates or mocks Antoninus, on a metatextual level rabbinic embryology that theologizes Greco-Roman embryology might very well in the process of imitating it make a mockery of it precisely because it overlooks God as the arbiter of life and breath, or soul.

As thoroughly as rabbinic embryology is infused with Greco-Roman embryology, almost to the point that it is frustrating to keep writing about them as if they are two distinct discourses, rabbinic embryology is equally shot through with theology, as I have repeatedly stated. Instead of fully exploring the ways postcolonial theory might illuminate the relationship between rabbinic and Greco-Roman embryology, which by definition would blur but not collapse the very distinction I am wary of making between the "two" constructs, I return to the more prevalent goal of this chapter: eliciting the theological aspects of rabbinic embryology. I leave open the question whether the rabbis, in addition to adapting late antique notions about fetal development and pregnancy, also "resisted" Greco-Romanness in the process. In order to substantiate a claim for rabbinic resistance would require reading this intent into rabbinic sources, and my reluctance to do so stems from the fact that in the end only two of the rabbinic traditions discussed in this chapter, albeit arguably the most fascinating ones, invite this speculation.[127]

In contrast, all of the rabbinic traditions set forth in this chapter link God and the fetus, and through it God and Israel, leading me to suggest that midrashic traditions about fetal development and pregnancy not only function theologically but were intended to do so.[128] These traditions communicate at least as much about the ways the rabbis constructed the relationship between God and Israel as they do about the developing fetus or about the relationship between rabbinic and Greco-Roman culture. My primary concern remains with the theological insights these sources provide not because theology is the "hidden transcript"[129] in these traditions, but because it is so baldly proclaimed at every turn in the texts presented—it frames and shapes their very contexts—yet still has remained either underarticulated or undertheorized by those who have written about rabbinic embryology in their own worry over whether the rabbis were too Greek or, conversely, not Greek enough.[130] In the majority of rabbinic traditions that shed light on embryology—excepting the two traditions with which I have been preoccupied—the Greco-Romanness does not, at least not explicitly, concern the rabbis themselves nearly as much as those who have written about them. Instead of superimposing the rabbinic concern about the Greco-Romanness of their embryology in the exceptional two traditions onto all other rabbinic traditions, the opposite turn should also be considered. In this case, what worries or preoccupies the rabbis is not so much Greeks, but God.

The traditions about ensoulment and the nonviability of the eighth-month child with which I began this chapter, and here belabored but still left open to further investigation, have their counterpart, if not analogue, in the topics saved for the end of this chapter: sex determination and facial resemblance. Here the Greco-Romanness of rabbinic theories on these topics is nowhere self-evident in Palestinian sources except in the fact that these sources, like Greco-Roman ones, consider the topics worthy of investigation. Bracketing off whether this lack presents rabbinic ignorance or adaptation of, or outright denial and thus resistance to, Greco-Roman theories—all of which are not without some difficulties[131]—what the texts surely represent is God's, and more or less only God's, control over these aspects of fetal development. These texts, along with all others presented in this chapter, use the discourse about fetal development and pregnancy to concretize God's relationship with Israel and God's involvement in fashioning Israel.[132] It's not that rabbinic traditions about embryology do not offer insight into how the rabbis were situated, and situated themselves, within late antique culture, but if primacy is shifted away from the exceptional, and exceptionally fascinating, two traditions that explicitly recognize and demarcate the intersection of rabbinic and Greco-Roman embryology to those that fail to do so, what remains primary to the sources themselves is God and the repeated message embedded in rabbinic traditions ostensibly about fetal development and pregnancy: God forms and sustains Israel—like a fetus in its mother's womb.[133]

Chapter 5
Reproductive Theology

A tradition in *Genesis Rabbah* compares the formation of *shamayim* (heaven), interpreted to mean "laden with water," to a bowl of milk that quivers until a drop of rennet is placed into it, causing the liquid to solidify.[1] This same comparison appears in *Leviticus Rabbah* describing the creation of the embryo in a woman's womb, which shakes with blood until—by the will of God—a "white drop" is placed into it.[2] These two traditions juxtapose the creation of the cosmos and the creation of the embryo, illustrating that both are the work of God and that each reflects the other.

Rabbinic traditions that theorize the creation of the embryo and the care of the fetus are most rewarding when read for both micro- and macrocosmic meanings.[3] In addressing the specific questions that rabbinic theories about procreation invite—including how God contributes to procreation, what roles are ascribed to men and women in the process of coming into being, whether women have seed, and how rabbinic theories about the creation of the embryo themselves come to be—I illuminate the ways in which rabbinic theories of procreation engage with far broader questions such as how the rabbis conceived the relationships between God and Israel, women and men, themselves and the broader cultural contexts in which they wrote, and, finally, themselves and, fittingly, their biblical ancestors. In other words, I demonstrate that the rabbis used an image as small as an embryo to reflect upon issues that loomed quite large for them—in this case theology, gender, self-fashioning amid hegemonic cultures, and continuity or lineage.

Rabbinic traditions that theorize procreation, like Greco-Roman theories and most likely drawing upon them, set forth more specific details about human, bodily contributions to procreation than those explicitly articulated by biblical authors, and in these traditions *male* seed takes on a significant role.[4] At the same time, these traditions consistently emphasize God's roles in procreation,[5] articulating rabbinic distinctiveness vis-à-vis

Greco-Roman "medical" writers in that seed(s), without God, do not make an embryo.[6]

I suggest that a primary focus on seeds instead of on God, while fruitful for contextualizing rabbinic sources within their broader geocultural milieu, ultimately distorts any understanding of how the rabbis imagined procreation; it grants Greco-Roman theories about generation *too much* influence over the rabbis, and it allows our own notions about "the facts of life" to get in the way of explorations into the rabbinic past. Taking seriously the extent to which rabbinic theories of procreation implicate God in this process illustrates the influence that biblical sources, in addition to Greco-Roman cultural notions, exert over rabbinic traditions. Furthermore, focusing on God's primary roles in the creation of the embryo and the care of the fetus reveals how the rabbis constructed the fetus as a bridge between themselves and their biblical past, establishing continuity between biblical and rabbinic Israel insofar as both are children of God, perhaps not exactly literally, but more concretely than one might expect.[7]

The fourteenth chapter of *Leviticus Rabbah* both illustrates the rabbinic construction of Israel as God's children and makes manifest rabbinic efforts to bring together notions of seed(s) and God, thereby theologizing procreation. Since *Leviticus Rabbah* 14 sets forth the most prolonged and deliberate discourse on procreation in all of Palestinian rabbinic literature, and one that is itself infused with biblical, extrabiblical, and even cosmic notions about the creation of the embryo and the care of the fetus, it provides an apt place from which to begin an examination of rabbinic theories of procreation and any subsequent exploration into the origins of such theories.[8]

In the pages that follow, I foreground a detailed examination of *Leviticus Rabbah* 14, paying particular attention to how rabbinic conceptions of Israel, God, and gender are all interarticulated in the process of theorizing, and theologizing, procreation. I then set forth theories of procreation that appear in other rabbinic compilations, situating *Leviticus Rabbah* in its larger rabbinic context, and from there I proceed to locate the origins of rabbinic theories of origins in both biblical and late antique notions about the process of coming into being. Finally, I briefly point out some of the similarities between rabbinic and patristic theories of procreation, focusing on the underlying commonalities instead of their more obvious and well-rehearsed points of departure. Through it all, I hope to illustrate that as much as the rabbis imagine the heavens as laden with water in the tradition with which

I began this chapter, the fetus, tucked away in rabbinic traditions about its own—and Israel's—beginnings is freighted with meaning.

Leviticus Rabbah 14: (Pro)Creation

The fourteenth chapter of *Leviticus Rabbah* sets forth the most extended rabbinic presentation of traditions about the creation of the embryo and the care of the fetus.[9] From its first section to its last, the chapter presents a theory of origins, using Lev. 12:2, *When a woman emits seed [tazria'] and gives birth to a male*, as its jumping off point. And jump off it does, such that an investigation that could have highlighted women's contributions to procreation, spurred on by the seemingly peculiar mention of woman's seed in this biblical verse, becomes instead an opportunity to expound upon male seed and ultimately, even more important, to extol God's works in (pro)Creation.

In its rabbinic context, *Leviticus Rabbah* 14 is not at all unique in imagining male seed as instrumental but God as primary in creating the embryo,[10] although it is exceptional in its explicit and repeated ascription of the care of the fetus to God over and against the pregnant woman.[11] The uniqueness of this chapter lies in its deliberation and details, as well as in its culling together perhaps once disparate traditions and passing them off precisely as inquiries into the possible meanings of Lev. 12:2.[12] Yet, as Burton Visotzky has suggested for *Leviticus Rabbah* more generally, this chapter functions less as a full elucidation of Lev. 12:2 than it does to set forth "aspects of a rabbinic agenda."[13] Explicating God's primary roles in the creation of the embryo and the care of the fetus and juxtaposing those with God's work in creating and caring for the world and Israel are this chapter's agenda. Nevertheless, Lev. 12:2 hardly remains uninterpreted; to the contrary, the persistent insistence on the woman's passivity in procreation—she does not actively emit seed but "conceives"—is never far from view, even if it apparently ceases to be the central focus.[14]

That an extended rabbinic inquiry into procreation and human origins should, and perhaps must, begin with God and recall God's "crowning" creation, *'adam,* is evident from *Leviticus Rabbah* 14's very beginning. The chapter's first interpretation of *When a woman* tazria' *and gives birth to a male* immediately turns away from the woman, and moreover humanity, as active in procreation, pointing instead straight to God. *Lev. Rab.* 14:1 opens with Ps. 139:5, midrashically understood as *You have created me behind and before*.[15] At this point, the midrash begins to expound upon God's creation of *'adam*. But in the context of *Leviticus Rabbah* 14, the citation of Ps. 139:5 functions to reflect not only on God's creation of *'adam* but also on God's creation of each individual in utero, as Ps. 139:13–16, suggests.[16]

The use of Psalm 139 to "open up" Lev. 12:2 sets forth, and encapsulates, that which becomes apparent throughout the chapter: procreation is God's work, not woman's, as Lev. 12:2 might suggest—and not even primarily man's, or both man's and woman's, as Greco-Roman theories might suggest. Although Lev. 12:2 might appear to present, or at least could have been read as presenting, a procreation theory where women are central and men and God are absent, rabbinic interpretations of this verse establish that the opposite is in fact the case. From the very beginning of *Leviticus Rabbah* 14, the chapter introduces its central lesson: God creates the embryo just as God created *'adam*; the creation of *'adam*—and according to other traditions the world—is reiterated through each embryo.

Lev. Rab. 14:2 makes it clear that God creates the embryo with male seed—not female seed. Using Job 36:3, midrashically understood as *I will lift up my thought to that which is afar, and to my Maker I will ascribe righteousness,* this tradition again emphasizes that God is one's creator.[17] In a passage that begins shortly after the text recalls God's continuous works in Creation—here not of *'adam,* but of the world—pointing out that while a person sleeps, God makes the winds blow, raises clouds, brings down rain, and causes plants to grow, the text turns to God's work in creating the embryo and caring for the fetus. In three statements attributed to R. Levi, the passage first presents a theory of procreation that imagines the creation of the embryo without any contribution from the woman and then asserts that God sustains the fetus while in its mother's womb and releases the fetus from the womb, further displacing the woman in procreation. The passage begins, "R. Levi said: It is customary in this world that when someone deposits an ounce of silver with his friend in secret and the friend returns to him a litra of gold in public,[18] will he not praise him? So too men deposit to the Holy Blessed One a white drop in secret and the Holy Blessed One returns to them complete and beautiful living beings in public.[19] And is this not worthy of praise? Thus, I will ascribe righteousness to my Maker, [as it is said] *and to My maker I will ascribe righteousness* (Job 36:3)."[20] This text overturns Lev. 12:2, shifting attention to male seed, and leaving it implicit, albeit abundantly clear, that the woman has no seed that she could possibly emit; there simply is no mention of female seed, or blood. Moreover, the woman is completely absent from the text, again leaving her involvement in procreation to inference. However, male seed contributes to procreation, but in and of itself it does not create the embryo—God does. So too God cares for the fetus and births the fetus, as R. Levi's following two statements make clear:

R. Levi said another thing: It is customary in this world that when someone is confined in prison and people do not watch over him one person comes and lights a lamp for him there. Will he not praise him? So too the fetus rests in his mother's womb and the Holy Blessed One lights a lamp for him there. Like that which Job said, *When his lamp shone upon my head* (Job 29:3).[21] And is this not worthy of praise? Thus, I will ascribe righteousness to my Maker, *and to my Maker I ascribe righteousness* (Job 36:3). R. Levi said another thing: It is customary in this world that when someone is confined in prison and people do not watch over him, one comes and releases him and sends him forth from there. And is this not worthy of praise? So too the fetus rests in its mother's womb and the Holy Blessed One releases him and sends him forth from there. And it is better if it is a male.[22] *When a woman conceives and bears a male child* (Lev. 12:2).

According to *Lev. Rab.* 14:2, God not only creates the embryo, but God continues to watch over the embryo while in the womb and to set the fetus free at the time of birth.[23] The passage does not ascribe the care, or apparently even the birth, of the fetus to the woman, but solely to God.

Lev. Rab. 14:3 continues to credit God alone with the care of the fetus, de-emphasizing if not downright denying any female contribution to procreation, either active or passive, and constructing the woman not as she who nurtures and protects the fetus, but as the one who endangers the fetus. Job 10:12, *You have granted me life and favor, and Your providence has preserved my spirit,* provides the verse through which Lev. 12:2 is now interpreted. As in *Lev. Rab.* 14:1 and 14:2, God "grants life" and here God also preserves the fetus in the womb. Three traditions attributed to R. Abba bar Kahana repeatedly point out that God protects the fetus, in contrast to the woman, who presents certain dangers to it.

First, since the woman's womb is shaped like an upside-down purse from which coins would fall out and scatter, so too, if it were not for God's providence, the fetus would "fall out and die."[24] The two other traditions attributed to R. Abba bar Kahana contrast the woman's physiology with that of other animals: since the woman walks upright, again the fetus might, but for God's protection, "fall out and die"; God has granted "life and favor" in placing the woman's breasts in a "place of honor," not in a "place of shame," like other animals. And, as a statement attributed to R. Eleazar explains it,

"If one is in an oven for even a moment, does he not die? But the womb of a woman boils and the fetus is placed inside her womb and the Holy Blessed One guards it so that it is not miscarried.[25] Is this not *life and favor*? (Job 10:12)."

Lev. Rab. 14:3 has the cumulative effect of simultaneously highlighting God's role in the care of the fetus and erasing any contribution that the woman might have, even that of nurturing the fetus, and all this is offered as interpretations of Lev. 12:2, which at the very least opens up the possibility of a very different conception of women's contributions to pregnancy and birth. Lev. 12:2 could have been mobilized to argue for women's active contributions to procreation; instead, *Lev. Rab.* 14:3, and for the most part the chapter as a whole, has the effect of erasing women from the process, and in the process, casting her at best as passive and at worst as actively harmful to the fetus.

The extent to which *Lev. Rab.* 14:3 obfuscates women's roles in procreation becomes even more striking when one considers these traditions within the broader Greco-Roman context of *Leviticus Rabbah*.[26] In its entirety, 14:3 fails to mention any positive female contribution to nurturing and sustaining the fetus. In contrast, even Greco-Roman "one-seed" theories maintain that the fetus is nurtured by the woman via her blood. Lesley Dean-Jones writes, "there was a general consensus among the Greeks that menstrual blood was indispensable in procreation. In some manner it formed the fabric of the child's body and also its staple diet when it first came into being."[27] She further writes, "During pregnancy a mother's monthly blood ceases to appear, but the Greek theorists did not infer that it was no longer present in her body; pregnancy did not change the nature of the digestive system that produced menstrual blood. Pregnancy modified a woman's body only in so far as the embryo absorbed the blood." She cites the Hippocratic work *Diseases of Women* (1.25): "Blood comes down from all the body when a woman is pregnant and gradually enters the womb, encircling that which is inside it; the blood makes it grow."[28]

In contrast, *Lev. Rab.* 14:3 removes menstrual blood from the fetus, since, according to a statement attributed to R. Meir, during the nine months of pregnancy God "raises it up to her breasts and makes it milk so that when the infant goes forth there will be food for him to eat."[29] This tradition does not maintain that menstrual blood ceases to be seen because the fetus needs it; blood does not make the fetus grow.[30] God does not bring the blood *to* the womb in order to nurture the fetus, but God brings it *away* from the womb to provide for the infant when it comes forth. Contrary to Greco-Roman authors who imagine menstrual blood, and thus women, as instrumental to the fashioning and nurturing of the fetus, rabbinic traditions never suggest that menstrual blood or women provide sustenance for the fetus. Instead, the traditions here maintain that while the woman endangers her fetus, God nurtures it.

Still other differences present themselves when *Lev. Rab.* 14:3 is juxtaposed with Greco-Roman sources. R. Abba bar Kahana's reference to God granting life and favor by placing women's breasts far from a "place of shame," may be contrasted with Galen, who writes: "In the female [Nature] has located the uteri below the stomach, because she found that this place is best for sexual intercourse, for receiving the semen, and also for the growth of the fetus and its birth when it has been perfected. For you would not find any place in the whole body of the animal more suitable for any of the uses I have mentioned; . . . most opportune for the growth of the fetus because it can be very greatly distended without pain, and most useful for birth because the fetus will emerge more easily if its exit is directed downward and is near the legs."[31] Additionally, R. Eleazar's remarks about the dangers of a boiling womb may be contrasted with Greco-Roman sources that also mention the heat of the womb. Helen King writes, "In classical Greek imagery, whether women were seen as 'hot' or 'cold,' the womb was seen as 'hot,' its role being to cook the seed. In a powerful analogy, retained even by Aristotle, for whom women were 'cold,' the womb was likened to an oven (*kaminos*; GA 764a12–20). In the Hippocratic *Generation/Nature of the Child* the womb is seen successively as an oven in which the seed is 'baked.'"[32] According to these theories, heat is *necessary* for the embryo's development, but *Lev. Rab.* 14:3 sees it as a danger to the fetus, *necessitating* God's protection.

Building upon the previous statements about the woman's physiology in *Lev. Rab.* 14:3, one that, in addition to those cited above, imagines the woman's innards[33] as made of cavities, coils, and bands, *Lev. Rab.* 14:4 likens the pregnant woman to a house, with doors, keys, and hinges as the text pauses to consider the word "doors" in Job 38:8, *Who shut up the sea with doors.*[34] This midrash opens up the metaphor of woman as house, already found in tannaitic sources, which has been previously investigated by Charlotte Fonrobert and Cynthia Baker.[35] Whether or not the metaphor of a house renders the woman an inanimate object—one should note that the house in this text is "*a* house," not "her house" or "his house"—the text renders the pregnant woman passive;[36] the doors may be unlocked, and the woman simultaneously confined to her body and unhinged from pregnancy and the birthing process. Indeed, the two proof texts brought to support that the woman has doors (Job 3:10) and keys (Gen. 30:22) again point to God's active roles in pregnancy and birth, to which *Lev. Rab.* 14:4 will turn with full force shortly after laying bare, and dispensing with, the woman. Furthermore, the text constructs the woman as a house, wherein the fetus surely dwells, in that she has cavities, coils, bands, doors, keys, and hinges, but she has no seed.[37] This text, like *Leviticus Rabbah* as a whole, is concerned with "the reproduction of Jewish bodies and rabbinic culture"[38] but such a (re)production takes place at the cost of the woman; any animation and dynamism in this text is taken up by God and the fetus, as the continuation of *Lev. Rab.* 14:4, which interprets the last part of Job 38:8, makes clear:

[*Who shut up the sea with doors,*] *when it broke forth and issued out of the womb* (Job 38:8). Because it [the fetus] raised itself up to go forth. *When I made the cloud its garment* (38:9)—this is the amniotic sac [which covers the fetus like a garment]. *And darkness its swaddling band* (38:9)—this is the placenta.[39] *And prescribed bounds for it* (38:10)—these are the nine months [of pregnancy]. *And set bars* (38:10)—these are the first three months [of pregnancy]. *And doors* (38:10)—these are the three middle months [of pregnancy]. *And said, Thus far shall you come, but no farther* (38:11). These are the last three months [of pregnancy].[40]

Here the fetus's actions are matched, and of course surpassed, by God's. The fetus rises up, but God swaddles it, keeping it at bay until the time of birth. Similar to *Lev. Rab.* 14:1, this section reiterates the cosmic context of (pro)Creation, here juxtaposing God's confinement of the sea with that of the fetus.

Writing about Job 38 as it appears in another *petihta* in *Leviticus Rabbah* (25:5), Galit Hasan-Rokem points out that "The text stresses God's domination of the world and his special care to every single detail of creation and its sustenance."[41] She further writes, "The Job chapter articulates a cosmic perspective of a complex mechanism of growth that sets off the planting of the old man as a miniscule event in a much larger, centrally dominated, scheme." In this context, I substitute Hasan-Rokem's focus on a tradition that emphasizes the planting of fruit trees by an old man with the "planting" or "seeding" of the embryo, and I suggest that *Lev. Rab.* 14:4's use of the same chapter from Job articulates a cosmic perspective of a complex mechanism of growth that casts the creation of the miniscule embryo in a much larger, centrally dominated scheme: the creation of humanity, Israel, and the world. In *Leviticus Rabbah* 14, pregnancy and birth recall and repeat, even recreate, Creation, as God births the fetus like God birthed the sea.

Structurally read, *Leviticus Rabbah* 14 has at least as many coils and bands, and surely openings, as the woman it purports to describe. Already Lev. 12:2 has been "opened up" to multiple readings, each of which has the effect of foreclosing upon the woman's active roles in procreation even as they end with the citation of the verse, *When a woman* tazria' [= conceives] *and gives birth to a male.* The (re)citation of this verse almost always comes right on the heels of the incessant claim "it is better if it [the offspring] is male," which, all androcentrism aside, also functions as a textual link back to the end of Lev. 12:2, *gives birth to a male*—as if the redactor knows how far he has strayed from its beginning. Thus each section, each *petihta,* has the effect of drawing the reader's attention away from the textual "problem" of the word *tazria'* by refocusing attention to men and, even more, God. At the same time, *tazria'* is over and over interpreted to mean that the woman conceives, or receives seed, but she does not emit or produce it.

Moreover, the chapter as a whole circles back unto itself. As seen above, *Lev. Rab.* 14:1 frames human origins in the cosmic context of Creation. *Lev. Rab.* 14:2 briefly mentions male seed and then shifts the focus to God's care of the fetus while disembodying the womb from the woman (or vice versa), 14:3 elaborates upon God's care of the fetus—despite the woman—and 14:4 first further objectifies the woman, making her into a house that the fetus occupies, only then to return to God's Creation, here the birth of the sea/fetus. The following traditions circle back to male seed, picking up on the first statement attributed to R. Levi in *Lev. Rab.* 14:2, "men deposit a white drop to God in secret and God returns to them complete and beautiful living beings in public."

Lev. Rab. 14:5, 6, and 9 all imagine God working with male seed to create the embryo. *Lev. Rab.* 14:5 is unique in all the sections of the chapter because it ceases to speak of procreation in general terms and focuses instead on one particular conception, that of David. Here Lev. 12:2 is opened up with Ps. 51:7, *Behold I was brought forth in iniquity, and in sin did my mother conceive me*:

Behold I was brought forth in iniquity (Ps. 51:7). R. Aha said, *'Iniquity'* is written *plene.*[42] Even the most pious of the pious,[43] it is impossible that he has no [sinful] side.[44] David said before the Holy Blessed One, 'Master of all the worlds, my father Jesse had no intention of having me, he only intended [to satisfy] his own needs. Know that this is such because when they were taking care of their needs, one turned his face this way and the other turned her face the other way.[45] And You inserted each and every drop [into my mother's womb].' Like that which David said, *Though my father and my mother have forsaken me, the Lord will gather me in* (Ps. 27:10).[46]

Setting aside the possible allusion to "original sin" that the invocation of Ps. 51:7 might carry with it, some more basic, even mundane, reasons for the juxtaposition of Ps. 51:7 and Lev. 12:2 should be made explicit.[47] To begin with, the mention of "brought forth" (*holalti*) in Ps. 51:7 can be juxtaposed with "gives birth" (*v'yalda*) in Lev. 12:2, and "conceived me" (*yehemtani*) in Ps. 51:7 can be juxtaposed with "conceives" (*tazria'*) in Lev. 12:2, reiterating, as apparent throughout *Leviticus Rabbah* 14, that the woman does not emit seed but conceives—or perhaps here "heats"—the embryo.[48] I suggest that taking into consideration the overall context of *Leviticus Rabbah* 14, Ps. 51:7, and its apparent gesture to "original sin," is not the point; rather Ps. 27:10, *Though my father and my mother have forsaken me, the Lord will gather me in*, delivers that point.[49] The passage emphasizes and concretizes that verse—God literally gathers David in when God inserts the semen into his mother's womb—in keeping with the emphasis placed on God's, not one's mother or father's, role in procreation set forth in almost the entirety of *Leviticus Rabbah* 14. Psalm 51:7 is the exegetical stepping stone, which explicitly, though somewhat peculiarly mentions birth and conception, like Lev. 12:2 (but in reverse order), and makes the later citation of Ps. 27:10 more readily contextually relevant and apparent.

It is not that I am averse to entertaining the possibility that some notion of "original sin" and some degree of anti-Christian polemic could be operative in this text; it's simply that not only is the mention of iniquity and sin in Ps. 51:7 out of place in the context of *Leviticus Rabbah* 14, but the verse's own placement of procreation in the human realm is also at odds with, or at least exceptional in, the chapter. Ps. 27:10, on the other hand, summarizes *Lev. Rab.* 14:1–4, and the chapter as a whole, quite aptly: God, not, or certainly not only, one's human parents, gathers one in; God creates the embryo. Moreover, God creates the embryo with male seed,[50] not any sort of female seed. Again, the woman does not contribute to the creation of the embryo; David's mother is a "vessel," receiving semen but not emitting it, as the second part of *Lev. Rab.* 14:5 makes clear: "*And in sin did my mother conceive me* (Ps. 51:7). R. Hiyya bar Abba said, 'A woman never receives [seed] except after her menstrual flow or near.'"[51]

The mention of sin in the second part of Ps. 51:7 is squarely laid upon the woman's menstrual flow, here separated both textually and presumably bodily from the male seed. Menstrual blood, which potentially could have been construed as the material substance from which the embryo takes shape, is, in this tradition, removed from the creation of the embryo and reconfigured as sinful.[52] Granted, here the dual interpretation of Ps. 51:7

mentions male seed and menstrual blood, a pair commonly found in Greco-Roman theories of generation. However, in this rabbinic tradition, blood contributes to neither the creation of the embryo nor the nourishment of the fetus. The woman's reception of seed is thought to take place only in the absence of menstrual blood, perhaps after the woman has been cleansed of her blood, or "sin."[53]

In its context in *Leviticus Rabbah* 14, I suggest that this passage, like those before and after, with the possible exception of *Lev. Rab.* 14:9, sets forth a rabbinic theory of procreation that certainly introduces or inserts male seed into the mix, all the while clearing away the woman's blood—and any contribution of the woman to procreation—and yet nevertheless primarily functions to highlight God's roles in procreation. As Margulies states, "the intent is to teach that the creation of the embryo is the work of heaven [God]."[54]

Lev. Rab. 14:6 is entirely concerned with male seed, further implicitly denying the possibility of female seed in Lev. 12:2. This passage returns to Psalm 139, cited previously in *Lev. Rab.* 14:1, but now focuses on an earlier verse, Ps. 139:3, midrashically interpreted to refer to either God's winnowing or scattering semen in order to create the embryo. The text asserts that an embryo is created only from male seed, stating, "God does not create the embryo/*ha-'adam*[55] except from a white drop that is *in him*."[56] Again, the juxtaposition of Lev. 12:2 in light of this interpretation of Ps. 139:3 here subverts the possibility that women have seed and instead shifts the focus onto men's seed—seed that is "in him," *not in her*. The text then proceeds to consider precisely how, or how much, *male* seed God uses in the (pro)creative process:

You sift/scatter [zerita] my seed; You are acquainted with all my ways (Ps. 139:3).[57] R. Yohanan and R. Shimeon ben Lakish [interpret this verse differently]: R. Yohanan said, "The Holy Blessed One creates an embryo only from the white drop that is in him." How does R. Yohanan interpret the word *zerita*?[58] [God sifts the semen] like a man who winnows [*zoreh*] and places straw by itself and chaff by itself so that the grain will be at its finest. R. Shimeon ben Lakish said, "God[59] does not allow any drop to be wasted, but God scatters part of the drop to the marrow, part of the drop to the bones and part of the drop to the sinews."[60] And it is better if it is a male. *When a woman receives seed and gives birth to a male* (Lev. 12:2).

Both R. Yohanan and Reish Lakish agree that God creates the embryo from male seed, but they differ concerning whether God's process is one of distillation or "dissemination." For R. Yohanan, God distills the seed to its finest, but according to Reish Lakish, God disseminates all of it to appropriate body parts.

The text does not address questions that occupied Greco-Roman authors, such as from where in the body semen originates or how it is produced, perhaps leaving it implied that God provides the seed. However, traces of such late antique theories might be present in the text. Noteworthy would be the mention of "marrow" in the interpretation attributed to Reish Lakish, perhaps alluding to the ancient linkage between the brain, spinal marrow, and semen, or even suggesting a "pangenetic" theory of seed, where seed comes from all of the parts of the body such as bones and sinews.[61] But again, in the statement attributed to Reish Lakish, the emphasis is not on the question of from where seed originates, but to where seed goes.[62] Of equal note is the absence, perhaps for the rabbis even the inconceivability, of another theory about the origin of semen, namely that it originates in blood, which has been "concocted."[63] The focus of the text is not on the bodily origins of semen, but on the origins of (male) embryos from, or in, men. Despite the fact that, or one must at least begin to wonder if precisely *because*, this passage expounds Lev. 12:2, this text never leaves any traces of women's active contributions to the creation of the embryo. The woman contributes nothing positive—or positively nothing—to procreation, according to this tradition and thus far in *Leviticus Rabbah* 14 in its entirety.[64]

The last section of *Leviticus Rabbah* 14, however, offers a brief shift in focus, not to women's seed, but to the woman's womb churning with and churning out the blood within: "The womb of the woman is always full of blood and from there menstrual blood goes forth from its source.[65] And by the will of the Holy Blessed One, a drop of white falls into it [the womb] and immediately, the embryo is created.[66] [This may be compared] to milk that was put in a bowl. If one puts a curdling agent in it, it coagulates and stands. And if not, it moves and shakes" (Lev. Rab. 14:9).[67]

According to the standard reading of this tradition, which always presents it in isolation from the rest of *Lev. Rab.* 14:9 and the chapter as a whole, the "white drop" falls into the womb and acts as a curdling agent upon the unwieldy blood.[68] The (active) male seed acts upon the (passive) blood. In this reading, the difference between *Lev. Rab.* 14:9 and all others in the chapter is that here the woman's contribution to procreation—through blood—is at last, and at least, imagined.

I would like to suggest an alternative reading that takes into consideration other traditions in *Leviticus Rabbah* 14, especially 14:3, which removes menstrual blood from the fetus during gestation and 14:5, which removes menstrual blood from the creation of the embryo.[69] Here, too, it seems possible that the creation of the embryo takes place once "menstrual blood goes forth from its source," and thus in a womb that is emptied of its blood.[70]

In either reading it remains abundantly clear that, in keeping with all other traditions in *Leviticus Rabbah* 14, the woman receives seed, she does not emit—or have—it. God's role in depositing the seed and ultimately creating the embryo appears equally consistent and becomes even clearer when this passage's immediate context is considered.

Lev. Rab. 14:9 begins with a debate between the houses of Hillel and Shammai about whether creation in this world mirrors that of creation in the next. This passage appears more organic and original in the parallel from *Gen. Rab.* 14:5 as an interpretation of *And God formed ha'adam* (Gen. 2:7). There, the extra *yod* in the Hebrew word for "formed" indicates two creations, one in this world and one in the future, or resurrection. In *Lev. Rab.* 14:9, however, there is no explicit exegetical link to Lev. 12:2; instead, the link is implicit in the content of the passage since it pertains to the formation of the embryo and God's role in it—the topic of central concern to *Leviticus Rabbah* 14. According to Beit Hillel, the two creations mirror each other: in this world and the time to come God creates humanity first with skin and flesh and then with sinews and bones, as Job 10:10–11 demonstrates. These verses, read in context, reflect upon the process of the creation of the embryo in this world: *Have you not poured me out like milk and curdled me like cheese. You have clothed me with skin and flesh and knit me together with bones and sinews.* However, due to their grammatical structure, the verses also teach about creation in the future when they are midrashically rendered, *You will pour me out like milk. . . . You will clothe me with skin and flesh and knit me together with bones and sinews.* The following verse, Job 10:12, previously used at length in *Lev. Rab.* 14:3, is by implication also doubly read: *You have granted me life and favor* becomes "You will grant me life and favor"—in the future.[71] Again, *Lev. Rab.* 14:9 asserts God's centrality to the process of procreation, but here it takes on the added concern of equating God's creation in this life and the next. In this juxtaposition, the message that God creates the embryo is reinforced, since beyond doubt God resurrects the dead.[72] *Leviticus Rabbah* 14 thus returns to where it begins, with a tradition paralleled in *Genesis Rabbah* that extols God's—not humanity's—roles in (pro)creation.[73] The chapter also moves from Creation to redemption or resurrection, encompassing the cosmic cycles of birth and rebirth, which are reiterated and (p)reenacted with the creation of each embryo.

Lev. Rab. 14:9, in its entirety, might very well function as a "messianic peroration" for the chapter as a whole.[74] According to *Lev. Rab.* 14:9, just as God fashions the embryo from a drop, which acts as a curdling agent, and then forms the embryo with skin and flesh and sinews and bones, so too God fashions humanity in the time to come. Although the tradition as it appears in *Gen. Rab.* 14:5 harks back to Creation, based on an intertextual link with *Genesis Rabbah* (4:7) that describes the creation of the heavens in precisely the same language as the creation of the embryo—a drop of liquid placed in the heavens causes them to solidify, forming the dry land—*Lev. Rab.* 14:9 further reflects upon the future to come. After the mention of the woman's womb always full of blood, *Lev. Rab.* 14:9 continues, and the chapter concludes: "R. Abbahu said, 'The Holy Blessed One did a great good for women in this world in not beginning with sinews and bones. If God began with sinews and bones, the fetus would have burst through her belly and come forth. For in this world, a woman gives birth in pain but in the future to come, what is written? *Before she travailed she gave birth; before her pains were upon her, she delivered a male*' (Isa. 66:7)."[75]

In yet another way, *Leviticus Rabbah* 14 ends where it begins: with a verse about the birth of a male child, but this one explicitly infused with miraculousness. In doing so, the text brings into relief the infusion of the miraculous into rabbinic interpretations of Lev. 12:2 set forth throughout the chapter. From beginning to end, God's involvement in procreation, and the rabbinic persistence in theologizing procreation, drives *Leviticus Rabbah* 14; such reproductive theology is at the expense of the woman, and to a lesser extent the man, since his seed bears some significance, but it takes God to make an embryo. According to *Leviticus Rabbah* 14, God creates the embryo like God created the world and *'adam* and like God will create in the future, when women will give birth—but still not emit seed—without pain.

Leviticus Rabbah 14 in Its Rabbinic Context

I have offered this protracted reading of a unique chapter in rabbinic literature not because it closes the book on how the rabbis theorized procreation, but because it provides a window through which to view other rabbinic traditions that in turn further illuminate *Leviticus Rabbah* 14. In a compilation at the heart of Palestinian rabbinic literature, and in the very place where the rabbis (some rabbi, even one rabbi) could have opened up Lev. 12:2 to construct women as active in creating the embryo, the assembled traditions rhetorically function to render women *at best* passive not only in the embryo's creation but also in its protection and care. Locating such vehement denial of women's roles in procreation precisely as interpretations of Lev. 12:2 looks deliberate—and maybe it was. However, without intending to undermine the feminist critiques that *Leviticus Rabbah* 14 invites, and perhaps adding to them, I suggest that before and even into fifth-century Palestine, the rabbis simply could not conceive of Lev. 12:2 as meaning anything other than *when a woman receives seed*. Nowhere do extant Palestinian compilations use this verse, or anything else, to suggest that both male and female seed contribute to the *creation* of the embryo because these sources assume women's passivity in this process from the beginning.[76] The displacement of women is thus more fundamental than deliberate.

Leviticus Rabbah 14 shows remarkable consistency with rabbinic *assumptions* about procreation found in other Palestinian sources, which further fail to attribute any role to women in the creation of the embryo. *Genesis Rabbah*, to focus on the Palestinian compilation with which *Leviticus Rabbah* 14 has the most direct parallels, constructs male seed as the only human substance involved in procreation—when it considers human contributions to this process at all.[77] For example, *Gen. Rab.* 63:8 states, "A *matrona* asked R. Yosi bar Halfota, 'Why did Esau issue forth first?' He said to her, 'The first drop was Jacob's. He made a comparison for her: If you put two pearls in a tube, does not the one that you put in first come out last? So too, the first drop was Jacob's.'"[78] *Gen. Rab.* 99:6 teaches that Reuben was Jacob's "first drop," when interpreting the verse *Reuben, you were my firstborn, my might, and the beginning of my strength* (Gen. 49:3).[79] Finally, according to *Gen. Rab.* 46:2, Abraham is circumcised prior to Isaac's birth so that Isaac would come forth from a "holy drop."[80] In stark contrast, an earlier statement in *m. Avot* 3:1 locates the origins of people in a "fetid drop." Despite the exceptionally negative characterization, this text still imagines male seed as the only substance that contributes to procreation.[81]

None of the traditions just cited directly addresses the question of how an embryo comes to be,[82] which accounts for why God is not mentioned and also why I do not consider these traditions as full-blown *theories* of procreation.[83] However, in their seemingly self-evident construction of male seed as the only substance involved in the process of coming into being, they reveal a fundamental rabbinic assumption about procreation, specifically that men are the primary (human) agents in this process.[84] I think they also indicate that when confronting Lev. 12:2 for its insights into procreation, as *Leviticus Rabbah* 14 does, the rabbis begin with the assumption of women's passivity in the process of coming into being, which begets an automatic rendering of *tazria'* as "conceives," connoting that she *receives* seed and foreclosing the possibility that she *produces* it.

A passage in the *Mekhilta of Rabbi Ishmael,* which is earlier than *Leviticus Rabbah* 14, already imagines the creation of the embryo as an affair between God and men. At the end of an extended passage highlighting the differences between divine and human powers to (pro)create, which again juxtaposes creation on cosmic and embryonic scales, the *Mekhilta* states, "God gives to man a son from a drop of liquid and he resembles the image of his father."[85] Once again, male seed is imagined as the only substance in procreation, and, as in *Leviticus Rabbah* 14, it is the substance with which *God* creates and fashions the embryo.

One final set of rabbinic traditions needs to be considered both to further situate *Leviticus Rabbah* 14 in its broader Palestinian rabbinic context and to appreciate more fully rabbinic theories of procreation in their own right.[86] In contrast to the traditions discussed up to this point, these next traditions, of which I cite only a couple of examples, appear content to attribute pregnancy entirely to God, without any mention of seed—either male or female.[87] *Gen. Rab.* 53:6 states, "*And God visited [paqad] Sarah* (Gen. 21:1). R. Isaac said, 'It is written, *And if the woman is not defiled, but is clean; then she shall be free, and shall conceive seed* (Num. 5:28).[88] This woman [Sarah] who had entered the house of Pharaoh and the house of Avimelech, and came out clean, is it not logical that she should conceive?' R. Yehudah in the name of R. Shimon said, even though R. Huna said there is an angel appointed over desire, Sarah had no need for such things. Rather, God, in God's glory, [gave her pregnancy], *And God visited Sarah.*"[89] This text attributes Sarah's pregnancy solely to God, "in God's glory,"[90] but rabbinic traditions do not confine God's granting of pregnancy only to the matriarchs or other biblical heroes. For example, *Gen. Rab.* 34:10, along with attributing the ensoulment of each embryo to God, also attributes conception to God, as the text states, "From when did you place the soul in me? From the time that You conceived me."[91] Finally, *Gen. Rab.* 14:5 and *Lev. Rab.* 14:9 also credit God alone with the creation and development of the embryo: God first forms the skin and flesh, and afterwards, sinews and bones.[92] In more general terms, God's necessity in procreation is aptly captured in the rabbinic statement "Three keys are in the hands of the Holy Blessed One: the key to the grave [resurrection], rain, and the womb."[93]

If, in the context of seeking to illuminate rabbinic theories of procreation, one places a primary emphasis on seeds rather than on God, the traditions just cited and the many like them are easily overlooked. But working from the opposite paradigm, which is what I am suggesting the rabbis did, the traditions that attribute pregnancy and fetal development solely to God emerge as additional places where the rabbis theorize procreation. These traditions, along with those that construct male seed as the only human substance that contributes to procreation, are interwoven into the very fabric of *Leviticus Rabbah* 14.[94] Moreover, *Leviticus Rabbah* 14, which cannot seem to conceive of both male and female seed coming together to create an embryo, deftly weaves together rabbinic traditions that attribute procreation solely to God and those that construct male seed as the sole human substance involved in procreation.

Leviticus Rabbah 14's extended discourse about the creation of the embryo is itself born out of the very productive tension between rabbinic assumptions about procreation. Or perhaps *Leviticus Rabbah* 14 is a product of the creative tension between what the rabbis assume or believe about procreation and what they know about it. They assume that man's contribution overshadows, even eclipses, woman's and that male seed contributes somehow to procreation; but they know that God creates the embryo. One could claim that the rabbis know that semen contributes to procreation, and they certainly assert this often enough; but "knowledge" about the specifics of male and female contributions to the creation of the embryo remained speculative well beyond late antiquity, and even now assumptions about gender (and miracles) pervade.[95] Likewise, one could claim that the rabbis simply assume or believe that God contributes to the process of coming into being, and that too was speculation—not "knowledge." But I am suggesting that the belief in God not only holding "the key to the womb" but also playing a rather "hands on" part in the process by which the embryo comes to be was so strong that it should be seen as the place from which rabbinic theorizing about procreation starts—not a quaint by-product. It is certainly the place from which *Leviticus Rabbah* 14 began.

When *Leviticus Rabbah* 14 gets down to the business of theorizing the creation of the embyro and the care of the fetus to an extent unprecedented in Palestinian rabbinic literature, finally using Lev. 12:2 as its point of entry, it is laden with, even weighed down by, other Palestinian traditions. These traditions, which fail to construct women as active in the creation of the embryo and instead emphasize either male seed or God's role, exercise a profound influence both upon the ways in which *Leviticus Rabbah* 14 understands Lev. 12:2 and how it theorizes the process of coming into being—leaving no room for the one Palestinian tradition from the *Yerushalmi* that might imagine procreation otherwise.

In the context of a discussion about animal husbandry and the inherited traits governing the size of mules' ears, ears apparently believed to be passed on by the female, *y. Kel.* 8:3(31c) states, "The white is from the man, because from it are the marrow and bones and sinews. The red is from the woman, because from it are the skin and the flesh and the blood. And the *ruah* and *nefesh* and *neshamah* are from the Holy Blessed One. And the three of them are partners in him."[96]

The *Yerushalmi* here maintains that women pass on the "red" parts of the body to their offspring. Either this tradition presents a theory about the creation of the embryo that runs counter to all other Palestinian rabbinic traditions, or it reflects a theory about inherited traits, like the size of ears, as it is set up to be when read in its immediate context. If the latter, then this tradition could acknowledge women's contribution to procreation but still not imagine her as an actual creative "force" behind the embryo's creation, which this tradition attributes primarily to God, who animates the embryo. If the former, then implicit in this theory is that women produce the "red" parts from their menstrual blood,[97] and men contribute the "white parts" from their seed.

I do not know why *Leviticus Rabbah* 14 does not incorporate this tradition.[98] Perhaps *Leviticus Rabbah* reads it as a tradition about inherited traits and thus deems it less relevant, or it purposefully leaves it out precisely because it runs counter to all other traditions it presents, both insofar as women actively contribute to procreation and in that blood is presumably absorbed by—not removed from—the embryo and developing fetus. Or, and much more simply, perhaps *Leviticus Rabbah* does not know the *Yerushalmi* passage. For some uncertain reason(s), this *Yerushalmi* passage lies dormant until the *Bavli* recontextualizes an expanded version of it in the other extended presentation of traditions about the creation of the embryo in rabbinic literature: "Our rabbis taught: There are three partners in [the creation of] a person:[99] the Holy Blessed One, his father, and his mother. His father emits the white [*mazria' haloven*],[100] from it [come] the bones, sinews, nails, marrow that is in the head,[101] and white that is in the eye. His mother emits red [*mazra'at 'odem*], from it [come] the skin, flesh, hair and black of the eye.[102] And the Holy Blessed One places in him *ruah* and *neshamah* and the facial features,[103] and the sight of the eye and the hearing of the ear, and the speech of the mouth and the movement of the legs, and wisdom and understanding" (*b. Nid.* 31a).

Despite the *Bavli*'s claim to this passage's tannaitic origin, this tradition does not appear in tannaitic sources.[104] Moreover, the *Bavli*'s use of the words *mazria'/mazra'at* suggests that this more detailed version is unique to the *Bavli*. Even the *Yerushalmi* passage, upon which the *Bavli* almost certainly draws, stops short of using *mazra'at* when it maintains that the woman contributes "red" parts of the body to her offspring, and Palestinian compilations prior to the *Bavli* never use *mazria'/mazra'at* in the context of procreation.[105] Such a lack is particularly striking in *Leviticus Rabbah* 14 since it interprets Lev. 12:2, which contains the word *tazria'*.[106]

If the *Bavli* here sets forth a theory of female "seed" that contributes to the creation of the embryo, it is one that is unprecedented in all of rabbinic literature.[107] Not only is this tradition unique to the *Bavli*, it is also exceptional *in* the *Bavli*.[108] In other places, the *Bavli*, like Palestinian sources, imagines male seed as the primary substance in the creation of the embryo, without mentioning any contribution from the woman.[109]

Decontextualized and read as a freestanding statement, which is how this passage has been presented in scholarly literature,[110] the "three partners" tradition looks almost entirely unrelated to those presented in *Leviticus Rabbah* 14. But *b. Nid.* 31a as a whole has more in common with *Leviticus Rabbah* 14 than in contrast.[111] For example, it too interprets Ps. 139:3 as *You sift my seed*, indicating that only the purest part of "the drop" is used, implicitly by God, in creating the embryo.[112] *B. Nid.* 31a also credits God with protecting the fetus since the woman's womb is open and turned downward.[113] The same page of the *Bavli* also sets forth a tradition that constructs male seed as primary, imagining that God watches over the *"seed" of Israel* (Num. 23:10) and wonders, "When will the drop come from which the righteous will be created?" And *b. Nid.* 31a consistently highlights God's role in the creation of the embryo when it repeatedly states, "God creates (*tsar*) the embryo in the woman's womb" and contrasts this with something that humanity does.[114]

There is hardly a rabbinic theory of procreation that the *Bavli*, on this one page, does not entertain. Still, the "three partners" tradition has been singled out as the dominant rabbinic theory of procreation, not only in the *Bavli*, but for all of rabbinic literature.[115] It warrants a close examination, not only for the differences it exhibits when compared with traditions in *Leviticus Rabbah* 14 but also for the similarities.

The "three partners" tradition is consistent with *Leviticus Rabbah* 14's repeated stress on God's necessity for the creation of the embryo. However, the uniqueness of this tradition lies in the extent to which it elaborates upon both men's and women's contributions to the embryo's creation *and* the consequences that such a redistribution of procreative power has on God's involvement in the process. That which *Lev. Rab.* 14:6 attributes more primarily to God, the dissemination of male seed to form the marrow, bones, and sinews, the "three partners" tradition allocates to the man. And the development of skin and flesh and bones and sinews, which *Lev. Rab.* 14:9 attributes solely to God, is distributed between men and women's contributions to the embryo in the "three partners" tradition.[116] In the "three partners" tradition, God does not work with semen to create the embryo, God works with the other partners in procreation to animate what they have provided. As a consequence of rendering both men's and women's contributions to the creation of the embryo more concretely, God's roles in procreation become not less potent but less material—excepting the facial features, which God still provides, perhaps as a remnant of other traditions signaling that although God's role is here more of the spirit than of the flesh, God still uses God's hands to fashion the embryo.[117]

Contextualized among other rabbinic traditions about the creation of the embryo, the "three partners" tradition appears unique not only because it imagines women's contributions to the creation of the embryo but also because it theorizes men's contributions to a point heretofore obscured. In *Lev. Rab.* 14:2, men deposit a "white drop" to God and God gives them children, and in *Lev. Rab.* 14:6 God creates the embryo from the "white drop" that is in men.[118] In both cases, male seed is necessary, but in and of itself it does not create the embryo—only God does. In the "three partners" tradition, men and women, along with God, *create* the embryo. This perhaps subtle difference profoundly nuances the question that should be put to all rabbinic sources that reflect upon the process of coming into being, not just the "three partners" tradition. Instead of asking how men and women contribute to the creation of the embryo, the question that should be asked is how do God, men, and women—in that order—contribute to procreation.

The varying ways in which the rabbis imagine God's roles in the creation of the embryo carry with them rabbinic assumptions about and constructions of gender. When male seed is assumed to be necessary but insufficient to create the embryo and no mention is made of women's contributions to procreation, the rabbis simultaneously construct men as more instrumental to and more active in the process of coming into being and displace women from any active contribution to the creation of the embryo. Whether assumptions of male primacy permeate the "three partners" tradition has been the subject of some scholarly debate. Lawrence Hoffman reads a clear gender hierarchy in the text, which Daniel Boyarin vehemently rejects.[119] Joshua Levinson, more attentive to God's presence in the text, asserts, "The contributions of the respective partners are hierarchized according to a clear scale of perfection."[120] If the "three partners" tradition by itself is made to bear the weight of all that the rabbis had to say, or believed, about the process of procreation, the stakes in any answer are inordinately high. Contextualized among other rabbinic theories, however, either the "three partners" tradition assumes the same hierarchy or it departs from it, but the stakes are at least a bit lower.

My own sense is that once contextualized among other rabbinic traditions and not presented as a self-contained, ahistorical, even ungenealogized theory of genealogy, multiple hierarchies, including those of gender, are operating in this tradition. My point has not been to dismiss the construction of gender along predictable hierarchical lines in either all or almost all rabbinic theories of procreation, but to demonstrate that this is a by-product of rabbinic traditions concerned with theorizing the process of coming into being born out of fundamental assumptions about gender that, while clearly at issue in the traditions from my own partial perspective, can only partially begin to engage rabbinic traditions more on their own terms. Gender inequity—or parity—is not the point of these traditions; theology is. The rabbis excel not at accurately reflecting twentieth- and twenty-first-century beliefs about "the facts of life,"[121] and perhaps not even accurately portraying third-through-sixth-century beliefs—or knowledge. Rabbinic traditions that theorize procreation are part of a theological discourse. The rabbis know that women become pregnant and that the fetus develops in women's wombs arguably better than they know that, or at least how, semen contributes to the embryo's creation—though not better than they know men's superiority. But when they theorize procreation, they have more than gender, and even sex, on their minds. They have God and the ongoing relationship between God and humanity—and God and Israel—on their minds. Because of this, asking only what men and women contribute to the creation of the embryo, or whether, according to the rabbis, women have seed, cannot provide the only lens through which these traditions are viewed.

The Origins of Rabbinic Theories of Origins

Both *Leviticus Rabbah* 14 and *b. Nid.* 31a present relatively extensive discussions about the process of coming into being. Each incorporates and builds upon other rabbinic traditions about the creation of the embryo. But the question remains, how do rabbinic traditions about the creation of the embryo and the care of the fetus themselves come to be? Answering this question requires that rabbinic traditions be contextualized among both late antique and biblical notions about coming into being, since rabbinic sources bring together insights gleaned from both when they theorize the creation of the embryo.

Previous scholarly inquiries into rabbinic theories about procreation have emphasized the Greco-Roman contributions, divvying up the rabbinic evidence along the lines of "one-seed" or "two-seed" theories of generation.[122] Summarized briefly,[123] the two-seed theory maintains that both men and women produce seed, which contributes equally to the creation of the embryo.[124] The one-seed theory maintains that only men produce seed, which acts upon women's menstrual blood used in the creation of the embryo. Hippocratic authors adhere to the two-seed theory,[125] while Aristotle is the major advocate for this particular version of the one-seed theory.[126] For Aristotle, it is not that the woman has no role in generation, but that her role is less valued.

These theories continue to be debated, and adapted, over time. Galen, in his theory of generation, draws from both the Hippocratic authors and Aristotle.[127] He thus maintains the two-seed theory of human generation, like the Hippocratics, but achieves some sort of synthesis with Aristotle's theory, since Galen assumes that the male seed is perfected and thus stronger.[128] Furthermore, he agrees with Aristotle that blood is the origin of seed.[129] The one-seed theory also lives on, but eventually erases any active contribution from the woman to the creation of the embryo—even the lesser contribution from menstrual blood. In other words, whereas for Aristotle menstrual blood was necessary for human generation, it seems that for some it was considered unnecessary for the creation of the embryo, but necessary for nutriment.[130] This view seems to have been accepted by Soranus.[131]

At stake in the "one-seed" and "two-seed" theories is, in part, the conceptualization and characterization of women's contribution(s) to generation and heredity as more active or more passive.[132] However, even the two-seed theory does not amount to a statement about the equality of men and women in general or, more specifically, in their roles in the creation of the embryo—nor was it meant to achieve this end. Lesley Dean-Jones points out that the Hippocratic authors were as convinced of female inferiority as Aristotle was, and she explains, "Their theory of female seed did not in any way amount to saying that women were equal to men (note their description of female seed as weak seed); it was merely the most obvious way of explaining the undeniable resemblance many children bore to their mothers."[133]

If one (super)imposes the Greco-Roman "one-seed/two-seed" distinction onto rabbinic traditions, it becomes apparent that a one-seed theory is by far the most prevalent one in rabbinic literature. The only question where *Leviticus Rabbah* 14 is concerned is whether the traditions there set forth a one-seed theory that leaves out any female contribution or whether, in one instance (14:9), female blood *might be* the passive matter upon which male seed acts.[134] As for the "three partners" tradition in the *Bavli*, this too is not simple evidence of a two-seed theory because the woman has no "seed" distinct from her blood; she "seeds red," which means that her contribution to the creation of the embryo derives from her blood, more akin to Aristotelian notions than Hippocratic ones.[135] However, the idea of men contributing to the material creation of the embryo, as the "three partners" tradition insists, would have been scorned by Aristotle but not other proponents of a more extreme one-seed theory apparently adopted by Soranus, a closer contemporary of the rabbis.[136] In turn, rabbinic traditions seem to have considered the origin of semen from blood, also found in Aristotle among others, impossible.[137] The difficulty in precisely lining up rabbinic theories about procreation with Greco-Roman theories about generation could be taken as a clue that, while not entirely off track, an additional context needs to be considered.

In a very palpable sense, the one- and two-seed theories of generation are both always already insufficient because of the consistent emphasis on God in rabbinic traditions about the creation of the embryo. This emphasis on God simultaneously articulates rabbinic distinctiveness amid what has come to be seen as representative of hegemonic Greco-Roman ideologies about generation and illustrates rabbinic continuity with biblical notions of coming into being.[138]

Neither the Greco-Roman nor the biblical context, in and of themselves, account for rabbinic theories of procreation because they are the product of the intermingling of both. The language of seeds itself—irrespective of any "one-seed" or "two-seed" distinctions—situates rabbinic traditions about the creation of the embryo within late antique culture; Israel and Rome are twin brothers still struggling here not within one womb, but over what happens within wombs. The theological language, however, locates the rabbis still within—or at least a product of—the biblical world, among their ancestors. It is as if the rabbis say to Greco-Roman influence that which God says to the fetus in its mother's womb, "Until here, but no further" (*Lev. Rab.* 14:4); seeds, without God, do not make an embryo.

Locating the discourse of seeds within late antique culture instead of biblical sources does not necessarily mean that the Hebrew Bible lacks *any* notion of seed in procreation. It does, however, call attention to the relative paucity of biblical sources that focus on seeds in contrast to the number of sources that attribute both pregnancy and the creation of the embryo to God.

When the Bible imagines the creation of the embryo, most explicitly and elaborately in Job 10:8–10 and Ps. 139:13–16, it posits God as the embryo's sole creator.[139] In fact, except for God's involvement in biblical pregnancies, the Bible lacks any explicit theory of precisely how pregnancy occurs.[140] Of course, sexual intercourse is often—but not always—alluded to or mentioned, but the Hebrew Bible never explicitly acknowledges the substances involved in bringing about pregnancy, at least in the context of recorded pregnancies.[141] By far the dominant theory of procreation in the Hebrew Bible—though it is not often cast as a procreation theory—is that God grants pregnancy, or, in biblical parlance, God opens, or closes, women's wombs.[142]

Most obviously, biblical sources credit God with granting pregnancy to barren women.[143] God restrains Sarai from childbearing (Gen. 16:2), but then God does that which God has promised for Sarah and she becomes pregnant and gives birth (Gen. 21:1). God listens to Isaac's prayers on behalf of Rebekah and she becomes pregnant and gives birth (Gen. 25:21). God opens Rachel's womb (Gen. 30:22). The previously barren wife of Manoah gives birth to Samson (Judg. 13:3). And God remembers Hannah and she becomes pregnant (1 Sam. 1:19–20 and 2:20–21). All of these women are explicitly labeled barren in the Bible, but they eventually become pregnant with God's help.[144]

Although God's participation in procreation may be most obvious in biblical sources about barren women, God's necessity for procreation is far more pervasive than this single motif. For example, God closes up the wombs in Avimelech's house (Gen. 20:18);[145] God opens Leah's womb, though there is no previous mention of her being barren (Gen. 29:31). Later, God listens to Leah and she becomes pregnant (Gen. 30:17). God gives Ruth pregnancy (Ruth 4:13). God promises that if Israel obeys God it will be blessed and there will be none among Israel who miscarry or who are barren (Exod. 23:26). God strips the people of Ephraim of their glory, giving them no birth or pregnancy (Hos. 9:11). God makes the barren woman a joyful mother of children (Ps. 113:9). Children in general are considered the heritage or inheritance of God (Ps. 127:3). Finally, God promises to make Abraham's offspring (seed) as numerous as the dust of the earth (Gen. 13:6) and Hagar's offspring (seed) beyond counting (Gen. 16:10). One could add to these verses the instances where biblical women credit God with their pregnancies, as Eve says, *I have acquired a man with God* (Gen. 4:1).[146] Leah repeatedly credits God upon the birth and naming of her sons (Gen. 30:32–33 and 35). Male biblical figures also credit God with the granting, or withholding, of progeny: Avram says to God, *Behold, to me you have given no seed* (Gen. 15:3), and Jacob states, *Am I in God's place, who has withheld from you the fruit of the womb?* (Gen. 30:2).

All of these examples function to drive home the notion that, according to by far the majority of biblical sources, without God there is no procreation—there is no genealogy of Israel.[147] Stated differently, the dominant theory of procreation evident from biblical sources could be called a "no seed" theory of coming into being. The Hebrew Bible never sets forth a theory of procreation that explicitly mentions semen (*shikhvat zera'*) as contributing to pregnancy;[148] although Lev. 12:2 states that a woman "emits seed" (*tazria'*), it remains unclear what this means, and it also remains unclear from where such seed might come and how it might contribute precisely to pregnancy. Nowhere are the man's contribution of semen and the woman's contribution—be it from menstrual blood or the aforementioned seed—linked together to form a theory of human generation.[149] Instead, the Bible announces most pregnancies with the phrase "she became pregnant and gave birth" (*vatahar vateled*) or something similar, at least grammatically construing the woman's role in pregnancy and birth as active; in the Hebrew Bible, the woman is God's primary partner in bringing forth Israel.[150]

As demonstrated above, rabbinic traditions address scripture's lack concerning the human substance(s) involved in coming into being, incorporating Greco-Roman notions about generation—particularly a more fully developed notion of *male* seed—into their own theories of procreation, but never completely straying from the biblical theory that God creates the embryo. However, except for the "three partners" tradition, rabbinic sources leave behind the biblical conception of women actively participating in procreation.

The relatively little attention rabbinic traditions attribute to women in the creation of the embryo and fetal development by way of their blood can be contrasted with earlier Jewish sources of the Second Temple period, which also draw from Greco-Roman notions in order to fill in the biblical record.[151] Pieter van der Horst and Michael Satlow have noted the "Aristotelian" influences evident in postbiblical Jewish sources.[152] Van der Horst particularly focuses on the woman's contribution through her blood in such texts, citing Wisd. of Sol. 7:1–2, *In my mother's womb I was sculpted into flesh during a ten months' space, curdled in blood by virile seed and the pleasure that is joined with sleep,* and 4 Macc. 13:20, *There do brothers abide for a similar period and are molded through the same span and nurtured by the same blood and brought to maturity through the same vitality.*[153] Although 4 Macc. 13:20 focuses on women's blood nurturing the fetus, the previous verse states, *You are not ignorant of the affection of family ties, which the divine and all-wise Providence has bequeathed through the fathers to their descendants and which was implanted in the mother's womb,* which presumably alludes to male seed being implanted in the womb. Van der Horst also cites Philo, who, like Aristotle, both insists on the primacy given to men's contribution of semen and maintains some role for women's menstrual blood: "The matter of the female in the remains of the menstrual fluids produces the fetus. But the male (provides) the skill and the cause."[154] Although van der Horst cites these traditions in order to emphasize that their mention of woman's blood indicates the Aristotelian tendencies of these postbiblical Jewish texts, the sources themselves also remain consistent with Aristotle's, and others', emphasis on male seed as the primary substance behind the creation of an embryo.

The significance of these earlier sources lies not in an imagined distinction between these proponents of a one-seed theory against the later rabbinic propensity for a two-seed theory.[155] Rabbinic traditions emphasize male seed, most often to the utter exclusion of female seed, as well. Rather, what these sources illustrate is that although Second Temple Jewish authors, consonant with Greco-Roman theories, seem more likely than not to ascribe some importance to blood in the creation of the embryo and, subsequently, nurturing the fetus, rabbinic traditions are less likely to do so. In at most two rabbinic traditions, blood contributes, actively in the "three partners" text and passively in *Lev. Rab.* 14:9, to the creation of the embryo. But I have not found a rabbinic tradition that imagines women's blood as instrumental at any point later in gestation, imagined as further contributing to the development and nurturance of the fetus.[156]

The Greco-Roman context simply cannot account for the overall rabbinic resistance to fully mobilize blood as important for the development of the fetus any more than it accounts for the rabbinic emphasis on God in the creation of the embryo; both run counter to Greco-Roman theories of generation. I suggest that both God's role in the creation of the embryo and the near absence of women's blood are related. The former is a continuation of biblical materials, the latter an outgrowth of them.

When *Lev. Rab.* 14:2–4 repeatedly displaces women from the care and sustenance of the fetus, rendering explicit what is implicit not only in *Leviticus Rabbah* 14 as a whole but also in almost the entirety of rabbinic traditions about procreation, the rabbinic proclivity of theologizing procreation provides a partial explanation. In the context of rendering unto God what is God's, which is what *Leviticus Rabbah* 14 does with Lev. 12:2, perhaps as perturbed by the androcentrism of the verse—the very humanity of it—as perplexed by the possible gynocentrism, the rabbis seek to set the record straight. And if God creates the embryo, then God cares for the fetus.

Attending to the theocentric perspective born out of biblical sources evident in both *Leviticus Rabbah* 14 and in other rabbinic traditions that reflect upon the creation of the embryo not only provides a more accurate rendering of how the rabbis imagined the process of coming into being but also allows for a more nuanced reading of the constructions of gender operating in these traditions. This does not result in any way in gender parity when all traditions are considered. It does, however, make more noticeable the fact that along with the utter displacement of women's roles in caring for and nurturing the fetus, men's roles in creating the embryo have been not entirely erased but diminished. Male seed, despite its consistent presence in the texts, does not—in and of itself—create the embryo. Furthermore, the actual appearance of the common designation of semen in other contexts— *shikhvat zera'*—is even more absent than women's blood in traditions that theorize the creation of the embryo. In these traditions, semen itself has been distilled, even reduced, to its purest part—the "white drop"—suggesting that in addition to setting forth a theological message, rabbinic concerns about (im)purity might explain the relative lack of both blood and semen.[157]

In sum, rabbinic traditions about the creation of the embryo and the care of the fetus cannot be fully explained by appealing to Greco-Roman theories of generation. Such theories provide a partial context that contributes to the rabbinic emphasis on male seed, but they fail to account for the rabbinic emphasis on God, the almost utter displacement of women from contributing to the care of the fetus, and even the extent to which men's contributions through seed are de-emphasized relative to God's. That which cannot be explained by Greco-Roman influence reflects the influence biblical sources exert over rabbinic traditions, as rabbinic traditions expand the one explicit biblical theory of coming into being to include a notion of male seed and to imagine God as not only the creator but also the caretaker of Israel already in the womb. The rabbis are thus heirs to and progenitors of the belief that God creates and cares for Israel—in the present as much as in the past, from its very beginnings and throughout time.

Reproductive Theologies

Although the emphasis that rabbinic traditions about the creation of the embryo place on God distinguishes the rabbis from Greco-Roman (medical) writers, this very emphasis brings the rabbis and patristic authors into close relation. To take an example from one of the church fathers whose close connection to the rabbis on anything having to do with procreation might be greeted with some surprise, Elizabeth Clark, summarizing Augustine, writes, "If God were to withdraw his good action in producing seeds, caring for them, and quickening the fetus, there would be no begetting."[158]

A full exploration of patristic theories of procreation is beyond the scope of this book.[159] My aim in what follows is simply to juxtapose rabbinic traditions with some patristic sources about the creation of the embryo for the purpose of further situating rabbinic sources in their late antique context. I focus on the writings of Clement and Augustine, who since separated chronologically and geographically, provide at least an interesting "sample" that highlights not only what they share between each other in spite of their differences but also what patristic and rabbinic sources of a broad range have in common.[160] In particular, I point out that despite some significant differences between rabbinic and patristic attitudes *about* procreation, sexuality, and marriage within which theories of the creation of the embryo are indelibly enmeshed, both rabbinic and patristic interpreters—and inheritors—of the Bible agree that God creates the embryo.[161]

Clement of Alexandria (ca. 150–211 CE), whose primary metaphor for procreation is that of a farmer sowing seeds,[162] writes, "If someone is a farmer or the father of a child, he is an assistant in depositing the seeds, but it is God who provides the growth and completion of all things in order that he might bring that which is born into accordance with nature."[163] In *Paidagogos* 2.83, Clement again uses this metaphor, explaining that the farmer who sows seeds in a living field "plants through God." He continues, "For God said 'Multiply yourselves' [Gen. 1:28] and it is necessary to obey. And in this way, man is an image of God since man collaborates in the creation of a human."[164] In the same passage, Clement further explains, "We should not sow on rocks; nor should we mistreat the seed, the leader and essence of generation which contains Nature's principles sown into it."[165] As Elaine Pagels writes in connection with another of Clement's passages about procreation, "Clement might well have added, 'when I say *nature*, I mean *God.*'"[166] Finally, in a passage that makes it clear that women are the fields into which seeds are planted, not farmers in and of themselves, Clement further involves God in creating the embryo: "Now the womb thirsts with desire for the seeding to make children . . . and after the seeding it now completely excludes licentiousness by shutting its mouth. The appetites which were previously spent in the excitement of affectionate embraces are diverted and busied internally with the making of children *in cooperation with the Creator.*"[167] For Clement, like the rabbis, both the creation of the embryo with male seed and the development of the embryo in the womb require God. Moreover, in terms of a partnership between humanity and God, Clement implies that God's actions carry more weight, while people assist, or cooperate with, God.

The specific procreative metaphor of a farmer sowing his seed into fertile ground is not well attested in rabbinic literature, but some rabbinic traditions do use agricultural images to describe both nonprocreative and procreative intercourse. For example, a tannaitic tradition, roughly contemporaneous with Clement, recommends nonprocreative intercourse between a husband and a nursing wife: "R. Meir says, 'he threshes inside and scatters outside.'"[168] According to *Gen. Rab.* 98:4, Jacob states, "All the furrows that I plowed in your mother (Leah), I was only supposed to plow them in Rachel."[169] And *y. Yev.* 1:1 states, "R. Yosi bar Halfota levirately married his brother's wife. He plowed five furrows and planted five plants and he had intercourse by way of a sheet."[170] Both rabbinic traditions refer to sexual intercourse by using the language of a man "plowing his furrow."[171] In the *Yerushalmi* passage, offspring are explicitly referred to as plants the father has planted.

In its rabbinic context, such agricultural imagery reinforces the construction of men as active and women as passive in procreation. It also suggests, although more subtly than the rabbinic traditions examined above, God's involvement in the process, since successful planting—be it of women or the earth—requires God.[172] The juxtaposition of the earth's and humanity's fertility, which rabbinic traditions bring together through agricultural metaphors for procreation, can be seen as part of what the rabbis inherit from biblical sources. Just as procreation in the Hebrew Bible remains largely in the purview of God, so too does the earth's fruitfulness. Both are linked, for example, in Deut. 7:13, *And he will love you, and bless you, and multiply you; he will also bless the fruit of your womb, and the fruit of your land, your grain, and your wine, and your oil*, and in Exod. 23:25–26, *You shall serve the*

Lord your God, and He will bless your bread and your water. And I will remove illness from your midst. No woman in your land shall miscarry or be barren, and I will give you the full count of your days.[173]

The rabbis bring God's power over both human and earthly fertility together in a passage that states, "Three keys are in the hands of the Holy Blessed One: the key to the grave (resurrection), the key to rain, and the key to the womb.... The key to rain, *God will open his treasure, the heaven, to give the rain* (Deut. 28:12). The key to the womb, *And God opened her womb* (Gen. 30:22). And some say also the key of sustenance, *You open your hand and satisfy every living thing with favor* (Ps. 145:16)."[174]

Although the above passage refers in general terms to God's control over earthly and human fruitfulness, *Gen. Rab.* 63:5, interpreting Gen. 25:21, *And Isaac entreated God for his wife, because she was barren; and God was entreated of him and Rebekah his wife conceived*, links procreation and agriculture imagery in more specific, and colorful, ways. First, a statement attributed to Reish Lakish interprets *And Isaac entreated [vaye'tar] God* as meaning "He overturned the decree [that Rebekah be barren], and therefore they call a pitchfork *'atrah*, because it overturns grain [*'idrah*]." Here Reish Lakish interprets Isaac's pleas as affecting God so that the divine decree of Rebekah's barrenness is overturned like grain. The text later interprets *And God was entreated of him [and Rebekah his wife conceived]*: "R. Levi said, this may be compared to a son of a king[175] who was digging to his father to take a litra of gold, and one (the king) dug from within, while the other (the son) dug from without."[176] Now the text alludes to the double-pronged action of God (king) and Isaac (king's son) digging together, from within and without, to make the embryo (the litra of gold).[177]

When rabbinic traditions use agricultural language to refer to procreation, here, too, they imagine God as necessary for the creation of the embryo, either because God is in control of agriculture or, even more specifically, God "digs" from within—God creates what is within.[178] This seems to be consistent with Clement, who, while favoring the "farmer" metaphor for procreation, nevertheless suggests that the farmer *assists* God in creating the embryo but does not in and of himself create the embryo.

Leviticus Rabbah 14 mobilizes agricultural imagery only once, demonstrating that it is not as central to rabbinic depictions of procreation as it is for Clement.[179] The chapter does, however, turn on the issue of seeds. In what follows, I return to *Leviticus Rabbah* 14, situating it in the broader context of inter-Christian disputes raging during the first part of the fifth century CE.

Elizabeth Clark writes that, by the year 418 CE, "'Seeds' are now manifestly on his [Augustine's] mind."[180] The context of Clark's statement is her exposition of the heated exchange between the bishop of Hippo and Julian of Eclanum that revolves around "issues pertaining to sexuality, marriage, and the transmission of original sin"[181] and raises "questions of anthropology, late ancient biology, and the status of Jesus."[182] If, as Clark points out, "As the debate proceeded . . . seeds became an increasingly important topic,"[183] and both Augustine and Julian, despite their differences, agree that "God makes all humans from seed,"[184] one can only wonder about the possible synchronicity between these authors and the fourteenth chapter of *Leviticus Rabbah*, compiled during the same period and turning on the issue of seed(s) and God's involvement with them.

It is not my intention to suggest an exegetical encounter between Augustine and the rabbis, nor between the Pelagian Julian and the rabbis, since despite the contemporaneity[185] of the sources, a direct exchange would be difficult to establish due to both different geographical locations and "the language barrier."[186] I merely point out some parallel concerns, first about the overarching notions of late ancient biology, gender, and theology operating across, and between, the lines of these sources and then about the more specific issue of *Leviticus Rabbah* 14's possible engagement with original sin and the status of Jesus. Finally, I consider whether, despite the ultimate denial of original sin articulated in *Lev. Rab.* 14:5, the chapter as a whole might nevertheless demonstrate some rabbinic anxiety and ambivalence about matters pertaining to procreation and sexuality, thereby suggesting some further contiguity between *Leviticus Rabbah* 14 and its fourth- and fifth-century patristic counterparts.

The notion of women passively conceiving and the man more actively generating is as dominant in Augustine's writings as it is in *Leviticus Rabbah* 14.[187] Augustine, at least in the *Contra Julian* or *Opus imperfectum*, never appeals to Lev. 12:2, suggesting that for him, as much as for the rabbis, imagining that women actively contribute to the creation of the embryo based on this verse—or apparently any other—is quite alien.[188] In the context of his debate with Julian about the interpretation of Rom. 5:12, which hinges upon whether sin was sexually transmitted through "one man," Adam, or passed on by imitation,[189] Augustine, a strong proponent of the former, writes, "For everyone knows that the parent who sows the seed is the one who most of all or first of all generates a child and that the woman either does not generate, but bears a child—or, if bearing a child is correctly called generation, she first conceived from the man who generates the child and afterwards generates the child she has conceived."[190] Except for the explicit concern about the transmission of sin through sex (or male seed),[191] Augustine's statement mirrors not only many of the rabbinic traditions in *Leviticus Rabbah* 14 but also one of the main lessons of *Leviticus Rabbah* 14, in my reading, as a whole: women do not have seed with which to generate the embryo but receive that seed from men.

The significance that Augustine attributes to male seed, however, does not signal Augustine's adoption of a Greco-Roman one-seed theory of generation any more than it does in rabbinic traditions. For Augustine as well, the importance of male seed is overshadowed by God. As Clark explains, "Augustine holds that the seed is created by God directly and does not receive its formation from 'lust.' Thus the child that results is a divine work, not a human one. If God were to withdraw his good action in producing seeds, caring for them, and quickening the fetus, there would be no begetting."[192] Most, if not all, of these statements would be well placed within *Leviticus Rabbah* 14 where it is assumed that God creates seed in men,[193] and it is repeatedly stated that God is responsible for the creation of the embryo and the development and care of the fetus.[194] The force of *Leviticus Rabbah*, as an elucidation of Lev. 12:2, is to make it clear that humanity does not create the embryo—God does. According to *Leviticus Rabbah* 14, like Augustine, without God, there would be no begetting.

The strongest commonality between Augustine's anti-Pelagian writings and the traditions in *Leviticus Rabbah* 14 is their consistent articulation of a "theology of reproduction."[195] For Augustine and the rabbis, in *Leviticus Rabbah* 14 and in other places, Greco-Roman theories of generation are infused with theology,[196] as both rabbinic and patristic traditions build upon biblical precedents.[197] Although Clark maintains that Augustine would have preferred to rest his arguments on biblical examples and theological grounds, Julian's insistence on his opponent's faulty biology set the terms of the debate.[198] *Leviticus Rabbah* 14, however, does not come about in answer to any explicit external challenges; it seeks to interpret, or at least presents itself as concerned with interpreting, Lev. 12:2. And that verse, which locates procreation within the human and even female realm, needs to be redressed. Having demonstrated that in the midst of such an unrelenting rabbinic (re)reading of Lev. 12:2, *Leviticus Rabbah* 14 incorporates—to a certain extent—late antique notions about the heightened importance of male seed for the creation of the embryo, I now consider if *Leviticus Rabbah* 14 *as a whole* is best conceived as remaining perfectly isolated not only from inter-Christian debates about original sin and the status of Jesus but also from much broader patristic disputes about the relative goods or ills of marriage, sexuality, and procreation.[199]

In order to open up the larger topic of a possible engagement with Christianity in *Leviticus Rabbah* 14 as a whole, I revisit *Lev. Rab.* 14:5, now returning to its use of Ps. 51:7, *Behold I was brought forth in iniquity and in sin did my mother conceive me.* Certainly, the citation of Ps. 51:7 raises the distinct possibility that *Lev. Rab.* 14:5 has original sin on its mind.[200] The text, however ultimately rejects such a notion, only going so far as to espouse a belief in universal iniquity.

Lev. Rab. 14:5 interprets the first part of Ps. 51:7 to teach that even the most pious is not without some iniquity. The example is Jesse, and his iniquity is having nonprocreative intercourse, as the text imagines that he and his wife have sex without the intent of bringing forth David.[201] While the text illustrates that David's human parents have forsaken him, it insists that his Father in Heaven gathers him in (Ps. 27:10). In other words, God brings forth David, *removing* him from any "taint" of *his parents'* iniquity.[202] The rabbinic interpretation of the second part of Ps. 51:7, *In sin did my mother conceive me,* further removes David, and all embryos since the text now speaks more generally, from being born in or with sin, which the text links with menstruation—not intercourse—and the embryo is created in a womb emptied of blood.

Lev. Rab. 14:5, while positing universal iniquity, denies original sin. David's iniquities remain his own, not those passed on through his parents, as Psalm 51, which focuses on David's iniquity insofar as he satisfied his own needs with Batsheva, makes clear.[203] But why does *Lev. Rab.* 14:5 choose to deny original sin (and virgin birth) through David? Visotzky provocatively suggests that David is a stand-in for Jesus, and the parents in the text are none other than Joseph and Mary. According to Visotzky, *Lev. Rab.* 14:5 unleashes a "vulgar parody" of *Jesus'* coming into being, and he concludes, "Original sin, immaculate conception, virgin birth and begetting by the Holy Spirit are ribaldly reduced to the crudest possible terms. *There is no room for theology here, only scorn.*"[204] If, as I maintain, *Leviticus Rabbah* 14 as a whole is largely a theological endeavor, which consistently theologizes procreation by attributing the creation of every embryo ultimately to God, then *Lev. Rab.* 14:5 should also be read as referring to David, as it presents itself as doing. This tradition might be taking a stand against virgin birth and begetting by the Holy Spirit, but only insofar as where Jesus is concerned, there is no sexual intercourse and semen, and further, the notion that the Holy Spirit—*not God*—takes on the role of "artificial inseminator," to use Visotzky's term.[205] However, it is neither denying nor even parodying the belief shared by both patristic and rabbinic sources that God creates embryos. The polemic I detect, my answer to why David is the concern of this text, in addition to the obvious one that Psalm 51 is attributed to him, has everything to do with theology, which throughout *Leviticus Rabbah* 14 far outweighs anthropology, biology, *and* polemic. David, the ancestor of Jesus, *Lev. Rab.* 14:5 proclaims, was "begotten" by God, and David, along with Jesus and everyone else, like *'adam* (*Lev. Rab.* 14:1) is created by God and born without sin.[206]

Rabbinic rejection of original sin is nothing surprising; it is, rather, almost axiomatic. It would be far more surprising if, when the rabbis seem to be directly engaging the notion, they did anything different. However, building not upon the reified differences between rabbinic and patristic attitudes about sex and procreation but instead upon the sources' common foundation of attributing the creation of the embryo to God, I want to explore whether *Leviticus Rabbah* 14, and rabbinic traditions that theorize the creation of the embryo more generally, might betray some rabbinic anxiety and ambivalence about sex—within the very context of [theologizing] procreation—which places these rabbinic sources in a different sort of dialogue with fifth-century Christian sources.

David Biale and Daniel Boyarin have explored the cultural tensions, the anxieties, appearing within rabbinic "dialectics of desire."[207] Biale frames his chapter on rabbinic materials with a concern about renunciatory tactics. He begins the chapter with the rabbinic portrayal of Moses' celibacy and he ends with the rabbinic interpretation of the Song of Songs as a theological allegory that simultaneously renounces this biblical book's erotic play between human partners and eroticizes the relationship between God and the rabbis.[208] By such framing, he complicates any overly simple assertion that the rabbis everywhere and always renounced sexual renunciation. Toward the end of his chapter Biale writes, "In the culture of late antiquity, the competition between holy abstinence and the duty to produce children created a deep anxiety to which the rabbis were not immune."[209] Boyarin begins his chapter by stating, "Far from being a simple legacy of its cultural heritage, the rabbinic insistence on the positive valence of sexuality seems to have been hard won and contested," and toward the end he writes, "The 'carnality' of rabbinic Judaism did not enable the faithful simply to bypass the sexual anxieties whose spiritual and social dimensions Peter Brown explores in his great work."[210]

Reproductive Theology   123

I suggest that rabbinic theories of procreation, especially as they appear together in *Leviticus Rabbah* 14, further express the anxieties about sex and procreation previously explored by Biale and Boyarin.[211] The very move to theologize procreation, to bring God into bed—where, according to Boyarin, rabbinic control could not enter[212]—and *into the womb*,[213] should be seen in the larger context of rabbinic anxieties not about the limits of their own knowledge or understanding of the process of coming into being, for these anxieties are for the most part not evident in rabbinic traditions,[214] but about their disbelief that *this* (the embryo, and ultimately the child) can come from *that* (sex, semen, all the more so blood). I find it particularly interesting that, although Boyarin points out, "Perhaps the most arresting fact about the discourse of sexuality throughout the talmudic literature is that desire is nearly always concatenated with having children," the obverse does not bear out. In *Leviticus Rabbah* 14, which I consider to be the most extensive rabbinic discourse of procreation, there is hardly any sex.[215]

Leviticus Rabbah 14, a chapter that goes to great lengths to describe the process of coming into being in ways that bear enormous cultural and cosmic significance, produces an encomium to God as the creator of the embryo and caretaker of the fetus—and Israel—that simultaneously displaces men and women and thus disassociates sexual intercourse from the procreative process.[216] Sexual intercourse is implied; any reader knows it is, just like the rabbis know that each time one of their biblical ancestors becomes pregnant it was as a result of God—assisted by male seed—though the contribution of seed is more often than not left implicit. But sex and its bodily by-products hover in the background of *Leviticus Rabbah* 14, barely making an appearance in the chapter. In a culture that ultimately insists on "the positive valence of sexuality" and also shows little evidence of shying away from bodily effluence, including sexual emissions, the textual omissions of blood and semen qua semen (*shikhvat zera'*), along with women and men, have given me pause and have led me to consider at least a possible rabbinic anxiety about sex, shared among patristic authors, surfacing in this otherwise quite expansive rabbinic chapter on procreation.[217] Interestingly, the one tradition in *Leviticus Rabbah* 14 that explicitly mentions sexual intercourse is *Lev. Rab.* 14:5, where Jesse and his wife's interest is nonprocreative sex, or their own lust.[218]

Leviticus Rabbah 14's inclination to discourse about the creation of the embryo and the care of the fetus without focusing on blood or semen, preferring to refer simply to the (purest part of the) "white drop" and consistently removing blood from the developing fetus and the creation of the embryo, could be more internally motivated by rabbinic concerns—even anxieties—not about the transmission of sin, or moral impurity, but about the contracting of ritual, bodily impurity.[219] In other words, one need not imagine—and I am not suggesting—that the only or even primary explanation for rabbinic uneasiness about sex and its fluids stems from the chapter's possible engagement with Christianity. Semen and blood, specifically female blood, both transmit ritual impurity, alone, and even more so in concert.[220] But if these two impure substances interact to create the embryo—or even if semen alone contributes to its creation—how does the fetus emerge "pure"?[221]

Lev. Rab. 14:4, decidedly ascribing neither ritual impurity nor moral iniquity to the newborn, nevertheless presents an interesting tradition. In a statement attributed to R. Aibu,[222] Job 38:11, *And here shall your proud waves [bige'on galeikha] be stayed*, is interpreted to mean, through a Hebrew pun, "in the iniquity of your filth [be'avon gelaleikha]."[223] The text continues, "Even though this child comes forth full of excrement and foulness, everybody hugs him and kisses him." It is as if the text, while affirming the newborn's purity, also articulates some doubt since it is born with such foulness, which accompanies birth and renders the woman ritually impure.[224]

A statement in b. Nid. 9a more explicitly voices some doubt that semen, which is impure, can create the pure embryo.[225] In the context of a debate about how breast milk is produced, R. Meir's theory that milk is transformed from blood is supported by Job 14:4, *Who can bring a pure thing from an impure? Not one.*[226] The midrashic reading of the verse is that no one but God can achieve the enormous task of transforming that which is impure (blood) into something pure (milk). But what of other rabbis, who do not maintain that the origins of breast milk are in blood? How do they interpret the verse from Job? For them, Job 14:4 refers to semen (*shikhvat zera'*), "which is impure, but the person created from it is pure." By implication, both from this statement's immediate context and from other rabbinic traditions set forth throughout this chapter, once again, only God can create the embryo, transforming that which is impure (semen) into that which is pure (the embryo). Although such a concern about the ritual impurity of semen is not explicitly found in *Leviticus Rabbah* 14, such anxiety about impurity might explain why semen is always referred to as "the drop" or "the white drop." Furthermore, the concern about (im)purity might further explain why *Leviticus Rabbah* 14 never imagines women's blood contributing to the development and nurturance of the fetus, but allocates this to God as well. The focus on God in *Leviticus Rabbah* 14, which brings with it not only the displacement of women and to a lesser extent men but also the downplaying of both blood and *shikvat zera'*, might be a way of sidestepping concerns about impurity that any mention of blood and semen would naturally invite, given the pervasive rabbinic concern about (im)purity.

Alternatively, *Leviticus Rabbah* 14 lacks any concern about (im)purity and imagines semen as "the drop" or the "white drop" simply to highlight the miracles that God performs in creating the embryo, matched by those that God, not women's blood, performs in caring for the fetus. In this case, that God continues to create Israel with just a drop of liquid—like God created the heavens—and that God cares for the fetus in its mother's womb—like God cares for Israel—remain the point of *Leviticus Rabbah* 14.

My goal has not been to decide definitively what drives *Leviticus Rabbah* 14's displacement of women and to a far less extent men, or to determine its exact reasons for shifting the focus away from blood and semen and to God when it theorizes (Israel's) origins, but to bring these aspects, previously left underarticulated, of *Leviticus Rabbah* 14 out into the open. Whether or not inter-Christian disputes during the fifth century and rabbinic concerns about (im)purity play a part in *Leviticus Rabbah* 14—and I think that they do—exploring both as possibilities situates *Leviticus Rabbah* 14 in its late antique cultural contexts, which extend beyond the already posed and still important question of "how much Greek in Jewish Palestine."[227] Once *Leviticus Rabbah* 14 is itself opened up to multiple, close, layered, and even opposing readings, in a fashion modeled upon the chapter's own deliberate rereadings of Lev. 12:2, larger cultural issues and contexts emerge as part and parcel of rabbinic attempts to explain (Israel's) origins, which is the work that theories of procreation often do, not only in cultures but also across them.[228] A careful reading of *Leviticus Rabbah* 14, which highlights not only what it says about procreation but also how it says it and what it does not say, brings into the open the cultural, and largely theological, work theories about procreation enact—in both rabbinic and patristic sources.

Conclusion

Rabbinic traditions that theorize the process of coming into being build upon—and weave together—both biblical notions of procreation, which emphasize God's roles in the process, and late antique theories about generation, which have a more developed concept of seed(s) than biblical sources. When one asks of rabbinic traditions only how many seeds it takes to create an embryo, the sources overwhelmingly answer one seed—that which is from the male, demonstrating that the rabbis, like their late antique counterparts, wrote hierarchical constructions of gender into the very nature of things. However, as illuminating as rabbinic traditions about the process of coming into being are vis-à-vis contemporary concerns about both the relationship between men and women and the relationship between the rabbis and late antique culture, these sources have some more primary concerns of their own: concretizing the relationship between God and Israel and articulating the connection, the continuity, between biblical and rabbinic Israel. Just as God was necessary for the coming into being of Israel's biblical ancestors, so too God continues to bring into being each member of rabbinic Israel.

Rabbinic traditions that theorize the creation of the embryo, moreover, make Creation itself—of humanity and the world—ongoing through the creation of each embryo. Procreation recalls, reiterates, and continues Creation. Just as God created the heavens with a drop of liquid, so too God creates each embryo with a drop of liquid. Rabbinic traditions about coming into being thus imbue procreation with cosmic significance. A later rabbinic tradition makes this explicit: "The creation of the embryo is like the creation of the world because a person is a small world" (*Midrash Tanhuma, Pekudei* 3).[229] Rabbinic traditions about procreation bring together the macrocosm (cosmos) and the microcosm (embryo), and attribute the creation of both to God.

Finally, like the traditions in the first part of the book that internalize and eternalize the Exodus from Egypt and the Revelation of Torah at Sinai by projecting them onto the fetus, rabbinic traditions about procreation internalize and make timeless Creation. Reading rabbinic traditions about the fetus as important textual sites where the rabbis reflect upon that which constitutes Israel reveals that the belief in a God who created the world and Israel—both the collective body and the individual one—is as foundational to rabbinic constructions of Israel as the belief in a God who delivered Israel out of Egypt and gave Israel its Torah.

Epilogue

Over the past twenty years, feminist scholarship has probed beneath the surface impressions of contemporary fetal images and illuminated the processes by which the (free-floating) fetus has become a powerful symbol for "life itself."[1] Such scholarship has exposed the ways that cropped, enhanced, or even doctored photographs and manufactured images produced by sound waves—that often still require interpretation and translation by those trained to read them—not only reveal the constructed nature of the once hidden though now public fetus but also bring into sharp relief the constructed, partial nature of vision itself.[2] Rosalind Petchesky writes, "Fetal imagery epitomizes the distortion inherent in all photographic images: their tendency to slice up reality into tiny bits wrenched out of real space and time."[3] She points out that any visual image "relies on our predisposition to 'see' what it wants us to 'see' because of a range of influences that come out of the particular culture and history in which we live."[4] Barbara Duden argues that in the time and space between 1965 and 1990,[5] we have become captivated—and held captive by—our own desire not only to see what was once hidden but also to be shown how and what to see. She writes, "We are told what to see.... Our readiness to see *on command* has grown tremendously in the intervening twenty-five years"; and further, "Now, we see what we are shown. We have gotten used to being shown no matter what, within or beyond the limited range of sight."[6] And Valerie Hartouni writes that "our vision is mediated by much more than the eye" and it is "trained in the fullest sense of the word." She continues, "to be able to 'see' the world at all is already to be making sense of it, or making it make the sense it seems a priori to possess."[7]

Rabbinic narratives about fetuses require a retraining of the eyes and a recalibration of vision. I have endeavored, to the extent possible, to see—and to show—how the rabbis envisioned the fetus and, through it, Israel. I continually had to look through and beyond the barrage of ascribed meanings to contemporary fetal images and find ways to meet the rabbinic textual images in their own contexts, on their own terms, and in their own language. These textual images, in their contexts and on their terms, shed light on how, in rabbinic narratives, the fetus is a symbol not for "life itself" but of Israel itself. When the rabbis cast fetuses as participants on their world stage, imbuing them with the power to speak along with, on behalf of, and for Israel, we best prick up our ears and hear what they are being made to say.

The mixing of visual and auditory language is intentional. As I have endeavored to see and show the rabbinic fetus, rabbinic fetuses, I have had to strain my ears as well as my eyes first to listen and then to articulate and to translate their meaning(s). Like a sonogram projected back through time with a transducer sending out pulses and picking up echoes carried within rabbinic sources—not women's abdomens—I have created a portrait and a moving picture of Israel. I have not, however, "colonized the past" by seeing fetuses and claiming that the rabbis saw fetuses too; the fetus as object of inquiry and subject or site of—and symbol with—profound meaning appears in the sources themselves.

In her book *Disembodying Women,* Barbara Duden eloquently traces the path she traveled, back and forth, between the twentieth century and its fetus and the eighteenth century, when women were "with child." She does this in order to come to know better how women in previous centuries experienced pregnancy and to illustrate how the experience of pregnancy has changed over time. My own travels to an even more distant, textual past do not give voice to women's experiences of pregnancy. I have neither attempted to read women into these rabbinic texts that, in large measure, leave them out, nor have I tried to read these texts "against the grain" in search of a sentient female subject who is, after all, "with child."[8] I have, instead, followed the rabbinic gaze as it has fixed upon fetuses.

Having trained my sights on rabbinic narratives about fetuses, this book has offered a further historicization of the "free-floating" fetus that is conjured and cast about today. However, as others have amply illustrated, contemporary imaged or manufactured fetuses, albeit often pictured disembodied from women, do not so much float freely but are instead caught up in a tangle of cultural meanings. In late twentieth- and early twenty-first-century U.S. contexts, the web within which the visible, public fetus is most often and obviously, though somewhat superficially,[9] entangled is contemporary clashes over abortion. This comes quickly to the surface in what Faye Ginsburg characterized as a "popular [pro-life] quip," which states, "If there were a window on a pregnant woman's stomach, there would be no more abortions."[10]

Whereas a window on pregnant women's stomachs opens directly into the issue of abortion and questions about "life itself" for many today, when the rabbis rendered women's wombs transparent they saw Israel—its creation and care. Rabbinic traditions that imaginatively turned pregnant women's bellies into glass and rabbinic traditions that imagined the creation, development, and care of the fetus thus opened a window through which I examined how the rabbis articulated Israel. Having, throughout this book, situated rabbinic narratives about fetuses amid the larger themes of rabbinic theology and gender and explored the insights these traditions provide into how the rabbis negotiated the relationships between biblical and rabbinic Israel as well as rabbinic Israel and its late antique "others," I now use these traditions as a vantage point from which to reflect briefly upon some of the broader methodological issues in scholarly attempts to reconstruct rabbinic (constructions of) Israel.

When I claim that rabbinic narratives about fetuses require a retraining of the eyes and a recalibration of vision, I mean much more than the need to see beyond the proliferation of fetal images in the context of contemporary concerns about abortion. Hand in hand with my attempts to see and bring to light how the image of the fetus operates in its narrative rabbinic contexts without allowing these textual images to be overshadowed by contemporary questions about abortion, I have also had to make my way through and see beyond the constructs of rabbinic Judaism and even rabbinic "Jewishness" in order to return to the language—and the focus—of rabbinic sources themselves: Israel.[11] I have, where possible, used the rabbinic self-appellation, Israel, instead of our more common terms in an effort to resist—and challenge—the ease with which we often conflate the two.

The paucity of rabbinic sources that use the term "Jew" (*yehudi*) or its correlates, along with the ubiquity of the term "Israel" in these same sources, makes it clear that the rabbis conceived themselves as Israel.[12] If, as Shaye Cohen aptly points out, "Jewishness is in the mind,"[13] it needs to be recognized that Jewishness, designated as such, is not at the forefront of the rabbis' own minds. To continue to impose the terms "Jewishness" and "Judaism" on rabbinic sources, which overwhelmingly neglect to embrace them or terms like them fully, contributes to and even encourages a reading of rabbinic literature that makes it make the sense it seems a priori to possess from our perspective.[14] That the rabbis gave birth to, or served as midwives for, "Judaism" need not be disputed, but it needs to be recognized that they did this by conceiving themselves as *Israel*. This is more than a semantic difference. The language that we use to portray one of the most central objects—and subjects—of rabbinic inquiry has profound implications for both the questions posed to these sources and the findings drawn from them; in other words, language shapes our field of vision—what we are willing and able both to see and to be shown.[15]

Remaining within the frame of rabbinic sources themselves, taking seriously their choice of language and terminology, has encouraged me to downplay the degree of—though in no way dismiss—the impact Christianity or the Christianization of Rome exercised upon the rabbis in antiquity. If Christianity invented Judaism, or if *Christianismos* and *Ioudaismos* need each other in order to invent themselves,[16] I find it significant that, as Cynthia Baker has pointed out, "The earliest rabbis, by and large, seem not to have had much use for 'Jews.' 'Israel' is the designation they most commonly apply to themselves and members of their imagined, covenanted community. 'Jews,' the term widely used by Gentiles and all Greek writers to describe the same community, appears hardly at all in classical talmudic literature."[17]

The ramifications of reorienting our language, and thus our vision, back to what is intrinsic to the sources themselves are far-reaching. While reaching back to the language and scope of the sources themselves, I do not wish to return us to a moment in the history of rabbinics scholarship where any and all contact with early Christian or patristic sources, except perhaps for the most obvious of polemics, is denied; nor do I wish to discount the more recent scholarship that illuminates the complexities of the interrelationship between and among "Judaisms" and "Christianities," which nuances our understandings of late antiquity. I do, however, wish to challenge, or at least offer an alternative to, the reading of rabbinic sources that places the confrontation with Christianity "at the very heart of Midrashic and Talmudic Judaism."[18] That rabbinic sources neither fully embraced the term "Jew" (*yehudi/Ioudaios*) nor incorporated or invented a word for "Judaism" or "Jewishness" (*Ioudaismos*)—despite the presence of such terms in nonrabbinic sources—in other words, the grammar of rabbinic literature cautions against overestimating the presence of "Christianity."[19] It is, moreover, untenable to maintain that the rabbinic self-appellation, Israel, arises primarily—if at all—in response, or as resistance, to competing claims to that title instead of arising first and foremost from biblical sources.[20] Highlighting the continuity in language between biblical and rabbinic Israel is also important precisely because it keeps the relationship the rabbis are constructing with their biblical past in view—even as they navigate their place in late antiquity.

Focusing attention back on rabbinic Israel instead of "Jewishness" has ramifications that extend beyond revisiting, yet again, questions about the relationship between rabbinic "Judaism" and "Christianity" in late antiquity. Because I have focused on rabbinic sources, I have asked not "who was a Jew," but who and what constitutes (an) Israel.[21] This not only retains the language of the sources themselves, but it also opens up new textual sites, in addition to those about lineage and conversion, that should capture our attention and ignite our imaginations on our ways to answering such a central question. Furthermore, what it means to be Israel, according to the rabbis, far exceeds the matter of descent. This has been demonstrated, albeit to varying degrees, by scholarship about converts and conversion in rabbinic sources.[22] My point is that rabbinic narratives about fetuses also illustrate this.

On the one hand, rabbinic traditions that imagine fetuses as always already participants in Israel seem to reinforce a rabbinic emphasis on birth, or genealogy, as definitive of being Israel. One is, quite literally, born "Jewish." On the other hand, what both marks the fetus as an individual Israel and makes it emblematic of Israel itself is not—or at least not only—its pedigree, but its practices and beliefs. There is more to being Israel, these traditions proclaim, than simply being born. Being Israel, even when projected onto fetuses and thus internalized and imaginatively made innate—written and woven into the very fabric of one's being—is more than genealogy as typically understood.[23]

Christine Hayes has pointed out that birth, or what she calls "genealogical filiation," was "a common *minimum* definition of Jewish identity" shared by all Jewish groups in the Second Temple period.[24] Hayes's point is significant because when we ask how the rabbis imagined Israel, a *minimum* definition cannot be all we see or show. If asked what constitutes and defines (an) Israel, the rabbis would not have answered "Jewish" parents, much less a "Jewish" mother, *and left it at that*.[25] For such an unequivocal definition, Shaye Cohen turns to a fourth-century Latin church writer, known as Ambrosiaster, who writes, "from a Jew a Jew is born."[26] Hayes, however, maintains that for some Jews, the rabbis among them, "genealogical filiation was a sufficient (though not necessary) condition of Jewish identity."[27] Rabbinic narratives about fetuses, while assuming genealogical filiation, ultimately demonstrate that this is insufficient to encompass all that being Israel meant for the rabbis.

Asking who is (an) Israel and what it means, according to the rabbis, to be Israel is a far broader question than who is a Jew by birth. The rabbis realize this, and therefore they not only formalize a process of conversion *and* open a door through which converts can become genealogically linked to Israel,[28] but they also use their fetuses to illustrate that being Israel means acknowledging God as one's maker and deliverer and accepting, learning, and keeping God's—and Israel's—Torah precisely because these beliefs and practices are what make Israel Israel.

Floating in the belly of late antiquity and confounding our contemporary distinctions between Judaism as a religion or ethnicity, Jewishness as either primarily covenantal or genealogical, lie the rabbinic fetus *and* rabbinic conceptions of Israel.

* * *

Scholarly representations of rabbinic Israel, and all the more of late antique Judaism(s), are, by necessity, cropped and enhanced portraits of an entity that both invites interpretation and requires speculation, still to remain simultaneously within our sights and in need of constant revision. I have aimed a spotlight on rabbinic traditions about fetuses, highlighting the ways that these sources play a small but significant part in rabbinic articulations of Israel.

Despite the fact that rabbinic narratives about fetuses appear across rabbinic documents—each time illuminating rabbinic constructions of Israel—these sources have been left underexposed if not almost entirely hidden from view. Ironically, they have been brought to the surface mainly, if not exclusively, in the context of questions about abortion and Judaism, where they are briefly invoked only to be immediately dismissed—as if at best quaint and at worst embarrassing. Fifty years ago, Immanuel Jakobovits assembled an impressive list of these traditions in such a context, ultimately concluding, "All these passages occur in purely aggadic contexts and are not related to legal issues."[29] Roughly fifty years before Jakobovits, Julius Preuss asserted, "The not infrequent expressions found in the sermonizing sections of the Midrash such as 'the children began to sing hymns in their mother's wombs, and they praised the Lord, etc.' are naturally not to be taken literally."[30]

What both Jakobovits and Preuss do not ask, and we as a community of scholars have further neglected, however, is once having asserted that these "purely aggadic" and "sermonizing" traditions are neither related to legal issues nor to be taken literally, to what issues are these traditions relevant, and how should they be taken? The absence of any detailed examination of rabbinic narratives about fetuses makes it seem as if, once removed from questions about abortion, these traditions have no meaning, or that, so ensconced are we in our own historical situations, we cannot see past them to examine these rabbinic traditions in their own narrative-historical contexts. But these traditions are deeply relevant not only insofar as they are enmeshed in broader discourses about rabbinic constructions of gender and collective identity and illustrate ways that rabbinic Israel was simultaneously embedded and distinct in its late antique settings, topics increasingly at the forefront of rabbinics scholarship, but also because rabbinic narratives about fetuses and traditions about embryology confirm, complement, and challenge some of the ways that rabbinic Israel has been portrayed.

Rabbinic traditions about embryology and procreation confirm the androcentrism, and at times misogyny, amply attested to in rabbinic sources and already noted by other scholars.[31] Even if, as I have suggested, the primary purpose of rabbinic traditions about embryology is to attribute the creation and care of (each) Israel to God—thereby affirming God's continued active involvement in Israel—rather than to establish a hierarchical relationship between men and women, the latter is utterly apparent. These same traditions also confirm that the rabbis were deeply situated within Greco-Roman culture, as they, and their Christian counterparts, adapted embryology to suit their theological purposes.[32] Again, I have suggested that the primary relationship being articulated throughout traditions about rabbinic embryology is that between God and Israel, not the rabbis and Greco-Roman culture, but the latter is apparent and most often assumed in the sources themselves.

Rabbinic narratives about fetuses challenge the extent to which we can superimpose our distinctions and bifurcations both between genealogy and covenant and between practices and beliefs back onto rabbinic constructions of Israel. The projection of quintessential rabbinic practices, done in the service of espousing fundamental or even "essential" rabbinic beliefs, onto the fetus—(an) Israel as it takes shape—again exemplifies the ways that both genealogy and *covenant*—which emphasizes relationship and not "law"—are woven into the fabric of being Israel and into rabbinic Israel's very being.

Rabbinic narratives about fetuses also challenge the ease with which we emphasize the construction of the collective self primarily in terms of the simultaneous constructions of its "others." To be certain, the scholarship that has focused on how rabbinic sources deal with those who occupy external, liminal, or interstitial spaces vis-à-vis rabbinic Israel has greatly enhanced our knowledge of how the rabbis constructed Israel. Rabbinic narratives about fetuses, however, precisely by providing an image of a hyperinternalized location, complement the work being done from that other angle. Rabbinic narratives about fetuses remind us that at least as much as rabbinic Israel constructs itself amid its late antique surroundings, in terms of both difference and sameness, rabbinic Israel—through the image of the fetus—also constructs itself in radical contiguity, and at times parity,[33] with biblical Israel. Furthermore, rabbinic narratives about fetuses, traditions about embryology, and theories of procreation suggest that, more than taking shape in relation with external others, Israel articulates itself in relationship—and through its relationship—with God.

I am, like many, suspicious of essentializing discourses. And in many ways, rabbinic literature is antiessentializing: it values debate and argument, offers multiple interpretations of scripture, canonizes dissent, and so on.[34] Such antiessentialism is, wherever it is found, cause for celebration. But when we find a motif, or an image, that does elicit and invoke an appeal to fundamentals or essentials, as I believe the fetus does for the rabbis, we need to see it for what it is, or might be, and allow it to be heard. I have emphasized the essentializing aspects of rabbinic narratives about fetuses knowing full well that the image of the fetus might invoke notions of liminality and interstitiality—even feelings of precariousness. It is more than likely that the rabbis knew the fetus, and life itself, to be frail, precarious. On a metatextual level, thinking with, or through, an image as small as a fetus about something as cumbersome as being Israel, as the rabbis did, invites a reading of these traditions that bespeaks the very precariousness of (being) Israel in late antiquity. However, the (image of the) fetus, as at once unstable and resilient, developing and enduring, permeable and insulated, vulnerable and protected—by the grace of God, according to the rabbis—makes the fetus a uniquely apt image through which to give testimony to Israel's eternal existence, its enduring right to life. On a textual level, despite the temptation to see the liminality of the fetus solely as a sign of precariousness, the rabbis grasp hold of this image to articulate and internalize much of what it means to be Israel.

Arguably the most important reason for deliberating and dwelling upon the relevance of rabbinic narratives about fetuses, even beyond noting how these traditions intersect with many key issues in contemporary rabbinics scholarship, is that the rabbis saw fit to reflect upon, and construct,

Israel through the image of the fetus. Should we not, then, incorporate these traditions into our scholarly endeavors to reflect upon and reconstruct the rabbis and their constructions of rabbinic Israel?

The understandable anxiety about bringing these narratives—and the visual images they conjure—to light, risking their exposure in our present historical circumstances where public images of embryos and fetuses are most often at the forefront of conservative "pro-life" agendas, should not translate into our continued disregard of these traditions. For the reasons just mentioned above, which provide only the broad strokes of arguments detailed in the preceding pages, rabbinic narratives about fetuses should capture our collective attention. It would be a failure of our imaginations to read rabbinic narratives about fetuses, and the rabbinic fetus, into our contexts and concerns without at first capturing and then magnifying the ways in which the rabbis drew upon the image of the fetus in their project of conceiving Israel.

I began this book with one textual image, or snapshot, of a fetus at rest in its mother's womb. That text goes on to say that, upon birth, that which was open is closed and that which was closed is opened.[35] I have not given birth to the rabbinic fetus, but I have opened up rabbinic narratives about fetuses in order to disclose the cultural work that I see them as doing, only to leave them open for further scrutiny.

Notes

Chapter 1

1. See Margulies's notes and manuscript variants (1993, 314). Unless otherwise indicated, all translations of rabbinic texts are my own. Translations of biblical passages are my own, in consultation with *The New JPS Translation* (Jewish Publication Society, 1985; hereafter cited as NJPS) and *The Holy Scriptures* (Koren Publishers Jerusalem Ltd., 1989; hereafter cited as Koren). Transliterations have followed the "General-Purpose Style" listed in the *SBL Handbook of Style* (Peabody: Hendrickson Publishers, 1999), 28 with some minor alterations.

2. According to *y. Nid.* 3:3(50d), *t. Nid.* 4:10, *b. Nid.* 25a, and a preceding tradition in *Lev. Rab.* 14:8, the fetus's mouth is stretched like a hair. See Lieberman's *Tosefet Rishonim* (1964, 267), and Margulies's notes in *Leviticus Rabbah* (1993, 313).

3. Cf. *b. Nid.* 30b.

4. I engage with feminist scholarship on fetal imaging below.

5. In the *Bavli*, the same question, "to what does the fetus resemble in its mother's womb" yields two different answers: a folded writing tablet (*b. Nid.* 30b) and a nut floating in a bowl (*b. Nid.* 31a).

6. Fetuses singing at Sinai appear in the tannaitic *Mekhilta of Rabbi Ishmael* (also cited as MRI); fetuses at Revelation appear explicitly in the medieval compilation *Midrash on the Ten Commandments*. See below for the chronological development in rabbinic narratives about fetuses; and see Chapter 2.

7. See Goodblatt 2006, 1–27, for a compelling defense of the term "nation" in ancient Jewish sources. See also Pardes 2000, 1–15.

8. See Morgan 2003.

9. The cultural significance of fetuses varies widely. See, e.g., Morgan 1997; LaFleur 1994; and Hardacre 1997. I discuss contemporary feminist analyses of the fetus and fetal imaging techniques below.

10. See Gen. 32:29 and 35:10. See Fishbane 1985, 377–78.

11. *Gen. Rab.* 63:6–8. See Chapter 3.

12. See, e.g., G. D. Cohen 1991; Yuval 2006, 3–20; S. Stern 1994, 18–21; and Boyarin 1999, 1–6.

13. Although it has become common to use the term "Jewishness" for late antique sources, I use "Israelness" here because I find it more accurate for rabbinic literature. Instead of discussing the ways that the rabbinic sources construct Jewishness, I have preferred to highlight how the rabbis constructed and saw themselves as Israel. See the Epilogue for more discussion.

14. See Addelson 1999.

15. Jon Levenson, writing about biblical traditions, points out, "Indeed, Israel exists only because of God's choice, and apart from God, it has no existence at all" (1996, 152–53).

16. Herr 1972; Fonrobert 2001; and Kalmin 2003. See also Schäfer 1990.

17. Porton 1988 and 1994.

18. Boyarin 2004.

19. Berkowitz 2006. See also Hayes 1998 and Gray 2003.

20. Boyarin (2004) deftly makes heresy central to the early rabbinic production of Israel, but the heretic in rabbinic texts often occupies the border spaces and even beyond.

21. The rabbinic propensity both to collapse time and to rabbinize certain tropes has been well documented, and rabbinic narratives about the fetus are to be seen in this broader context. However, rabbinic narratives about the fetus not only demonstrate the rabbinic tendency to rabbinize the past but also quite powerfully project a rabbinized Israel into the future.

22. On the word *pinaks*, see Lieberman 1994, reprint. DuBois (1988, 130–66) examines the metaphor of the writing tablet for the woman's body in Greek literature.

23. See G. D. Cohen 1991; Neusner, e.g., 1986a; Boyarin 1999, 1–6; and Yuval 2006, 13–20.

24. *Gen. Rab.* 63:6 applies Jer. 1:5, *Before I formed you in the womb I knew you* to Jacob/Israel, and *Gen. Rab.* 63:7 applies Mal. 1:3, *But Esau I hated,* implying Mal. 1:2, *But Jacob I loved.* Cf. Rom. 9:11–13. See Chapter 3.

25. At least insofar as that other almost always refers to an earthly other. It is possible that God emerges from these texts as the ultimate "Other" with whom—though not against whom—rabbinic Israel constructs itself, but I have not pursued this because I think that a significant point of these traditions is not that God is "Other" but God is "Thou" in a Buberian sense. Similarly, these traditions consistently assert the "sameness" between biblical and rabbinic Israel instead of emphasizing the otherness or distance between them.

26. The answers lie somewhere in between and vary according to context. See, e.g., Boyarin 1990, 11–19; Fraade 1991, 13–15; Hayes 1997, 17–20; and Berkowitz 2002, 743–44.

27. See, e.g., Neusner 1985b and Goldenberg 1994, which minimize the impact of Christianity on rabbinic sources, and see, e.g., Neusner e.g. 1986a–c and 1987a–b and Boyarin 1999 and 2004 for a more maximalist approach.

28. Irad Malkin cautions against reading such bipolarity into ancient constructions of "Greeks and Others" (2001, 12–13); see also S. Stern 1994, 135–38, and below.

29. Neusner 1989, 1.

30. Green 1985, 52. See also Porton 1988.

31. Green 1985, 52.

32. Ibid.

33. Boyarin 1999, 4–5. See *Gen. Rab.* 63:6.

34. Malkin 2001, 12–13.

35. Ibid., 13.

36. S. Stern 1994, 137, emphasis in original.

37. Ibid., 138, emphasis in original.

38. See Hall 1997, 47–51. Hall differentiates between oppositional and aggregative self-definition based on the former being "from without" and the latter being "from within" (1997, 47). Buell applies and expands Hall's formulation, writing, "In Hall's second discursive strategy, the aggregative, ethnicity is established through connections more than by distinctions" (2002, 442). She further writes, "When Christian authors devise or use genealogies to trace their roots to ancestors also claimed by Jews (such as Abraham), aggregative strategies are similarly in play" (2002, 443). Finally, Buell supplements Hall's emphasis on genealogies for aggregative strategies, demonstrating that "Religious practices could also serve as a means of aggregation" (2002, 444). My point is to emphasize that when the rabbis invoke the fetus they use both genealogy and religious practices as ways to trace their roots to their ancestors.

39. That rabbinic narratives about fetuses rend the fetus out of the woman's body such that the fetus, and not the woman, becomes the "sacrum" emblematic of Israel is discussed below. On the fetus as sacrum, see Duden 1993, 108–9, and Haraway 1997, 175.

40. For a discussion of the universal horizon in biblical sources, see Levenson 1996.

41. Chronologically this works in both directions. Earlier traditions that use the fetus to think about Israel inform later sources, and later sources that use the fetus to think about Israel confirm that such a reading is implicit, at least to later rabbinic interpreters, in earlier sources.

42. Lines before, Deut. 32:9 states, *For the Lord's portion is his people, Jacob his own allotment.*

43. *Mekhilta of R. Ishmael* (*Shirata* 8). The passage specifically comments on "fearful in praises" (Exod. 15:11). The passage continues to comment on "doing wonders," where the focus on Israel emerges quite clearly: "*Doing wonders.* It is not written here: 'Who did wonders,' but: 'Who does wonders,' that is, in the future as it is said: *Therefore, behold, the days come, says the Lord, that it shall no more be said: 'As the Lord lives, that brought up the children of Israel out of the land of Egypt.' But, 'As the Lord lives, who brought the people of Israel from the land of the north, and from all the lands where he had driven them'; and I will bring them back to their land that I gave to their fathers* (Jer. 16:14–15)." Translation follows Lauterbach 1933–35, 66, with some minor modifications.

44. Hirshman defines the word *ha'adam* as "a person in the most general and universal terms" (2000, 107). However, the word *'adam* at times functions in a much more particular way; to cite just one example, *m. Pes.* 10:5, "In every generation an *'adam* is obligated to see himself (herself?) as if he went forth from Egypt." I am hard-pressed to see how this statement, and what follows in the Mishnaic passage, does not use *'adam* in the specific sense of Israel.

45. Marc Hirshman has demonstrated that although there might be a universal strain in tannaitic sources that suggest that the Torah is for all the world's people, such a strain is not embraced in amoraic sources: "Rabbinic Judaism eventually moved more and more to a strain of particularism of the sort that may be observed in Akiva's school, banning the Gentile for the study of Torah. In the first centuries,

however, the rabbis were divided, with at least one school vigorously advancing a universalist approach—the path not taken in coming generations" (2000, 115). See also Hirshman 1999; and Goldenberg 1998, 105–8.

46. I am not suggesting that every *sugya* in the *Bavli*, simply by virtue of its being an elaboration of a mishnah, be seen as providing proof of the *Bavli's* sole concern with Israel. However, tractate *Niddah* seems to me to warrant the *presumption* of an underlying focus on Israel due to its specific topic, and therefore, establishing a more universal scope requires evidence that exceeds the use of the word *'adam*. *Bavli Kid.* 30b also records the teaching that "the the three of them are partners in him," but again, taking into consideration its exegetical context, a more specific focus on Israel emerges. The tradition juxtaposes biblical verses that mention honoring one's parents (Exod. 20:12) with honoring God (Prov. 3:9) and fearing one's parents (Lev. 19:3) with fearing God (Deut. 6:13). Although Prov. 3:9 makes no mention of Israel, Exod. 20:12, Deut. 6:13, and Deut. 5:16 (which again mentions honoring one's parents) are explicitly addressed to Israel. Cf. *Sifra Qedoshim* 1:7 (Weiss 1862, 86d); *Mekhilta of R. Ishmael* (*Bahodesh* 8); and *y. Kid.* 1:7 (61b).

47. When I discuss *Leviticus Rabbah.* 14 at length in Chapter 5, I emphasize how far the rabbinic interpretations seem to stray from a plain reading of the verse, specifically in the construction of gender that emerges in the traditions. Here, however, I take seriously *Leviticus Rabbah* 14's framing of these traditions by a verse that is directed to Israel.

48. *Leviticus Rabbah* 14 draws heavily on verses from Job. However, rabbinic traditions are divided as to Job's status as an Israelite or non-Israelite. See Baskin 1983, 8–14. *Lev. Rab.* 31:3 does read the mention of "the work of God's hands" (Job 14:15) as specifically referring to Israel, not humanity.

49. The rabbinic compilation often touted for its universalism is *Seder Eliyahu Rabbah*. Visotzky details *Leviticus Rabbah's* turn away from a focus on the Levitical priesthood to that of the rabbinic agenda and establishes that its program centers not upon polemic but "the doing of charitable works and performance of the commandments, the study of Torah and attendance upon rabbinic leadership" (2003, 76–89, 154–72, quotation from p. 172). Both of these findings support that *Leviticus Rabbah's* overall concern is with Israel in particular. Neusner, though differing from Visotzky insofar as Neusner maintains that *Leviticus Rabbah's* response to fourth-century events, primarily the Christianization of Rome, was in its silence to such events, stresses that *Leviticus Rabbah's* central, salvific message "declared that Israel remained Israel, wholly subject to its own law, entirely in control of its own destiny, fully possessed of its own land," thus also making Israel and its sages the central focus of *Leviticus Rabbah* (1986b, 94ff., quotation from p. 96). *Lev. Rab.* 1:11 strongly supports Hirshman's specific findings vis-à-vis the particularistic scope of Torah in amoraic compilations (2000, 113–15), and *Lev. Rab.* 1:11–13 calls attention to at least a particularistic leaning of the compilation. The praise of converts in *Lev. Rab.* 1:2 is noteworthy, and while such a tradition signals acceptance of others it does not translate into any type of comprehensive universalist stance.

50. See, e.g., Boyarin 1994, 228–60; J. Z. Smith 1996; Levenson 1996, 143–45; R. Schwartz 1997, 33–38, 88; J. Dunn 1999, 57–60; Buell 2002, 466–67, and 2005, e.g., 10–12, 138–65; and Mazusawa 2007.

51. Levinson 2000a, 345–48. Porton also connects the ethnic construction of Israel with genealogy and the religious construction with covenant (1994, 1). See also Stern 1994, 80–81, and Hayes 2002, 164ff., 193–98.

52. Levinson 2000a, 344.

53. On the problems of both defining religion and applying it to ancient (or premodern) sources, see, e.g., J. Z. Smith 1982, xi, and 1998, 269, and Asad 1993, 27–54. Daniel Boyarin has persuasively argued against the scholarly consensus that " 'religion' in the sense in which we use the term today is a post-Enlightenment concept and category produced within Protestant Christianity" (2004, 11 and 203ff.). He has demonstrated that fourth-century Christian texts exhibit a "robust notion of 'religion' " that is "something quite close to our modern notion of religion" (Boyarin, forthcoming). He does, however, maintain that "religion" is less applicable to rabbinic sources, specifically the *Bavli*. He writes, "In the finally hegemonic formulation of rabbinic Judaism in the Babylonian Talmud, however, the Rabbis rejected this option" (forthcoming; 2004, 224). I would add that I do not find the term "religion" useful or accurate for Palestinian midrashic sources either. Regarding both definitions and the applicability of the term "ethnicity," coined in the mid-twentieth century, to ancient sources, see, e.g., Brett 1996, 1–22; Hall 1997, 1–33; Malkin 2001, 1–19; Buell 2002, 432–35, and 2005, 13–21; and Lieu 2004, 15–17. It should be noted that these authors ultimately maintain that "ethnicity" can be applied to ancient sources and do so. See also S. J. D. Cohen 1999, 69–106 and 109–39; Porton 1988, 288–93; 1994, 1–3; and 1999, 201–6; and Lapin 1998, 8–28.

54. Levinson writes, "If the Bible and Second Temple literature contain various and conflicting models of identity (covenantal, biological, historical, territorial, tribal), in the period following the destruction of the Second Temple, this profusion was replaced by two dominant paradigms: the genealogical model of the sons of Jacob, and the covenantal model of Israel" (2000a, 344). To the extent that territory is important for ethnic formation, the fetus deterritorializes Israel and makes it even more of a "portable culture." See also Cohen 1999, 134, and Boyarin 1994, 251–59.

55. Levinson 2000a, 345–46, using the specific example of *y. Bik.* 1:4(64a): "It was taught in the name of R. Yehuda, a convert does bring [*bikkurim*] and recite. What is the reason, (because the verse says) '*for I make you the father of a multitude of nations*' (Gen. 17:5), in the past you were the father of Aram [*av-ram*], and from now on you are father to all the nations [*av-hamon*]. R. Joshua ben Levi said, the law is like R. Yehuda."

56. Buell 2005, 163.

57. Levinson describes the God-fearers, literally "Fearers of Heaven," as a non-homogeneous group who "felt a sufficient closeness to the Jewish community to adopt some of its beliefs and/or customs; but they did not convert, nor did they become an integral part of the Jewish community" (2000a, 356).

58. Ibid., 348.

59. Ibid., 351, quoting Arthur Darby Nock. And see Levinson 2000a, 362.

60. Levinson 2000a, 361 and 362.

61. Ibid., 361.

62. Ibid., 365.

63. Levinson's article consistently points out the gendered hierarchy apparent

when the narrative of affiliation is compared and contrasted with the dominant fictions of identity. In the former, the affiliation is through the maternal, transgressive body; in the latter, it is through the pure male body (2000a, 347 and 362–65). I attend to the "disappearance" of the pregnant female body in rabbinic traditions about the fetus below.

64. Even when the fetus in rabbinic narratives breaks the rules, for example in the rabbinic portrayal of prenatal Esau, it does so to articulate the positions, rules, and borders of rabbinic Israel.

65. Levinson 2000a, 365.

66. This emphasis on ethnic constructions of Israel is, of course, readily apparent in scholarship that posits one of the primary differences between early Christianity and ancient Judaism along an ethnic/nonethnic axis (see Buell 2005, 11–12; Buell and Hodge 200, 241–42; and Neusner 1995). Neusner locates this distinction in Paul, or more precisely in the "current interpretation of Paul" (1995, 304). See also Boyarin 1994, 228–60; and Cohen 1999, 134. Buell and Hodge (2004) complicate such a reading of Paul. I focus on rabbinics scholarship that has incorporated the distinction between ethnic and religious constructions of Israel. See, e.g., Porton 1994 and Cohen 1999.

67. Concerning the frequency of God-fearers in rabbinic sources, Levinson writes, "the number of explicit references is no more than a dozen (2000a, 359).

68. See Fraade 1994. See also Himmelfarb 2006, 184.

69. Porton, echoing J. Z. Smith, writes, "the scholarly dichotomy between religious and ethnic Jews is just that, a creation of the modern scholar (1999, 215).

70. Certainly there are obvious contenders and degrees of anxiety that vary according to time and place.

71. Levinson notes that one of the similarities between the genealogical and covenantal fictions of ethnicity is that they maintain that identity is belated. Using a passage from *b. Shab.* 145b–146a as his example, he writes, "Finally, and most surprisingly, it seems to me that both paradigms present identity as belated rather than indigenous. Whether the decisive moment is the revelation at Mt. Sinai or the birth of the twelve tribes, identity is achieved only through a detergent process, by the natural body purging itself of foreign elements. This belatedness, which stresses the acquired nature of identity, would seem to indicate a certain anxiety concerning the inconstancy of identity, which undermines the very distinctions these texts work so hard to construct" (2000a, 348). Rabbinic narratives about the fetus, I think, consistently make the opposite claim. According to the passage on *b. Shab.* 145b–146a, the "original" formation of Israel's identity is belated, but rabbinic narratives about the fetus suggest the very indigenousness of Israelness. The fetus that is always already Israel requires no "detergent," no purging of foreign elements; to the contrary, the rabbinic fetus manifests Israel quite immediately. Rabbinic narratives about the fetus do not remove the anxiety that, as Levinson notes, often lies at the center of concerns about identity—the very projection of covenantal expressions of Israel onto the fetus might arise in response to such anxiety—these narratives simply deal with such anxiety differently, wishing or washing it away.

72. Levinson 2000a, 345.

73. See Anthony Smith 1986, 211, quoted in Malkin 2001, 16.

74. This is consistent with the broader focused study by Kalmin (2003). See Chapter 2.

75. Buell briefly suggests a connection between the antithetical juxtapositions of ethnic/not-ethnic (particular/universal) and practice/belief when she writes, "I suspect that 'practice' often functions as a shorthand for 'ethnic' and 'belief' for 'universal'" (2005, 61).

76. I might be too optimistic about the discrediting of this distinction, which according to Buell remains "troublingly pervasive" (2005, 61).

77. Morgan 2003, 263–64. Morgan notes that "embryo" is again on the rise due to discussions about stem-cell research.

78. Duden 1999, 13.

79. Ibid., 20.

80. Ibid., 19. See also Keller 2000.

81. Keller suggests the seventeenth century as the time when embryos are first granted subjectivity (2000, 324). She writes, "Although the visual depiction of the fetus *at term* is a centuries-old device, the seventeenth century offers for the first time in its theories of embryology the personhood of the *embryo* and even, in one theory, of the generative germ" (2000, 330, emphasis in original). She cites a statement by George Garden, an English embryologist, written in 1691, "It is acknowledged by all, that the *foetus in utero* for some considerable time after conception has no connexion with the womb, that it sits wholly loose to it, and is perfectly a little round egg with the foetus in its midst, which sends forth its umbilical vessels by degrees, and at last lays hold on the uterus" (2000, 340), which conflicts with Duden's claim, based on her research about German physicians, that prior to the end of the eighteenth century, the fetus did not exist.

82. The concept of "fetal development," which Duden considers new at the end of the eighteenth century, was alive and kicking in ancient embryological writings, from Hippocrates and Aristotle to Soranus and Galen, to the rabbis. Rabbinic sources use the words *valad* and *ubar*, both of which I translate as "fetus" when accompanied by the phrase "in its mother's womb," and they use the additional terms *shefir, shefir merukam* and *sandal*. See G. Kessler 2001 for discussion of these terms.

83. See, e.g., *m. Nid.* 3:3, *t. Nid.* 4:10 and 4:12, *y. Nid.* 3:3(50d), and *b. Ber.* 4a, for impurity; see *m. Bek.* 8:1, concerning firstborns. See also *m. Ker.* 1:3 and 1:5 for the hypothetical consideration of whether a woman who miscarries any number of shapes would need to bring an offering to a priest had the Temple still stood. Whether or not such examinations actually took place, the texts still exemplify awareness of the idea of fetal development.

84. *Shefir merukam*, literally, "embroidered or variegated sac." I translate as "articulated fetus," but "a sac containing embroidered (articulated) matter" would be more precise. Cf. Albeck 1952–59 at *m. Nid.* 3:3, where he explains *merukam*: that the shape of the fetus was recognizable in the sac but it was unknown whether the fetus was male or female.

85. Literally, "at the beginning of its creation [it is] like a locust." See below.

86. Cf. Aristotle *History of Animals* 7.3.583b: "In the case of a male embryo

aborted at the fortieth day, if it be placed in cold water it holds together in a sort of membrane, but if it be placed in any other fluid it dissolves and disappears" (Barnes 1984, 914).

87. See *m. Nid.* 3:1–2 and *t. Nid.* 4 for other descriptions of miscarriages, all of which are at least reportedly in a matter-of-fact manner.

88. See Psalm 139 and Job 10.

89. *Gen. Rab.* 14:5 and *Lev. Rab.* 14:9. The Hebrew Bible, however, has no distinct word for fetus but uses the phrase "fruit of the womb."

90. *T. Nid.* 4:10; *y. Nid.* 3:3(50d); *Lev. Rab.* 14:8; *b. Nid.* 25a.

91. Parallels in *t. Nid.* 4:10, *y. Nid.* 3:3(50d), and *b. Nid.* 25a cite this description in the context of a discussion about the *shefir merukam,* not the form of the fetus. Interestingly, the rabbis reasoned from miscarried embryos long before Lennart Nilsson's photographic images of miscarriages were used to illustrate "life before birth." On Nilsson's photographs, see, e.g., Petchesky 1987; Berlant 1997; Newman 1996; and Michaels 1999.

92. Exod. 21:22, *When two men scuffle and deal a blow to a pregnant woman, so that her children abort-forth.* I have reproduced the translation by Everett Fox (1995) because other translations consistently render the passage as "so that her fruit depart." Although the phrase *p'ri ha-beten* is used in other places in the Bible, it is not used here. See, e.g., Gen. 30:2 and Deut. 7:13, 28:4, and 28:18.

93. Both words are used in reference to human and animal fetuses.

94. See, e.g., *m. Kid.* 3:12. In *m. Nid.* 3:3, 3:6, and 3:7, I think *valad,* though variously rendered as "child" or "valid birth," might appropriately be rendered as "fetus." In the Bible, however, in the one place it occurs, *valad* indicates "child" or "offspring" (Gen. 11:30). Cf. *Gen. Rab.* 82:7, which seems to have an alternate reading of 2 Sam. 6:23.

95. See Needham 1934, 77, for a schematic, albeit unsupported by the sources as a whole, that suggests such a reading.

96. See Morgan 1999, 59 n. 13. See also Michaels 1999, 114: "I should note from the outset that the term 'fetus' is radically ambiguous and has come to signify, outside of embryology, whatever is 'in there' from the proverbial moment of conception onward."

97. *Song of Songs Rabbah* 1:40 (on Song of Songs 1:6) uses the word for son, *ben,* but this is the exception that I have found in amoraic compilations. Medieval compilations do use the word *tinok,* along with *valad* and *ubar,* in reference to children in their mothers' wombs. See, e.g., *Midrash Psalms* on Ps. 8:4 and *Midrash Tanhuma* (Buber), *Tazria'* 1 and 4.

98. See Schiff 2002, 27. This is not to claim that the fetus has no "rights" in rabbinic sources, which again runs counter to Duden's bold assertion cited above, but it clearly does not have the status of a child.

99. See, e.g., *y. Sot.* 5:6(20c) for children singing at the sea; see, e.g., *Mekhilta of Rabbi Simeon* (hereafter cited as *MRS*) on Exod. 19:18, *Song of Songs Rab.* 1:4(1), *Midrash Mishle* 6, and *Exod. Rab.* 5:9 for children at Revelation.

100. See Duden 1993, 7.

101. Morgan 2003, 261.

102. Ibid., 262.

103. Though perhaps the presence of tails accounts for the description of some miscarriages as beasts, wild animals, and birds (e.g., *m. Nid.* 3:2; *m. Bek.* 8:1; and *m. Ker.* 1:3).

104. Morgan 2003, 289.

105. Ibid., 162. See also Addelson 1999.

106. This seems to point to a difference between rabbinic and some early Christian and patristic sources, which might call into question the extent to which these sources were actually engaged with each other.

107. Morgan 1999, 46.

108. Keller points out that embryology "needs to be read symptomatically, that its rhetoric is necessarily a register of the culture in which it functions" (2000, 343).

109. Morgan 1999, 46.

110. Beginning in the medieval period, rabbinic sources have been scrutinized for their insights into concerns about abortion. Nevertheless, elective abortion is not mentioned in the sources. For detailed analyses of abortion in Judaism, see Jakobovits 1959 and 1979; Feldman 1995; Aptowitzer 1924; Schiff 2002; and the numerous citations and bibliographies included in these works.

111. See, e.g., Rothman 1986; Petchesky 1987; Berlant 1997; Newman 1996; Hartouni 1997; Haraway 1997; Duden 1993 and 1999; and Michaels 1999.

112. Newman 1996. See also Duden 1999 and Morgan 1999 and 2003, discussed above. Duden's article is, in part, a critique of Newman's project, since Duden would trace the beginnings of the free-floating fetus only to the beginning of the nineteenth century.

113. Newman 1996, 25–26. The word of Duden that is implicated by Newman is her 1993 book *Disembodying Women*. Duden's 1999 article comes after Newman, in part in response to her critique.

114. Newman 1996, 27 and 33.

115. Latour 1986, 3.

116. Ibid.

117. Whether or not the *beit midrash* was actually the place where rabbinic interpretations were made, the *beit midrash* became a symbol for rabbinic interpretations that was projected back to biblical times by the rabbis imagining the *beit midrash* of Shem and Eber. See, e.g., Rubenstein 2007 and Hezser 1997 on rabbinic social structure and institutional settings.

118. See Fonrobert 2001 and Baker 2002.

119. It will become clear that the fetus is not exactly autonomous but dependent on God instead of its biological mother. And, as mentioned above, the fetus is not autonomous insofar as it serves as a figure for rabbinic ventriloquism.

120. This tradition simultaneously asserts women's presence at Sinai and absents them since they are there in order to highlight the future Israelites. For another rabbinic text that clearly attests to women's presence at Sinai, see *Exod. Rab.* 28:2.

121. Rhetorically, in the language of the texts, the woman is present insofar as most often the phrase used reads "the fetus [*valad* or *ubar*] in its mother's womb," but she consistently fades into the background while the fetus is foregrounded.

122. Petchesky 1987, 268.

123. Although biblical and early Christian sources are invoked in the context

of fetal rights, rabbinic traditions are too unknown and/or marginalized to themselves have any direct impact in such contemporary debates.

124. Although some ancient Greek theories about generation promote a notion of female seed, Dean-Jones points out that such an idea "did not in any way amount to saying that women were equal to men (note their description of female seed as weak seed); it was merely the most obvious way of explaining the undeniable resemblance many children bore to their mothers" (Dean-Jones 1994, 178). The relationship between rabbinic and Greco-Roman embryology is discussed at length in Chapters 4 and 5.

125. Petchesky 1987, 268.

126. Stormer 2000, 124. I focus less on the space of the womb than Stormer does because I think it is too backgrounded and even erased in the rabbinic traditions upon which I focus to consider in depth how the rabbis are locating the very beginnings of Israel in the womb and not through the fetus. Keller, writing about seventeenth-century embryological images points out that "although some of the images suggested her [the pregnant woman's] existence, they almost uniformly denied her *presence*" (2000, 328). It should be noted here that at least according to the grammar of biblical sources, where it is most commonly written that a woman "becomes pregnant and gives birth" (*vatahar vateled*), activity, rather than passivity, is ascribed to women.

127. This has been most explicitly documented by Emily Martin (1991). See also Delaney 1986. And for examples in seventeenth-century embryology, see Keller 2000, 339–43.

128. Delaney 1986, 503; 1991; and 1998b, 30.

129. At the same time, it is quite probable that the rabbinic discourse, and concern, about embryology, largely absent in biblical sources, contributes to the creation of rabbinic narratives about fetuses.

130. Lieberman 1994.

131. See *Midrash Tanhuma Pekudei* 3 for an explicit statement to this affect. However, the connection between Creation and (pro)creation is evident in earlier sources as well.

132. Keller 2000, 324.

133. Men's roles as the sole creators of the embryo are also displaced by God. See Chapter 5.

134. See *Gen. Rab.* 72:6, *y. Ber.* 9:5(14a), and *b. Ber.* 60a.

135. Since I have not found the word *ubar* used for anything but what I consider to be a fetus, I do not know why the word is also always followed by the phrase "in its mother's womb," but I think it signals the hyperbolic inclusion of fetuses. In narratives it most often appears in statements that assert that *even fetuses* do or know something.

136. In most cases, I assign the date of a tradition to the approximate redactonal date of the compilation in which it appears. For example, a tradition in *Genesis Rabbah*, even if attributed to a tanna, is treated as a fifth-century source provided no parallels are found in tannaitic compilations.

137. Halakhic sources are beyond the scope of this study.

138. Ellen Aitken has noted the paucity of sources about Jesus in utero, especially when compared with foundational figures in other religious traditions. She writes, "Jesus *in utero,* however, appears not to have attracted the imaginative or midrashic activity of early Christian storytellers and authors" (Aitken, forthcoming). Aitken's article focuses on Christian traditions from the first and second centuries CE. Interestingly, rabbinic traditions do not elaborate about Moses as a fetus, preferring to hook their prenatal musings onto Jacob/Israel, where scripture (Gen. 25:22) invites such expansions—and then only in the third century at the earliest. On Moses, see Sasson 2007.

139. Aitken writes, "A full exploration of how the unborn is imagined in Christianity as a whole would require an extensive collaborative project, examining many different historical periods and the multifold traditions of the eastern and western churches, as well as the spread of Christianity worldwide in recent centuries. Such a project would also take into account not only a wide range of written and oral texts, but also art and architecture. Prayer and other ritual practices related to pregnancy and childbirth would provide further material for analysis. Such research into the workings of Christian imagination would give considerable insight into lived religion and its conceptualizations, as well as into the interrelation between scriptural tradition, theological reasoning, and religious practice, but to our knowledge, no such study exists" (forthcoming).

140. *Gen. Rab.* 1:1. See Visotzky 1991, 212–24.

141. Morgan 2003, 289.

Chapter 2

1. *B. Sot.* 41b and *b. Sanh.* 91a–b. The Hebrew word used is *le'om* from Gen. 25:23. The word is used quite sparingly in the *Bavli;* in addition to the texts cited, it also appears only at *b. Avod. Zar.* 2b. I translate as "nation" and not "people," as is common in translations of Gen. 25:23, because I think in this instance "nation" is clearer. Furthermore, I think there is an implicit connection between *le'om* and *ha'umot* or *umot ha'olam,* often rendered as "nations" and "nations of the world." However, the only explicit connection between "the nations of the world" and *le'umim* (Isa. 60:2) that I have found in rabbinic literature appears in *Mid. Tanhuma* (Buber), *Tetsaveh* 5. I thank Professor Visotzky for this reference.

2. For a disagreement on the relevance of the covenant in tannaitic rabbinic literature, see Neusner 1980 and Sanders 1980. See also Segal 1985. For a comparison of the concept of covenant in rabbinic and Qumran writings, see Schiffman 2003. For my purposes here, I use the word "covenant" to signify the relationship between God and Israel begun at the Exodus from Egypt and Revelation at Sinai, and I am in agreement with Sanders about its importance for rabbinic Judaism.

3. Preuss 1978, 384.

4. *MRI, Shirata* 1; *MRS* (Epstein and Melamed n.d., 73–74; the text is not found in D. Hoffmann 1905); *t. Sot.* 6:4; *y. Sot.* 5:6(20c); *b. Sot.* 30b; *Mid. Tanhuma,*

b'Shalakh 11; *Mid. Psalms* 8:5 and 68:14. Cf. *b. Ber.* 50a and *b. Ket.* 7b for partial parallels that only record R. Meir's statement at the end of this text. *MRS*, in contrast to all other versions, does not record R. Meir's statement.

5. *MRI* (Horovitz and Rabin, 1970, 120–21; Lauterbach 1933–35, 2:11–12). This is the most elaborate version of the tradition in tannaitic and amoraic sources. It records a debate between R. Yosi the Galilean and R. Yehudah haNasi (Rabbi) about whether the Hebrew word *'olalim* refers to fetuses or to children. This debate is not preserved in the *Tosefta*, *Yerushalmi*, or *Bavli* versions, but it resurfaces in medieval versions in *Midrash Tanhuma* and *Midrash Psalms*. See Aptowitzer 1924 for a reading of this tradition in the context of rabbinic views about abortion.

6. Translated according to its midrashic interpretation.

7. Here *mimakor* is midrashically understood as "from the womb, or source." Cf. *t. Shab.* 9:14; *Sifra Tazria'* 3:6; *Lev. Rab.* 14:9; and *b. Nid.* 17b, 18a, 22a, 41b.

8. I have cut out the interpretation attributed to Rabbi that appears between those attributed to R. Yosi the Galilean and R. Meir. Rabbi maintains that *olalim* refers not to fetuses, but to "babes that are out in the streets" as in Jer. 9:20.

9. Aptowitzer (1924, 71 n. 60) suggests that the text should read R. Yosi, not R. Yosi the Galilean.

10. According to the *Bavli* (*Sot.* 30b), the fetuses see the Shekhinah after God turns their mothers' bellies into glass.

11. Quoted from *Midrash on the Ten Commandments* (Jellinek 1967, 1:68–9). Cf. *Midrash Psalms* to Ps. 8:3.

12. Later versions of the tradition about the fetuses singing at the sea also maintain that the women's bellies were turned into glass. Cf. *b. Sot.* 30b–31a and *Mid.Psalms* to Ps. 8:5. However, this tradition is the first to imagine a dialogue between God and the fetuses.

13. For rabbinic texts about women at Revelation, see *Exod. Rab.* 28:6 and *Pirkei Rabbi Eliezer* 40.

14. I follow the textual emphasis, which centers on fetuses, not the women's wombs.

15. Exod. 19:17: *And Moses brought forth the people out of the camp to meet with God.*

16. Hoffmann 1905, 100. Cf. Epstein and Melamed n.d., 143. Epstein is not certain that this text is original to *MRS*. The version printed in Epstein's *MRS* and the one in *Midrash HaGadol* (19:18), are longer than that of Hoffmann's. In that version, the Israelites offer their ancestors as guarantors after the heaven and earth have been rejected but before their children are offered. Cf. *Song of Songs Rab.* 1:4; *Midrash Mishle* 6; *Mid. Tanhuma*, *Vayegesh* 2. See Visotzky 1990, 41–42, for additional parallels. Even if this tradition is not original to the tannaitic *MRS*, its parallel in *Song of Songs Rabbah* suggests that it is at least an amoraic tradition, attributed to the tanna R. Meir.

17. *Song of Songs Rab.* 1:4 also cites Ps. 29:11, *And God gives strength [Torah] to his people.*

18. *Mid. Psalms* to Ps. 8:4 and 8:5.

19. Cf. *MRI*, *Shirata* 3. See Goldin 1990, 17 and 111.

20. The presumption of the fetus's maleness is discussed below.

21. Cf. *b. Ber.* 10a and *Mid. Psalms* to Ps. 103:3 where a similar tradition is applied to David. The word *k'ravai* suggests while inside his mother, as in Gen. 25:22, *And the sons struggled within her* [*b'kirbah*]. I have filled in "this is said," following Margulies (1993, ad loc.) and the *Bavli* parallel. *Lev. Rab.* 4:7 continues to mention the next four worlds that one sees. See also *Mid. Psalms* to Ps. 18:26.

22. I do not mean to equate the womb and the pit, however, *Lev. Rab.* 14:2, cited below, likens the womb to a prison and other traditions juxtapose the womb with the grave (e.g., *Qoh. Rab.* 3:2 and 5:11, *b. Ber.* 15b; *b. Sanh.* 92a), based on Prov. 30:15–16. Prov. 30:16 specifically mentions the "barren womb," but in the rabbinic interpretations, the womb is not barren. In contrast to these images, *b. Nid.* 30b maintains that no time is happier than that spent in the womb.

23. Paul's interpretation of the crossing of the sea as baptism in 1 Cor. 10 will be briefly discussed later in this chapter.

24. Pardes 2000, 27–28. In later chapters, I discuss how the rabbis imagine Creation as continuous, through God's roles in procreation. The rabbis do not explicitly equate the crossing of the sea with birth; however, by placing the fetuses there, as well as at Revelation, they imply that these events signal the "birth" of Israel.

25. R. Simlai is a second-generation amora who was born in Babylonia but taught in Israel.

26. The Hebrew states, "And they teach him/it ['*oto*, sing. masc.] all the Torah in its entirety." It is unclear, at this point, who precisely teaches the fetus Torah as the text simply states "they." I discuss the gender of the fetus below.

27. The *Bavli* (*Nid.* 30b) previously applied Job 29:3, *When his candle shone upon my head*, to the fetus. Cf. *Lev. Rab.* 14:2 and 31:8.

28. Solomon is referred to as a prophet at *b. Sot.* 48b and Job at *b. Bab. Bat.* 15b.

29. Alternatively, or additionally, the concern might be that neither Prov. 4:4 nor Job 29:2–4 explicitly refers, in their biblical contexts, to fetuses or the womb.

30. Rashi (*b. Nid.* 30b) points out that Job 29:2–3 was applied to the fetus earlier in the passage. Cf. *Mid. Tanhuma*, *Tazria'* 1. Job 10:10–12 is used to describe the formation of the embryo in *Gen. Rab.* 14:5 and *Lev. Rab.* 14:9, and it is applied to the fetus in *t. Nid.* 4:10 and *b. Nid.* 25a.

31. *Mid. Tanhuma* (Buber), *Tazria'* 2; cf. *Mid. Tanhuma*, *Tazria'* 1. This midrash interprets Lev. 12:2 in light of Ps. 139:5, midrashically understood as *You have created me after and before*. The text offers multiple interpretations of "after" and "before." In this section, the text imagines '*adam* saying, "*After* the Holy Blessed One created the beasts and living things, God created me?" Thus the text tries to understand why God created '*adam* after the beasts and other living creatures. The answer offered is that, presumably, God was busy commanding '*adam*, and so too all fetuses, the laws concerning which living creatures were permitted to be eaten and which were not permitted, or were unclean. Furthermore, God instructs '*adam* and every fetus all the mitzvot in the Torah, and, after that, they are born. Why Lev. 12:2 proves this lesson remains somewhat unclear. Perhaps this tradition is not directly connected to Lev. 12:2, and it is stated here because the rabbis are interpreting Ps. 139:5 with its mention of "after and before." Perhaps Lev. 12:2 is being interpreted as, "When a woman conceives and [after] gives birth to a male." I have referred to

the fetus as "he" because this tradition specifically comments on Lev. 12:2, which is concerned with the birth of a male child. The presumed maleness of the fetus in this and the previous *Bavli* tradition is discussed below.

32. See Urbach 1987, 246–48, for discussion about platonic elements of this tradition.

33. This mishnah literally states, "In every generation a man [*'adam*] is obligated to see himself as if he went forth from Egypt." Implicit in this statement is that the person is an Israel. Most likely the term *'adam* includes both men and women. See Goldin 1990 on the importance of the Exodus and the song at the sea for the tannaim. And cf. *MRI*, *Shirata* 3, discussed below.

34. See Goldin 1990, 123.

35. *Mid. Tanhuma* (Buber), *Yitro* 7. Although this tradition is attributed to the tanna Ben Zoma, I have not found it in earlier rabbinic compilations. However, cf. *Song of Songs Rabbah* 2, which interprets the mention of "this day" in Deut. 27:9 similarly. Hirshman (1996, 76–77) considers the tradition from *Song of Songs Rabbah*, attributed to R. Eliezer b. Jacob, tannaitic.

36. It seems implicit that the souls referred to are, or will become, part of Israel.

37. *Mid. Tanhuma*, *Pekudei* 3. The text continues, "*Who does great things past finding out* (Job 9:10)? These are the great things that the Holy Blessed One does in the creation of the embryo." Cf. *b. Shev.* 39a; *Exod. Rab.* 28:6; *Mid. Tanhuma*, *Nitsavim* 3 and *Mid. Tanhuma* (Buber), *Nitsavim* 8. In its biblical context, Deuteronomy 29 addresses the Israelites as they are about to enter the land of Israel. Rabbinic traditions interpret this verse to refer to Revelation at Sinai. See, e.g., *b. Shev.* 39a; *Exod. Rab.* 28:6; *Mid. Tanhuma*, *Yitro* 11; *Pirkei Rabbi Eliezer* 40. I discuss the time at which ensoulment occurs in the latter part of this book.

38. Note that *Mid. Tanhuma* (*Pekudei* 3) also locates all souls at creation. Cf. *b. Sanh.* 91b.

39. Herr 1972; Fonrobert 2001; Kalmin 2003. Herr provides a list of twenty-one prohibited practices (1972, 94ff.). Kalmin enumerates the prohibited mitzvot differently, examining the differences between the motif in Palestinian compilations and the *Bavli*. He notes the lack of prohibition on Torah study in Palestinian compilations, and its relatively frequent mention in the *Bavli* (2003, 40–41 and 47). His findings are echoed here, where it is only *Bavli* and post-*Bavli* traditions that explicitly claim that the fetus receives/studies Torah. On the particular esteem of Torah study in the *Bavli* as a specifically *stammaitic* contribution, see Rubenstein 2003, 31–38.

40. Fonrobert 2001, 398–99.

41. Ibid., 399. Kalmin writes, "What the rabbis describe as having been prohibited by the Romans, and/or as having been difficult or impossible to fulfill during 'the time of danger,' is for the most part what these rabbis viewed as most precious about Judaism" (2003, 22).

42. Herr 1972, 102.

43. There is, of course, notable overlap between that which is essential to rabbinic Israel evident in traditions about foreign prohibitions and about the fetus. See Herr 1972, 94ff.

44. Herr correctly notes that "it was extremely difficult to enforce full com-

pliance with these persecuting decrees in practice" (1972, 102). Although it seems reasonable to assert that it is harder to prohibit specific beliefs than practices, I am not suggesting that beliefs cannot be changed, nor that external practices can be easily kept in check. Certainly beliefs may be changed if a dominant culture exercises enough power. The difference is one of degree, allowing for many different variables, one of which would be the amount of time of any period of persecution. Still, contemporary postcolonial theory makes good use of the apparent tenacity of some aspects of minority cultures, problematizing any hard and fast divide between minority and majority cultures themselves. In a later chapter on rabbinic embryology, I suggest that such tenacity is exhibited when the rabbis bring together biblical sources and Greco-Roman embryological theories, ultimately producing a unique blend.

45. In the following chapter I discuss traditions that project Jewish practices onto prenatal Jacob.

46. Kalmin 1999 and 2003. On the particular esteem of Torah study in the *Bavli* as a specifically *stammaitic* contribution, see Rubenstein 2003, 31–38.

47. Kalmin 2003, 49.

48. Ibid.

49. See Chapter 3.

50. The distinction between the rabbinization of the fetus in the *Bavli* and other compilations is one of degree. For example, in *Genesis Rabbah* 63 Jacob is indeed reconceived as an ideal embodiment of rabbinic Israel, but he is not made into a rabbi. The projection of rabbinic practices, along with the projection of the Exodus and Revelation, onto the fetus is also part of the construction of rabbinic Israel that is being articulated in these sources.

51. Although this statement is attributed to a Palestinian sage, I have not found it paralleled in other compilations. Directly preceding the passage cited above, the *Bavli* states, "Rav Judah said in Rav's name: Whoever withholds a halakhah from a student, it is as if he had robbed him from his ancestors' heritage, as it is written, *Moses commanded us Torah, even the inheritance of the congregation of Jacob* (Deut. 33:4). It is an inheritance for all Israel from the six days of creation." If this tradition is connected to the one that follows about fetuses, then fetuses are included in the "congregation of Jacob." While the first part of the passage includes all Israel in the inheritance of Torah, the second part, with its concern over the transmission of halakhah to a student directs attention away from all Israel and to the rabbis and their disciples. Cf. *b. Sot.* 41b, where embryos curse those given to excessive flattery. The context of this tradition is not about the transmission of halakhah, but of etiquette. Both *b. Sot.* 41b and *b. Sanh.* 91b invoke Gen. 25:23 as proof texts for the fetuses' cursing.

52. See Kalmin 1999. See also Rubenstein 2003.

53. Part of the motivation for limiting the Psalm singing to David in the womb is the attribution of Psalms to David. But *b. Ber.* 4a reconceives David himself as a rabbi, making halakhic decisions and worrying about their correctness and this tradition about David singing psalms in the womb is part of an interpretation of Prov. 31:26, *She opens her mouth with wisdom and the torah of loving kindness is on her tongue,* which the text applies to David. Thus David not only sings psalms, but

he has wisdom and torah in his mouth. Recall that according to the *Bavli*, David is born circumcised (*b. Sot.* 10b). Still, why David is the *Bavli's* chosen figure for fetal narratives remains hard to determine, especially in light of Kalmin's claim that Babylonian traditions are more critical of David than Palestinian traditions are (1999, 83–93).

54. *B. Yom.* 82b.

55. For much of this discussion I confine myself to a small sample of Origen's interpretations for reasons delineated in Chapter 3.

56. Hirshman (1996, 67–81) stresses the orality of Origen's homilies, as opposed to the by and large literary form of rabbinic interpretations.

57. Origen *Hom. Exod.* 8 (Heine 1982, 316). Origen's focus remains, at most, on the Ten Commandments. His comments in this homily extend only to Exod. 20:1–6, and my main focus is on his remarks here on the Exodus. Rabbinic traditions would consider all mitzvot as revealed at Sinai (see, e.g., *Sifre Deut.* 1).

58. Hirshman 1996, 73.

59. *Hom. Exod.* 8 (Heine 1982, 320). For examination of Paul's categories of "flesh" and "spirit," see Boyarin 1994.

60. See also *Hom. Exod.* 6, "And therefore, if you cross the Red Sea, if you see the Egyptians drowned and Pharao destroyed and cast headlong into the depth of the abyss, you can sing a hymn to God; you can utter a sound of praise and say, 'Let us sing to the Lord, for he has been glorified magnificently; he cast forth horse and rider into the sea [Exod. 15:1]" (Heine 1982, 285). Origen teaches that the song at the sea continues to be sung as people continue to praise God.

61. *Hom. Exod.* 5 (Heine 1982, 276). See Hirshman 1996, 69ff.

62. *Hom. Ex.* 5 (Heine 1982, 283).

63. See Goldin 1990, 21–30.

64. See Chapter 4.

65. The claim to Revelation also appears in Origen's homily, cited above, but this is specifically confined to the ongoing relevance of the beginning of the Decalogue.

66. See Ruether 1991, 184ff.; Simon 1986; and Langston 2006, 189.

67. In the post-*Bavli* traditions, the texts would work against both Christian and Muslim supersessionist claims.

68. Cf. *Mid. Psalms* to Ps. 8:4. Contrast *Midrash Mishle*, redacted in the eighth century, which maintains "our children."

69. For circumcision as a prerequisite for seeing the divine, see Boyarin 1992 and Wolfson 1987.

70. This text seems to provide a countertext to the *zekhut* (merit) of the fathers pervasive in rabbinic literature. An earlier version in *Song of Songs Rabbah* also rejects Abraham, Isaac, and Jacob as fitting guarantors because of their failings.

71. To pursue this reading would require an extensive foray into Christian notions of original sin and the practice of infant baptism, topics far beyond the scope of the present project. Moreover, one would have to consider the relative lack of direct engagement with original sin in rabbinic sources and whether this changed in medieval Jewish literature. Shaye Cohen's discussion of circumcision in rabbinic

and post-rabbinic materials (2005) might serve as a guide, but again, this is beyond the scope of this book. For original sin in rabbinic sources, see Visotzky forthcoming and the bibliography cited there.

72. Langston 2006, 189, points out that even though Christians believed that the Law was insufficient by itself, when "followed within the context of Christianity, however, it could have positive benefits." He continues, "Origen thus speaks of the Decalogue as being the product of freedom, given to spiritual Israel (i.e., Christians) by Jesus. From this standpoint, the spiritual context (Jesus) took precedence over the physical one (the Israelite exodus from Egypt)."

73. It seems doubtful that any discourse about the fetus purely reflects the fetus in and of itself. See Morgan 2003.

Chapter 3

1. The Bible also dismisses this reconciliation insofar as Edom, who is Esau (e.g., Gen. 25:30 and 36:1), continues to be portrayed as one of Israel's enemies (e.g., Numbers 20; Obadiah 1; Lamentations 4). See Fishbane 1985, 377–78; G. D. Cohen 1991; Neusner, e.g., 1986a–c; Visotzky 2003, 154–60; and Yuval 2006, 3–10.

2. S. Stern 1994, 19. I have qualified Stern's statement in lieu of the important reminder by Bakhos (2007) that Esau is not always symbolic of Rome. See also S. Stern 1994, 18–21. I should stress, however, that in the passages discussed here from *Genesis Rabbah* 63, Esau does represent Rome—both "pagan" and Christian.

3. See, e.g., G. D. Cohen 1991; Ruether 1991; Simon 1986; Neusner 1986a–c and 1987a; Segal 1986; S. Stern 1994; Hirshman 1996; Boyarin 1999; and Yuval 2006. For early Christian sources that do not yet see Jacob as symbolic of "Church"/ "Christians" and Esau as "Synagogue"/ "Jews," including Paul's Epistle to the Romans, see G. Dunn 1998. The point is not that Esau always and everywhere in rabbinic literature signifies (Christian) Rome, as exceptions to the seeming absolute, hostile typology can surely be noted (see Stern 1994, 18–21, for some examples). Similarly, I am not claiming that everywhere the rabbis mention Jacob, the broader collective Israel is intended.

4. Hirshman 1996, 13. Hirshman notes the relative lateness of explicit rabbinic engagement with Christian claims, but suggests that "definitely by the fourth century, if not before, the rabbis were contending with this claim" (1996, 16).

5. For the connections between Jacob and Israel in the Hebrew Bible, see Fishbane 1985, 377–78.

6. See, e.g., Neusner 1986a–c, and 1987a. Bakhos (2007) points out that even in *Genesis Rabbah,* Esau is not always Rome.

7. Reish Lakish's explanation is based on a *notarikon*—a rabbinic hermeneutic that divides a word into two or more words. See Strack and Stemberger 1996, 29–30.

8. Theodor and Albeck 1965, 682. Theodor, in his comments to *Gen. Rab.* 63:6 explains, "That which is forbidden to Israel is permitted to the nations of the world and their laws which are forbidden to them (the nations), are permitted to Israel."

9. This statement makes a pun from *vayitrotsatsu*, interpreting that they each ran (*rats*) to kill each other. The word *ratsats*, meaning "to squeeze or crush," is also being punned here.

10. The twelfth-century midrashic compilation *Lekah Tov* elaborates, stating, "This one permitted the commands of this one. How so? This one (Israel) forbids [work on] shabbat and this one (Rome) forbids [work on] Sunday; this one forbids [the eating of] pork and this one permits it." See Theodor and Albeck 1965, 682, in the comments to *Gen. Rab.* 63:6. *Gen. Rab.* 63:7, discussed below, asserts that Jacob was born circumcised. Perhaps one of the *mitzvot* alluded to here that Israel permits but Rome prohibits is circumcision. Cf. *Ruth Rabbah*, proem 3.

11. Theodor and Albeck 1965, 682. Cf. *Pesikta de Rav Kahana* 3 (Mandelbaum 1962, 39). Translations for Ps. 58:4 vary, demonstrating the problematic rendering of *rekhem* and *beten* into English. Equally problematic is the rendering of *zoro* reflecting either "estrangement" or "defiance" and "oppression," here midrashically rendered as "making fists."

12. In contrast to the previous traditions, this one is unattributed.

13. Here *vayitrotsatsu* is read as related to the word "to run, or hasten." The Hebrew *batei avodah zarah* is also similar to *zoro* from Ps. 58:4.

14. Theodor and Albeck 1965, 682–83. Although current scholarly consensus points to the *beit midrash* as within the purview of the rabbis, more so than the synagogue, this text nevertheless juxtaposes the synagogue and house of study.

15. Jer. 1:5 continues, *and before you came forth out of the womb I sanctified you, and I ordained you a prophet to the nations.*

16. It is possible that the interpretations in *Gen. Rab.* 63:6 once existed independently of those in *Gen. Rab.* 63:7 and 63:8, where the national readings of Jacob and Esau as Israel and Rome are rendered explicit. However, these traditions, once incorporated into *Genesis Rabbah* 63—and they do not exist elsewhere in extant rabbinic compilations—should be read along with those that follow, since the passage as it appears quite consistent and cohesive.

17. See *Tanna debe Eliyyahu Zuta* 19, for Esau's part being this world and Jacob's part being the world to come. See also 4 Ezra 6:7–10, cited in G. D. Cohen 1991, 244.

18. Cf. Justin, *Dialogue*, chap. 134.

19. Because rabbinic traditions that theorize procreation overwhelmingly emphasize the male's activity in relation to the female's passivity in the process of coming into being, I do not see this text as making Rebekah pregnant with Solomon and Hadrian, but Jacob and Esau. Rabbinic theories of procreation are discussed at length in Chapter 5.

20. I am not sure why the text mentions Solomon instead of David.

21. Yuval reads these two interpretations of Gen. 25:23 as indicative of a period, before the official Christianization of Rome, of relative calm between Israel and Rome and even suggests a "strange solidarity" between the two during the third century CE (2006, 11–12; see also G. D. Cohen, 1991, for the similarities between Israel and Rome). I think the overall context of *Gen. Rab.* 63:6–8, and the statement that immediately follows that "those who hate your children," left uncited by Yuval, mitigates against this reading. Both interpretations are unattributed in *Genesis Rabbah*, and thus the safest date of the statements is the early fifth century CE, when

Genesis Rabbah was redacted, *after* the Christianization of the Roman Empire. Previous interpretations of Gen. 25:22 attributed to R. Yohanan and Reish Lakish in *Gen. Rab.* 63:6 could suggest a date for these traditions around the year 300 CE, but again, the more certain dating would be the redaction of *Genesis Rabbah*, especially since these traditions do not appear to exist elsewhere in Palestinian compilations.

22. Theodor comments, "Two nations that hate each other" (Theodor and Albeck 1965, 685).

23. Almost all manuscripts state "children." However, see R. Enoch Zundel b. Joseph of Bialystok in his *Etz Yoseph* and R. Jacob Moses Ashkenazi in his *Yede Moshe* and also Issachar Ber Ashkenazi in his *Matnoth Kehunah*, where all of these exegetes emend the text to "Creator." Theodor rejects this reading (Theodor and Albeck 1965, 685). Cf. *Song of Songs Rabbah* on 1:4 for another tradition that teaches that God hated Esau.

24. Cf. *Song of Songs Rabbah* on 1:4; *Ecclesiastes Rabbah* on 4:3.

25. Cf. Rom. 9:11–13, discussed below.

26. Theodor and Albeck 1965, 685. Jacob is one of a number of biblical figures said to be born circumcised. See S. Stern 1994, 64; G. Kessler 2001; Kalimi 2002; and S. Cohen 2005, 23–24. I return to the end of *Gen. Rab.* 63:7 below.

27. Presumably Esau remains uncircumcised, even after birth. *Ruth Rabbah*, proem 3, interprets *The way of man is crooked and strange* (Prov. 21:8) to refer to Esau: "*Man*, refers to the wicked Esau, as it is said, *And Esau was a man, a cunning hunter* (Gen. 25:27). *And strange [zar]*—because he estranged himself from circumcision and he estranged himself from mitzvot." *B. Sanh.* 59b apparently excludes Esau's descendants from the commandment of circumcision. *Pirkei Rabbi Eliezer*, chap. 29, however, claims that Isaac circumcised Jacob and Esau.

28. See Theodor and Albeck 1965, 686 for manuscript variants.

29. Theodor and Albeck 1965, 686. Cf. *Pesikta de Rav Kahana* 3 (Mandelbaum 1962, 39). According to *b. Nid.* 30b, the fetus must make an oath that it will be righteous. Contrast *b. Nid.* 16b, where God decrees the fate of embryos at (or before) conception—except for whether one will be righteous or wicked. See, e.g., *b. Meg.* 6a and 11a and *b. Sanh.* 39b for more on Esau's wickedness.

30. Parallels to some of the other traditions in *Gen. Rab.* 63:6–8 appear, but the passage as a whole, and the traditions that directly address prenatal Jacob and Esau, are lacking in other sources. (But see the fourteenth-century *Midrash HaGadol*, ad loc.) *Pesikta de Rav Kahana* 3 depicts prenatal Esau as wicked insofar as he wishes to hurt Rebekah while fighting with Jacob, but nothing further about prenatal Jacob is mentioned. Both the *Yerushalmi* and *Bavli*, as well as *Midrash Tanhuma*, which also often shares traditions with *Genesis Rabbah*, lack much in the way of parallels to the traditions about prenatal Jacob and Esau in *Genesis Rabbah* 63. Intertexts, however, exist, and these will be discussed below.

31. Boyarin also notes, in reference to Gen. 25:23, "Quite astonishingly, but understandably, not one of the three major medieval biblical commentators, Rashi, Ibn Ezra, and the Ramban, makes even an attempt to interpret this verse" (1999, 5).

32. Segal writes, "The prophecy about Jacob and Esau, Rebecca's twin children, in Gen. 25:23 was used by both Judaism and Christianity to further their competing

claims to divine favor (e.g., Midrash Rabba ad loc., Romans 9:6–13)," but he does not elaborate upon the texts (1986, 179).

33. Cf. Gal. 4:28–29; Heb. 12:16–17. Prior to Paul's letter, I have only found Hosea 12:4, which is rendered quite differently in the Koren and NJPS translations: *He took his brother by the heel in the womb, and by his strength he had strove with God* (Koren); *In the womb he tried to supplant his brother; grown to manhood, he strove with a divine being* (NJPS).

34. Scholars continue to debate the meanings of this passage, as well as Romans 9–11 as a whole both in its own setting and in patristic writings. Stowers (1994, 285–316) suggests that the supersessionist, traditional Christian reading is not borne out in Paul's letter itself. See also Dunn 1998 and Gager 2000. My interests lie in the third-to-fifth-century patristic interpretations of Romans 9, not its first-century context. On the uses of Romans 9–11 in Origen, John Chrysostom, and Augustine, see Gorday 1983.

35. I will explore possible avenues of transmission below, but at this point I am not in any way suggesting that the traditions in *Genesis Rabbah* serve as background for Paul.

36. See G. D. Cohen 1991, which does not cite *Genesis Rabbah* 63, and Boyarin 1999 and Yuval 2006, each of which briefly discusses only one tradition from *Genesis Rabbah* 63. Boyarin cites a section of *Gen. Rab.* 63:6 and Yuval cites a section of *Gen. Rab.* 63:7. I discuss rabbinic interpretations of the latter part of Gen. 25:23, *and the elder will serve the younger*, below.

37. As noted above, *Pesikta de Rav Kahana* 3 elaborates upon Esau's prenatal wickedness, but Gen. 25:23 is explicitly interpreted to teach only that Rebekah merited bringing forth the twelve tribes. Cf. *Gen. Rab.* 63:6; see Boyarin 1999, 6. Tannaitic compilations do not expound upon prenatal Jacob and Esau, and the one time that Gen. 25:22 (though not 25:23) appears in a tannaitic source, it is about not Jacob and Esau but God's powers to give birth (*Sifre Deut.* 319 on Deut. 32:18). The *Bavli* (Ber. 57b and *Avod. Zar.* 11a) cites Gen. 25:23, but in reference to Antoninus and R. Yehudah haNasi (see Yuval 2006, 11). And the *Bavli* (*Sot.* 41b and *Sanh.* 92a), rather remarkably in the context of this book, uses Gen. 25:23 to teach, "nations [*le'om*] only means fetuses." One could suggest that the relative neglect of rabbinic interpretations of Gen. 25:22–23 stems in part from the lack of a tannaitic compilation on Genesis; alternatively, such neglect could signal that either the rabbis were aware of early Christian interpretations of the verse and did not choose to engage them or that the rabbis remained unaware of such interpretations. See below.

38. I leave discussion of the finer points of this passage, and how it is to be best understood in the context of Paul's writings, to Pauline scholars. Here I only note the shared mention of righteousness in Romans 9 and *Gen. Rab.* 63:6–8.

39. Especially if Paul, in contrast to his later interpreters, does not understand "the elder" as the "Jews." See, e.g., Stowers 1994, 298–304; and G. Dunn 1998, 124–25.

40. I am not suggesting that the rabbis were reading patristic sources. For methodological considerations on the comparison of rabbinic and New Testament, early Christian, and patristic sources, see Visotzky 1995, 3ff. and 61–74, and 2008; and Hirshman 1996. See also Vermes 1982. My focus on the literary evidence of

an exegetical encounter between patristic and rabbinic sources does not preclude a broader cultural exchange between Christian and Jews. Hasan-Rokem 1998 argues compellingly to include such a reality in rabbinics scholarship.

41. G. D. Cohen 1991 and Yuval 2006. See also Simon 1986, 148, 171, and 188; and Boyarin 1999. Both Cohen and Yuval mention that the typology of Jacob and Esau is only implied in Paul and first fully articulated in Irenaeus (G. D. Cohen 1991, 252; Yuval 2006, 14). Cohen writes, "There is not the remotest suggestion in this argument that Paul considered the Jews to be the incarnation of Esau." See also G. Dunn 1998, 138ff. Whether the typology is even implied in Paul, however, is disputed. See Stowers 1994, 285–316; G. Dunn 1998; and Hodge 2007, 102.

42. Though the far majority of sources cited come from Western authors.

43. Yuval 2006, 13–20; G. D. Cohen 1991, 251–55.

44. G. D. Cohen 1991, 253. For Cohen, before the fourth century, such interpretations "bore no particular sting" for the rabbis (ibid.). See G. Dunn 1998 for the nuances among early Christian and patristic authors on Gen. 25:23 prior to, though not later than, Tertullian.

45. Yuval 2006, 18.

46. Ibid., 16–17.

47. See Visotzky 2008. See also Visotzky forthcoming (a), for the difference between a *Zeitgeist* and an "exegetical encounter."

48. On Origen and the Jews, see de Lange 1977; Brooks 1988; Blowers 1988; and Hirshman 1996. And see L. Levine 1975a, 80–85 and 119–24. Urbach (1971) and Kimelman (1980 and 1981, 230) have also written on the relationship between Origen's and rabbinic interpretations of Song of Songs. Gorday points out Origen's importance in the history of Romans interpretation, writing, "Origen is the first to deal seriously with the epistle and to construct self-consciously an alternative both to the Marcionite and Valentian perspectives" (1983, 45). For some difficulties in the transmission and reception of Origen in general, see Gorday 1983, 16–17 and 103–4. Although not pursued here because I cannot place Tertullian in close proximity to the rabbis due to different locales and languages, *De anima* 26 should be noted:

> Consider the wombs of the most sainted women instinct with the life within them, and their babes which not only breathed therein, but were even endowed with prophetic intuition. See how the bowels of Rebecca are disquieted, though her child-bearing is as yet remote, and there is no impulse of (vital) air. Behold, a twin offspring chafes within the mother's womb, although she has no sign as yet of the twofold nation. Possibly we might have regarded as a prodigy the contention of this infant progeny, which struggled before it lived, which had animosity previous to animation, if it had simply disturbed the mother by its restlessness with her. But when her womb opens, and the number of her offspring is seen, and their presaged condition known, we have presented to us a proof not merely of the (separate) souls of the infants, but of their hostile struggles too.

49. Gorday dates *Homilies on Genesis* to 239–42 and 246–47 and his *Commentary* to 243 (1983, 45). Origen already commented (ca. 229–30) on Jacob and Esau in Romans 9 in *On First Principles* 1.7.4, 2.9.5, 2.9.7, and 3.1.20.

50. Translation from Heine 1982, 177. As mentioned in the above note, Origen had already discussed Jacob and Esau via Romans 9 in *On First Principles*.

51. See Hirshman 1996, 67–81.

52. Heine 1982, 179, my emphasis. Later in *Hom. Gen.* 12:4, Origen explains that he does not deal with Romans 9 at length here because he does not want to strive with the "Philistines," presumably those from the schools of Marcion, Valentinus, and Basilides. Cf. *On First Principles* 2.9.5.

53. Heine 1982, 179.

54. E. Kessler points out, "An important study by de Lange suggests that Origen was involved in debates with Jews and, like Chrysostom, addressed congregants on a Sunday when they had been to synagogue the previous day" (2004, 16–17).

55. Gorday writes, "It is not clear just why Origen waited until such a late point in his career to compose a commentary on Romans, or for that matter to deal with any of the Pauline epistles. One may note, however, that the works associated with Origen's Alexandrian period are just those that are most related to the context of gnostic and of Hellenistic Jewish speculation.... By contrast, the works of the Caesarean period relate more clearly to issues of Christian piety and to questions that would arise in the context of debate with a less speculative, more historically minded audience, including the rabbis of Palestinian Judaism" (1983, 47–48).

56. Translation from Scheck 2002, 112.

57. Ibid. Origen uses "sons of God" instead of "of the promise."

58. See *Comm.* 7:18 (Scheck 2002, 120–21), where Origen, perhaps ill at ease about the apparent lack of "free will" in Romans 9, suggests that Jacob's soul had cleansed itself in order to become a vessel of honor, but Esau, made from the same mass, and whose soul was not pure, was made into a vessel of reproach. On Origen's difficulty with the lack of "free will" in Romans, see Trigg 1983, 117: "Most of the passages which seem to deny free will come from the epistles of Paul, and it was with Paul that Origen found it most necessary to struggle." See also Gorday 1983, 77. See below, note 63.

59. *Comm.* 7:19, cited from Scheck 2002, 129, my emphasis. I cannot pursue this passage in depth; I cite it only insofar as it complements the traditions in *Genesis Rabbah* 63, which make Jacob's—and thus Israel's—righteousness inborn.

60. See E. Kessler 2004 on the exegetical encounter. Origen's *Homilies on Genesis* might be more apt to have been known by Jews than his *Commentary,* but in trying to determine whether an *exegetical* encounter occurred, this does not present too much difficulty. Kessler explains, "By the term 'exegetical encounter' I mean that Jewish interpretation either influenced, or was influenced by, a Christian interpretation or vice versa. The term does not imply that Jewish and Christian exegetes met to discuss their interpretations...; rather an exegetical encounter indicates awareness by one exegete of the exegetical tradition of another, revealed in the interpretation" (2004, 1; see also 22–29).

61. The attributions in *Gen. Rab.* 63:6–7 are to third- and fourth-century sages (R. Yohanan and Reish Lakish, 250–90; R. Berekiah and R. Huna, 320–50). However, the compilation as a whole is dated to the early fifth century.

62. To my knowledge, Paul is the first to connect Mal. 1:2–3 with Jacob and Esau while in Rebekah's womb. Philo cites Mal. 1:2–3 in *Biblical Antiquities* 32, applying these verses to Jacob and Esau after their birth. On the uniqueness of *Gen.*

Rab. 63:6–8, see above. Origen's use of Mal. 1:2–3 also appears somewhat unique (cf. *On First Principles* 2.9.5 and 3.1.22). Although evident in Romans 9, mention of this verse is lacking in Justin (*Dialogue* 134) Tertullian (*De anima* 26 and *Adv. Jud.* 1), and Irenaeus (*Adv. haer.* 4). But see Augustine *Enchiridion* 98.

63. Origen had struggled with Paul's apparent disregard of merit in *On First Principles*, written about a decade before his *Homilies on Genesis* and *Commentary*. There he repeatedly explained, or justified, God's election of Jacob over Esau by suggesting that it was the result of older causes in their preexisting souls. See *On First Principles* 1.7.4, 2.9.5, 2.9.7 3.1.22, and 3.3.5. And see Trigg 1983, 115–20, and Gorday 1983, 77. It is perhaps significant, then, that in *Hom. Gen.* 12:1, while paraphrasing Rom. 9:11, Origen glosses, "before the children are born or do anything good or evil *in this world*," and again, in *Comm.* 7:15, he writes, "before the birth occurred, and before the boys had any good or evil *deeds among men.*" In this regard, the rabbis and Origen, with their shared concern about merit, were not as far apart as one would think. However, I think that such a nuanced understanding of Origen on Paul would have been missed by the rabbis, much as Origen might have missed nuances of rabbinic interpretations, which allowed him to thoroughly misunderstand or at least misconstrue the rabbis as literalists. See *Hom. Gen.* 12:4, where Origen does not want to open himself to malicious charges from the "Philistines," who, according to *Hom. Gen.* 13, are, among others, Scribes, Pharisees, and Jews buried under the weight of their own literal interpretations of scripture. On "Jewish literalism," see Clements 2005, 159.

64. This is implied in the text's citation of Mal. 1:3.

65. As noted above (note 63), Origen is also troubled by Paul's apparent disregard of merit. And Paul's disregard of "works" might well have been grafted back onto Paul. Stowers writes concerning related passages in Romans, "After fifteen hundred years of Christian theology, we tend as modern readers to overgeneralize the meanings of 'works' and 'faithfulness' here" (1994, 304). Gorday points out Augustine's influence upon subsequent interpreters that might contribute to this overgeneralization (1983, 15–24).

66. I take seriously Yuval's claim for Pauline priority when it comes to the topic of election, and I am suggesting that *Gen. Rab.* 63:6–8 is—to a certain extent—reacting to Romans 9 *via Origen*. However, since the typological link between Jacob and Israel is already readily apparent in biblical sources, I do not go so far as to entertain the notion that the rabbinic reading of Jacob as rabbinic Israel is completely "reactive and defensive": it is, rather, typical. What is unique in the passages from *Gen. Rab.* 63:6–8 is that the typology of Jacob as rabbinic Israel and Esau as (Christian) Rome is projected onto fetuses.

67. Direct engagement with the phrase *the elder will serve the younger* is lacking in tannaitic and amoraic compilations and appears only once in *Genesis Rabbah*. See also *Mid. Tanhuma* (Buber), *Bereishit* 31. The identification of Esau with Rome and the message that Israel will triumph over Rome in the future appears in earlier sources (Fraade 1991, 38–40 and 201), but Gen. 25:23 is not invoked.

68. Yuval 2006, 16.

69. Boyarin 1999, 4–5.

70. Ibid., 5.

71. I return to Yuval and Boyarin in the following section, when I consider the impact of patristic interpretations on *Genesis Rabbah* 63.

72. *Gen. Rab.* 63:7. Cf. *Sifre Deut.* 41. I have translated in keeping with the language of the verse. Neusner translates, "Said R. Huna, 'If he has merit, he will be served, and if not, he will serve'" (1987a, 108). This translation has the advantage of making clear that the words I render as "will serve" and "will enslave" are from the same word in Hebrew.

73. R. Huna is a fourth-generation Palestinian amora (320–50 CE)—considerably later than Origen.

74. Read in its immediate context, it is clear that the "elder" is presently Rome (Hadrian being mentioned a few lines above), but whether it is pagan Rome or more specifically Christian Rome cannot be determined since both are operating throughout the passage (the former more often and openly than the latter).

75. Theodor (Theodor and Albeck 1965, 692) notes that Siloni is a prominent Palestinian philanthropic family. Cf. *Lev. Rab.* 5:4.

76. Theodor and Albeck 1965, 692. See G. D. Cohen 1991, 244, where Cohen translates from the Apocalypse of Ezra, "From him sprang Jacob and Esau, but Jacob's hand held the heel of Esau from the beginning. The heel of the first age is Esau; the hand of the second is Jacob." Cohen continues, "Latin and Arabic versions of the book render the answer even more pointedly: 'For Esau is the end of this world, and Jacob is the beginning of the one which follows.'" Cf. *Sifre Deut.* 343.

77. The two traditions diverge in that the former also makes Israel's triumph contingent on its merit but the latter might not.

78. Theodor and Albeck 1965, 692.

79. Whether Rome is Christian Rome or pagan Rome is significant insofar as if the former, then *Genesis Rabbah* 63 stands not only in contrast with patristic interpretations but in direct opposition to them. See below.

80. It is here, where the rabbis turn *Jacob* into the elder, that Yuval's suggestion that the rabbis "internalized" the Christian reading becomes even more fascinating. Jacob still remains rabbinic Israel, but he is the "elder," as the Christians say. As exciting a possibility as this might be, especially in light of a postcolonial reading that would emphasize how the subjugated takes on—but alters—the dominant perspective, I do not pursue it here because it assumes that the rabbis are directly engaging with patristic interpretations of Gen. 25:23, having merely deflected them onto Gen. 25:25. For reasons laid out below, I am not convinced, despite some considerable evidence that I have added to the likelihood of an "exegetical encounter" between Origen and *Genesis Rabbah* 63, that the rabbis have Christianity that much on their minds, even here.

81. Boyarin compellingly suggests that one of the interpretations in *Gen. Rab.* 63:6 "effectively erases Esau" by incorporating him into the twelve tribes of Jacob (1999, 4–5). In *Gen. Rab.* 63:8, however, Esau is not incorporated into Israel but at least twice utterly erased from or blotted out of Israel.

82. Theodor and Albeck 1965, 687–88. See Origen *Hom. Gen.* 12:4

83. Another subtext of the interpretations here, which make Jacob the elder, would be Gen. 25:29–34 where Esau ceases to be the firstborn, elder son.

84. R. Halfota is a tanna, but this statement does not appear in tannaitic compilations and is unparalleled in other amoraic sources.

85. See G. D. Cohen 1991, 247, for the similarities between Israel and Rome. And see Yuval 2006, 11–12.

86. Cf. *Sifre Deut.* 31, 312, and 343.

87. Neusner 1986a, 27.

88. Or the very beginning of the fifth century, with the redaction of *Genesis Rabbah* and *Leviticus Rabbah*.

89. Yuval 2006, 23. I have quoted from the English translation of Yuval's book; the original Hebrew rendered more literally reads, "The confrontation with Christianity is the very breath of Midrashic and Talmudic Judaism" (2000, 37).

90. Schwartz 2001, 179.

91. E. Kessler 2004, 182.

92. Bakhos 2007, 260. This quite possibly distorts early Christian and patristic literature as well. My own excessive rhetoric here is meant to match the excessiveness of putting Christianity everywhere and always at the heart of rabbinic "Judaism."

93. See Neusner, e.g., 1987a, 106–13. However, G. D. Cohen argues compellingly for the mutual affinity, the kinship or brotherhood, of Israel and pagan Rome (1991, 247). I had also thought that the demarcation of difference vis-à-vis circumcision—Jacob being born circumcised in contrast to Esau—is better suited for Esau as Christian Rome, and perhaps it is. But pagan Rome was as uncircumcised as Christian.

94. The absence of the verse itself might be read as indicative of the rabbis' knowledge of the verse's usefulness to Christian claims, but previous scholarship has neglected to mention the lack of direct engagement with Gen. 25:23 in rabbinic sources, assuming instead that Christian interpretations were an issue. Boyarin comes closest to noting the lack of direct engagement with the verse, but he mentions this explicitly only in connection with medieval commentators (1999, 4–5).

95. Boyarin 1999, 3. See *y. Ned.* 3:8(38a).

96. *Gen. Rab.* 63:8, Theodor and Albeck 1965, 688–91. Theodor appears to reject connecting the two passages but does not offer a compelling alternative.

97. See Goldenberg 1994 for an argument suggesting the lack of difference Christianity made during the amoraic period. See also Neusner 1985b.

98. Or surfaced in their interpretations of other verses, e.g., Deut. 33:2 in *Sifre Deut.* 343.

99. Yuval suggests they are "reactive and defensive" (2006, 18); Boyarin writes, "it is not certain to me just how and when and where the Rabbis started to read the elder as Christianity. Is it in reaction to Christian readers, a cause of their reactive readings, or perhaps, as I have suggested, only a product of the historical succession of pagan Rome by Christian Rome?" (1999, 125–26).

100. Cf. Hosea 12:4. Kaminsky points out, however, that the contract Esau makes in Gen. 25:29–34 could be construed as under duress, and "would be enforceable neither by the legal standards of later rabbinic Judaism nor by most contemporary legal systems" (2007, 46).

101. What is internalized throughout *Gen. Rab.* 63:6–8 is not "the Christian position," but Israel itself.

102. See Alexander 1992; Boyarin 1999, 1–7; Yuval 2006. And see Neusner, e.g., 1986a.

103. Segal 1986, 179.

104. Boyarin 1999, 5–6, though Boyarin later suggests that such "kinship metaphors need to be abandoned" (8).

105. My point is not, of course, that "Christianity" was not a "proximate other" in these sources, and thus, as J. Z. Smith points out, "is, in fact, most problematic when he is TOO-MUCH-LIKE-US, or when he claims to BE-US" (1985, 47), but I do wish to emphasize that despite their location in Rebekah's womb, prenatal Jacob and Esau are being rhetorically configured as not at all alike.

106. See Neusner, e.g., 1986a and 1987a.

107. It is possible to see the rabbinization of prenatal Jacob, and through him all prenatal Israel, as a response to Christianity, but I have not found enough textual evidence to support this. Therefore, while not ignoring the possible exegetical exchange between rabbinic and patristic interpretations, I have sought to emphasize the link between biblical and rabbinic Israel that is central to these traditions.

Chapter 4

1. S. Schwartz 2001, 162. Boyarin, in turn, would prefer "to abandon language of 'influence' and simply understand that 'Judaism' is itself a species of Hellenism" (2004, 235 n. 73). He counts himself among "many if not most scholars of Judaism [who] currently do not operate with an opposition between Judaism and Hellenism, seeing all of Jewish culture in the Hellenistic period (including the anti-Hellenists) as a Hellenistic culture" (2004, 18). Visotzky (2003, 49 n. 3) suggests that, from a certain perspective, "Rabbinic Judaism is to be considered an hellenistic religion." See also Visotzky 2006. The broad question of the relationship between Palestinian rabbinic sources and Greco-Roman culture has engaged scholars for years. See, for example, Lieberman 1994, Fischel 1977, and Gruen 1998; and see L. Levine 1998, 1–32, for a recent overview and additional bibliography.

2. S. Schwartz 2001, 1.

3. Ps. 139:13–16 and especially Job 10:8–12 are the only examples resembling some sort of data about embryology. However, Psalm 139 is lacking much detail, and seems primarily to attest to the theological claim that God creates, and knows, the fetus. And both verses—at best—only deal with fetal formation, without mentioning any details about when the fetus is formed, how the biological parents contribute to its creation, and pregnancy in general.

4. Fonrobert 2000, 11 and 42.

5. In contrast to the presence of biblical laws pertaining to menstruants, the Torah does not deliberate upon embryology, and therefore, in contrast to rabbinic traditions about menstruation, where biblical precedents must play a primary role, no such explicit biblical constraints are operative on the topic of embryology.

6. S. Schwartz 2001, 1.

7. It is my assumption, here remaining largely unsubstantiated, that such

"uniqueness" is shared by patristic writings about embryology. However, I disagree with Schwartz's blanket statement that "quite a lot of the distinctive Jewish culture was, to be vulgar about it, repackaged Christianity" and his assertion that Jews "*appropriated* much from the Christian society around them" (S. Schwartz 2001, 179). What both rabbinic and patristic sources demonstrate is the simultaneous adaptation, which could be seen as appropriation or accommodation, of Greco-Roman embryology. I see no need here, in the case of embryology, to suggest that the rabbis are repackaging Christian embryology. Needham suggests, "The Patristic writers, who on the whole were careful to base their psychology on the physiology of the ancients, had little to say about the developing embryo. Most of their interest in it was, as would naturally be expected, theological" (1934, 75). Crego (1996, 22) supports this. Nevertheless, it is precisely the theological aspects of embryology about which I am concerned, and there seems to be an opening for further comparative study about patristic and rabbinic embryology as theology—one that examines more completely the ways both Christian and Jewish interpreters of scripture are repackaging both the Bible and Greco-Roman embryology—than I can pursue here.

8. Seth Schwartz points out, "For the rabbis, the world of the Hebrew Bible was at least as real as the world in which they actually lived" (2001, 166).

9. See, e.g., S. Muntner 1977; Kottek 1981; Newmyer 1985 and 1988; and van der Horst 1990. Geller (2000, 13) articulates some methodological problems specifically on the comparison of Greco-Roman sources and the *Bavli*. See Stol 2000a and 2000b for further contextualization and comparison with ancient Near Eastern sources.

10. Greco-Roman embryology is itself a construct that masks the divergence of opinions set forth by various proponents. See, for example, Dean-Jones 1994; Lloyd 1983; and Lonie 1981. Helen King (1998, 21) writes, "Creating an overview of 'Hippocratic gynaecology' is an artifice which always risks falsifying its object.... Of the texts which have come down to us under the name of 'Hippocrates,' possibly none was written by the historical 'Father of Medicine.' Instead, what has become the 'Hippocratic corpus' is a disparate collection in terms of geographical origin, date of composition and, most significantly for this chapter, theoretical position." Much the same can be said for the artifice of the rabbinic corpus or "the rabbis."

11. I do not focus on halakhic traditions in this chapter, but confine myself to citing some of the sources in footnotes. See G. Kessler 2001 for a more in-depth treatment of some halakhic traditions. The relationship between halakhic and aggadic/midrashic traditions is beyond the scope of this chapter.

12. There are divergent opinions about the point at which the embryo is formed, when the fetus first moves, and even on the duration of full-term pregnancy. For example, the Hippocratic treatise *Nutriment* 42 states, "For formation, 35 days; for movement, 70 days; for completion, 210 days.—Others, for form, 45 days, for movement 90 days, for delivery, 270 days.—Others, 50 for form; for the first leap, 100; for completion, 300 days.—For distinction of limbs, 40; for shifting, 80; for detachment, 240 days" (Jones 1995, 1:357). Needham (1934) cites *Regimen* 1:26, which also mentions a great deal of variation in fetal development. Galen, in his "The Construction of the Embryo," writes, "For there is no single time-frame for all embryos, whether for clarity of construction, for motion, or for birth" (cited from

Singer 2001, 177). For a recent overview of varied ancient opinions on ensoulment/ animation, see Kapparis 2002, 32–52. Kapparis also discusses some of the ambiguities surrounding the Greek and Latin terms used to describe the fetus in its mother's womb ranging from embryo, child, to person (2002, 36–39), which are all also ambiguously used in rabbinic traditions. See also Noonan 1965, 89–91, for a brief summary of ancient views on ensoulment. For an important discussion about the soul in ancient philosophy and the difference between such ancient views and contemporary ones, see D. Martin 1995, 7–15. See Feldman 1994, 271–75; and Schiff 2002, 42–44, for a discussion about ensoulment in the context of Judaism and abortion. The complex questions about the nature of the soul, what constitutes human life, and when life begins will not be pursued here.

13. For a general discussion of the soul in rabbinic literature, see Hirsch 1947, 150–207. Hirsch asserts that despite possible differences in the biblical uses of *neshamah, nefesh,* and *ruah,* "the Rabbis employed them synonymously, without distinction" (151). See also Visotzky 1999; Rubin 1988; and Urbach 1987, 214–54. See *Gen. Rab.* 14:9: *"And the Lord God formed 'adam of the dust of the ground, and breathed into his nostrils the breath of life': 'breath of life:* it is called five names: *nefesh, neshamah, hayyah, ruah, yehidah.'"*

14. That ensoulment occurs prior to birth and that the soul is given by God seem accurate for patristic sources as well. See, e.g., Huser 1942; Noonan 1965, 89–91; Connery 1977, 46–58; O'Connell 1987, 118–200; and Kapparis 2002, 32–52. See also G. Kessler 2001, 367–91.

15. Cf. *b. Kid.* 30b for a partial parallel. And see *Sifra Qedoshim* 1:4–7 (Weiss 1862, 86d) for the earliest record of this statement, without the elaboration upon it that appears in amoraic sources. See *b. Nid.* 30b for another mention that the soul is given by God.

16. The *Yerushalmi (Kelayim)* and the *Sifra* state, "and the three of them are partners in him/it." *Ecclesiastes Rabbah* states, "At the time that the embryo is formed/created [*notsar*], in its mother's womb, there are three partners in him." The *Bavli* states, "there are three partners in humans."

17. The *Yerushalmi* version covers all the bases in claiming that God provides the *ruah, nefesh,* and *neshamah.* The *Bavli* and *Ecclesiastes Rabbah* versions claim God provides the *ruah* and *neshamah.*

18. *Ecclesiastes Rabbah* might indicate at conception, but the Hebrew word used, *notsar,* is ambiguous, either referring to creation or formation. See also *b. Ber.* 10a, "He [R. Shimeon b. Pazi] said: Come and see: the rule of the Holy Blessed One is not like the rule among people. A person creates a shape on the side of a wall, but he cannot put in it spirit and soul, insides and intestines. But the Holy Blessed One can create a shape inside a shape and place in it spirit and soul, insides and intestines." See also *Mekhilta of R. Shimeon ben Yohai,* "A person creates a shape and he cannot give it a soul and insides, but the Holy Blessed One creates a person and gives to him a soul and insides (Ps. 103:1)" (Hoffmann 1905, 67). Both traditions, read in their context, assert that the soul is placed in the fetus by God, however no specific time is given. The last tradition might not be original to *Mekhilta of R. Shimeon ben Yohai;* it appears, though in slightly different form, in *Midrash HaGadol.* On the reliability of Hoffmann's text of *Mekhilta of R.*

Shimeon ben Yohai, and on the larger issue of the relationship between *Midrash HaGadol* and *Mekhilta of R. Shimeon ben Yohai*, see Nelson 2006.

19. Preceding this question about the soul, Antoninus asked Rabbi, "When is the evil inclination placed in humans?" In this case, the opinions originally set forth by Rabbi and Antoninus are reversed when compared with the question about the soul. Rabbi originally maintains that the evil inclination is placed in the fetus before birth but later agrees with Antoninus that this occurs at birth. Contrast *Pesikta de Rav Kahana* (Mandelbaum 1962, 460) and *Avot d'Rabbi Natan* 16, which both suggest that the evil inclination exists in utero. For bibliographic references on the Rabbi and Antoninus motif, see S. Cohen 1998, 141–72. See also Meir 1999 and 2006; Hezser 1997, 441–45; Herr 1971, 123–50; Wallach 1941. For the specifically Stoic elements of this encounter, see Kottek 1981, 310; and Newmyer 1988. However, Kapparis (2002, 41–44) notes that the opinion that the soul enters the body at birth, often seen as a sure indication of Stoic beliefs, exists in various ancient sources prior to the Stoics.

20. Cf. *b. Nid.* 31a where salt is used as a metaphor for the soul. Cf. *Gen. Rab.* 17:8, where the analogy of meat needing salt is said in reference to Eve's creation.

21. Hebrew: *mishenifqad*. Literally the word *paqad* means "visit," "remember," "deposit," or "decree." It can also euphemistically mean "to have marital connection with," as in *b. Yev.* 62b. Here it is best understood as "from the time that one is conceived." Cf. Gen. 21:1, *And the Lord visited Sarah as he had said, [and the Lord did to Sarah as he had spoken. For Sarah conceived and bore Abraham a son in his old age]*. Cf. 1 Sam. 2:21. See Feldman 1995, 271 n. 19; and Hirsch 1947, 188 n. 6. Rubenstein reads the use of the root *p.q.d.* as "visitation" following Rashi to *b. Sanh.* 91b, who cites *b. Nid.* 16b (2002, 166 and 287). However, Palestinian midrashic sources, especially in *Genesis Rabbah*, often use the root *p.q.d* to mean conception, and in most cases to indicate that God gives conception. See, e.g., *Sifre Num. Naso* 19 (Horovitz 1992, 23); *Gen. Rab.* 53:6, 56:2, 60:13, 72:6, and 73:1.

22. The specific attribution of this text to Rabbi and Antoninus might limit the exchange as one that occurs between officials, but other rabbinic traditions that less self-consciously display the interchange of ideas on embryology seem to indicate that such shared knowledge occurs for rabbis more generally. Furthermore, to see the text as indicative of the relationship between Rabbi and Antoninus seems to assume that such a conversation did take place. I see this text as more valuable for the insights it offers in terms of a rabbinic methodology on how to deal more broadly with the shared embryological notions in rabbinic and Greco-Roman sources.

23. Aptowitzer (1924, 69 n. 55) states that the text from *b. Sanh.* 91b "constitutes a transmutation of the legend [from *Gen. Rab.* 34:10] and an accommodation to the point of view of the editors of the Babli." Hirsch claims the exact opposite, and he asserts that the *Genesis Rabbah* version "can hardly be correct" (1947, 188 n. 6). I have not found a tradition in Palestinian compilations that explicitly maintains that ensoulment occurs after forty days of gestation. For formation at forty (or forty-one) days, see *m. Nid.* 3:7 and parallels. See also *b. Yev.* 69b and *b. Ber.* 60a, both of which are unparalleled in Palestinian sources. See below.

24. In the *Bavli*, only one proof text is given (Job 10:12), in contrast to *Genesis Rabbah*, where two proof texts are cited.

25. On Greco-Roman and patristic sources, see Noonan 1965; Huser 1942 49ff.; and Kapparis 2002, 48–49. The distinction between a formed and unformed embryo evident in patristic sources stems in part from the Septuagint's rendering of Exod. 21:22–24. Philo also upholds such a distinction (*De specialibus legibus* 3.108–9). See Feldman 1995 and Schiff 2002, 34–36.

26. Both R. Eleazar (ben Pedat) and R. Yohanan are second-generation Palestinian amoraim.

27. The *Bavli* Munich manuscript reads "the soul is given in forty days." The text, read either with the printed version's mention of "formed" or with the manuscript variant as "given," is at odds with the Rabbi and Antoninus text, though the version in the *Bavli* does mention ensoulment at formation as an option. It is possible, even likely, that the two opinions, ensoulment at conception or at formation, can stand in tension. However, it should be noted that *Gen. Rab.* 32:5, in a similar tradition to the one in *b. Men.* 99b, also possibly attributed to R. Yohanan, discusses the formation of the embryo at forty days, not that of the soul. (The attribution to R. Yohanan in *Gen. Rab.* 32:5, however, follows Albeck's emendation.) Furthermore, *Gen. Rab.* 32:5 uses both the Hebrew words *hatsurah* (form) and *nitnah* (given), similar to the words that appear in the different *Bavli* manuscripts. It seems possible that the *Bavli* tradition is either "corrupted" or modified to refer to ensoulment, not fetal formation, at forty days.

28. Alternatively, biblical support for the Torah being given at forty days serves as "proof" that the soul is given in forty days. I pursue a similar possibility below.

29. This text does not cite a specific proof text to support that the Torah was given in forty days, but this would have been obvious.

30. Aristotle maintains that a male embryo is formed at forty days, but a female sometime after ninety days (*History of Animals* 583b). The author of the Hippocratic work *On the Seven Months' Child* also maintains that the male is formed at forty days, but the female later (Kapparis 2002, 45). However, the Hippocratic work *Regimen* 1.26 states, "Some [fetuses] have everything visible in forty days, some in two months, some in three months and others in four" (Jones 1995, 265), without distinguishing between male or female embryos. See *m. Nid.* 3:7, *t. Nid.* 4:17, and *b. Nid.* 30a–b. See Kottek 1981, 305–6; and 1996, 80–85. These sources record a debate between the sages and R. Ishmael about the difference between the time of formation for male and female embryos. Ultimately, however, the rabbinic consensus maintains that formation for male and female embryos is completed at forty-one days. In the *Bavli* version, R. Ishmael supports his view that male embryos are formed at forty-one days and female at eighty-one days based on the differing lengths of a woman's impurity after childbirth (Leviticus 12). Cf. *The Nature of the Child* 18 (Lonie 1981, 9–10), which suggests a correlation between the after birth discharge and the formation of the fetus. The Gemara (*b. Nid.* 30b), however, states, "[The sages] said to [R. Ishmael]: 'Development of a fetus cannot be learned from [the time] of impurity" and they continue to assert that formation occurs at forty-one days, without providing scriptural support. I cannot account for the slight difference between halakhic sources that fix formation at forty-one days and the midrashic sources that attest to formation at forty days.

31. Cf. *Num. Rab.* 9:1 and *Midrash Tanhuma Naso* 4. See also Brown 1988,

20–21. Cf. *Gospel of Philip* trans. W. Isenberg in Robinson 1990, 156: "The children a woman bears resemble the man who loves her. If her husband loves her, then they resemble her husband. If it is an adulterer, then they resemble the adulterer. Frequently, if a woman sleeps with her husband out of necessity, while her heart is with the adulterer with whom she usually has intercourse, the child she will bear is born resembling the adulterer." It should be noted that *Lev. Rab.* 23:12 collapses the distinction between actual adultery and imagined adultery, making the parallels even more closely aligned.

32. I have rendered *tsayyar* as "sculptor," and I imagine the *icon* as a statue, taking advantage of the three-dimensionality of the parable. However, "painter" and "painting" are also accurate.

33. Although the text asserts that formation is completed at forty days, it also makes clear that God can re-form the embryo if God wishes. Stol writes, "Note that the Babylonians held it possible that the features of the foetus could still change during pregnancy; all references from Classical Antiquity only name the sexual act as the decisive moment for maternal imagination" (2000b, 62).

34. Tannaitic sources (see note above) already assert that the embryo is formed at forty-one days, without any scriptural support, which leads me to believe that they have incorporated one of the many options for formation from Greco-Roman culture. One could suggest that the rabbis come to this number by examining miscarried embryos or embryos during gestation, not from absorbing Greco-Roman notions, but such examination is specifically considered unreliable evidence in *t. Nid.* 4:18 and *b. Nid.* 30a–b. But perhaps such evidence is dismissed because R. Ishmael offers it in the name of Cleopatra of Alexandria (!). See Needham 1934, 65–66. And see *y. Nid.* 3:3(50d), *t. Nid.* 4:10, and *b. Nid.* 25a–b, where miscarried embryos are examined. It also seems difficult to imagine that the rabbis would have been able to determine the day of conception with enough precision to know the fortieth or forty-first day of gestation. The *Bavli* voices such uncertainty about reckoning the exact days of pregnancy in an unparalleled *baraita*, which after strongly condemning sexual intercourse during pregnancy on the ninetieth day of gestation asks, "How does one know?" and leaves the protection of the fetus to God (*b. Nid.* 31a).

35. The version of this tradition in *Leviticus Rabbah* remains ambiguous about whether or not God actually does change the embryo's facial features to expose the adulterous relationship. However, the parallel traditions are less ambiguous, suggesting that God does.

36. See Berkowitz 2006, 163–64, for another example of the use of Lev. 18:3 for "Jewish uniqueness."

37. Of course Greco-Roman embryology is equally ideological (Lloyd 1983; Dean-Jones 1994), but it is far less theological.

38. Cf. *Num. Rab.* 5:4. See *b. Bek.* 21b for mention of formation of the embryo at forty (not forty-one) days. See also *b. M. Kat.* 18b, *b. Sot.* 2a, and *b. Sanh.* 22a, which state, "forty days before the formation of the embryo a *bat kol* issues forth and says, 'This one will marry this one.'" Cf. *Lev. Rab.* 8:1.

39. It seems possible that this tradition might also connect the generation of the flood with what comes directly before in Gen. 6:4, and refers not to adulterous

unions in general, but the unions between and offspring of the "sons of God and the daughters of men." Cf. *Gen. Rab.* 26:7, cited in a note below. And see *Testaments of the Twelve Patriarchs (T. Reu.* 5:1–7). See Stol 2000b, 60–61.

40. The previous statement in *Gen. Rab.* 32:5 explains that God caused it to rain for forty days because they transgressed the Torah that was given in forty days. This reinforces that God forms the embryo, because certainly God gave the Torah. Cf. *b. Men.* 99b, discussed above.

41. See, e.g., the Hippocratic work *On the Nature of the Child* 15 and 19. See also Aristotle *History of Animals* 583b. For a detailed discussion about the differences between Hippocratic sources and Aristotle on the order of fetal development and the problems involved in reasoning that the fetus develops from "outside to inside," see Boylan 1986, 69ff. Rabbinic sources also consider from where the embryo develops. Kottek points out, "It should be emphasized that the Talmud does not deal with the problem of the first organ to be completed in embryogenesis (the heart, according to Aristotle), but is interested only in determining the topographic origin of the fetus' development" (1981, 308). Palestinian sources all maintain that the fetus develops from its navel (*y. Nid.* 3:3[50d] and *y. Sot.* 9:3[23c]), but they never cite a proof text. Some Greco-Roman sources maintain that fetal development begins from the navel (e.g., the Hippocratic *On the Nature of the Child* 15 and 29; Aristotle *History of Animals* 586a32 and *Generation of Animals* 740b9–10). However, the *Bavli* (*Yom.* 85a and *Sot.* 45b) debates whether fetal development begins from the navel or the head. Needham writes, "Some Talmudic writers held that development began with the head, agreeing with Lactantius, and others that it began at the navel, agreeing with Alcmaeon" (1934, 78). Kottek relies solely on sources from the *Bavli* when he asserts that the sages maintain that the fetus develops from its head. He explains, "The head is the noblest and highest part of the individual, and in the embryo and young child it is large in relation to the rest of the body. The Talmudic opinion on the source of the embryo had been defended by the pre-Socratic philosophers Anaxagors, Alcmaeon, and Hippo of Samos, all of whom held that the head was formed first in embryonic development" (Kottek 1981, 308). In contrast to the lack of any attempt to find biblical support for fetal development from the navel, the *Bavli* cites proof texts for fetal development from the head that theologize this point of embryology. Nevertheless, Palestinian sources maintain that fetal development begins from the navel, even without scriptural support, suggesting that they might have incorporated this from Greco-Roman culture.

42. R. Abbahu is a Palestinian amora reputedly well versed in Greek (see below).

43. *Gen. Rab.* 14:5, although lacking the passage attributed to R. Abbahu, is also quite clear that God forms the embryo, since it interprets Gen. 2:7, *And the Lord God created ha'adam.*

44. Hebrew: *tsurat havalad.* In the parallel traditions (*y. Nid.* 3:3[50d], *t. Nid.* 4:10, and *b. Nid.* 25a) the description is offered in answer to the question "what is the *shefir merukam* [articulated fetus]?" mentioned in *m. Nid.* 3:3. In *t. Nid.* and *b. Nid.* sources, Job 10:12 is cited instead of Ps. 139:16.

45. On the use of the word *pinaks* in rabbinic literature, see Lieberman 1994,

204–5 (*Hellenism*). The Hippocratic treatise *On the Nature of the Child* 28 states, "The child while in its womb has its hands tucked against its chin, while its head lies near its feet. However it is not possible to decide with any accuracy whether its head is above or below—not even if you actually see the child in the womb" (Lonie 1981, 18). Aristotle writes, "human embryos lie bent, with nose between the knees and eyes upon the knees, and the ears free at the sides" (*History of Animals* 586b3–4; Barnes 1984, 919).

46. Exceptions include Genesis 25 and 38.

47. *Lev. Rab.* 14:4, which demonstrates God's care of the fetus during each trimester, is discussed in the following chapter. See also *b. Nid.* 31a, which describes which part of the uterus the fetus occupies during each trimester.

48. See *b. Nid.* 31a: "Our rabbis taught: the first three months [of pregnancy] intercourse is difficult for the woman and for the fetus. The middle months [intercourse] is difficult for the woman but good for the fetus. The last months [intercourse] is good for the woman and for the fetus, because as a result the fetus is cleansed and strengthened." I do not discuss this tradition in the body of this chapter because I have not found any parallels in Palestinian sources, even though it is presented as a *baraita*. Nevertheless, it demonstrates that the rabbis, like Greco-Roman authors, consider the effects of sexual intercourse during pregnancy. See Soranus's *Gynecology*: "Sexual intercourse, however, is *always harmful* to pregnant women both on account of the tossing motion and because the uterus is forced to submit to a movement which is contrary to the process of pregnancy. *And even more so in the last months*, lest because of it the chorion burst and the fluid which has been prepared for use in parturition be evacuated before the proper time" (Temkin 1991b, 56–57, my emphasis). Mention of the possible dangers of sexual intercourse during pregnancy is also found in the Hippocratic corpus. Kottek and Baader cite *On Superfetation* 13 (Littré ed., 8:484) and write, "Hippocratic gynaecology holds that parturition is easier if the woman avoids intercourse altogether during pregnancy" (2000, 86). But see Rousselle 1988, 42. Aristotle succinctly writes, "Women who have connection with their husbands shortly before childbirth are delivered all the more quickly" (*History of Animals* 584a; Barnes 1984, 915). See also *History of Animals* 584b: "Of all animals the woman and the mare are most inclined to receive the commerce of the male during pregnancy; while all other animals when they are pregnant avoid the male." Thus, this rabbinic source on the benefits of intercourse during pregnancy stands in agreement with the opinion recorded by Aristotle (although Aristotle does not mention benefits to the fetus), and at least the later interpretation from the Hippocratic corpus recorded by Oribasius (see Rousselle 1988, 42). However, it stands in direct contrast with Soranus's teaching, even though Soranus is writing closer to the period in which this tannaitic statement ostensibly originates.

49. Other rabbinic traditions that refer to nine months of pregnancy as the norm include: *Sifre Num. Naso* 8 (Horovitz 1992, 15); *Gen. Rab.* 53:6; *Lam. Rab.* 1:11; *Eccles. Rab.* 12:10; *b. Sot.* 20b; and *Num. Rab.* 11:31. See Wasserstein 1985 and Kottek and Baader 2000 for exceptions.

50. Cf. *Lev. Rab.* 14:2 and *b. Nid.* 30b, with no mention of nine months.

51. Cf. *Lev. Rab.* 30:13.

52. The *Bavli* records no parallel to the Palestinian tradition about the shortest term for a viable birth being 212 days. In contrast, *b. Nid.* 38b (cf. *b. Yev.* 42a) interprets 1 Sam. 1:20 to teach that the shortest term for pregnancy is 202 days.

53. This does not mean, however, that all who are born after 212 days live, because the rabbis maintain the widespread belief in the nonviability of the eighth-month child (see below).

54. See, e.g., Aristotle *History of Animals* 583b, "Children that come into the world before seven months can under no circumstances survive. The seven-months' children are the earliest that are capable of life, and most of them are weakly" (Barnes 1984, 915). Hippocratic treatises discuss the viability of children born at seven months and nine months.

55. Cf. *y. Nid.* 1:4(49b); *y. Yev.* 4:11(6a); and *b. Nid.* 38a. The rabbis maintain that the seed could remain potent up to three (or four) days. Although the midrashic basis for this belief is not mentioned in this tradition, other rabbinic traditions establish that the seed spoils after three days based on Exod. 19:15, when Moses tells the Israelites, *Be ready by the third day, do not come near a woman.* Cf. *m. Shab.* 9:3; *y. Shab.* 9:3(12a); *y. Yev.* 4:2(5c); and Rashi on *b. Shab.* 86a, s.v. "three days." See Preuss 1978, 384. The parallels in *y. Yev.* 4:11(6a) and *y. Nid.* 1:4(49b) state, "R. Berekiah in the name of Shmuel: 'A woman only gives birth on the 271st, or 272nd, or 273rd, or 274th day." Perhaps this addition of the fourth day conflicts with the idea that seed disintegrates after three days.

56. Alternatively, the statement about 270 days of pregnancy is simply placed here because the text previously discusses the shortest term of pregnancy. I prefer to give the midrash the benefit of the doubt and find meaning in its placement as an interpretation of Gen. 3:16. *Gen. Rab.* 53:6 interprets Gen. 21:2, *At the set time of which God had spoken to him,* to teach that Isaac's birth was at nine months.

57. Perhaps the emphasis on the blessing of pregnancy and birth here could be seen in light of the overall rabbinic reading of what is taken to be the commandment to procreate, *And God blessed them and said to them, be fruitful and multiply* (Gen. 1:28). However, *Gen. Rab.* 20:6 later interprets the verse more in keeping with its biblical context: "*Your pain*—this is the pain of conception; *your pregnancy*—this is the pain of pregnancy; *in pain*—this is the pain of miscarriages; *shall you bring forth*—this is the pain of birth; *children*—this is the pain of raising children."

58. On the nonviability in of eight-month children in Greco-Roman sources, see Dean-Jones 1994, 209–11; King 1998, 112; and Jouanna 1999, 386. In Jewish sources, see Preuss 1978, 393–94; Wasserstein 1985; Lieberman 1994, 77 (*Hellenism*); van der Horst 1978; and Kottek and Baader 2002, 87–89. See also Tertullian, *De anima*, chap. 37.

59. The midrash interprets the "extra" *yod* in *vayyitser* to teach that there are two formations. The parallel in *y. Yev.* 4:2(5d) begins, "From where do we know that there are two formations? R. Zeira in the name of R. Huna: [*And the Lord God*] *formed*: formation for seven and formation for nine [months]." There exist a number of variations between *y. Yev.* 4:2, *Gen. Rab.* 14:2, and *Gen. Rab.* 20:6, both in printed versions and in manuscripts, that I cannot pursue here (see G. Kessler 2001). Instead of looking for the "correct" or "original" text, I take the variations as indica-

tive of the complexity sometimes, though not always, involved in rabbinic adaptation of Greco-Roman embryology.

60. Albeck's printed text at *Gen. Rab.* 14:2 states, "Rav Huna," but a manuscript variant here and in *Gen. Rab.* 20:6 reads, "R. Huna." I assume the text refers either to R. Huna, a fifth-generation tanna or a fourth-generation Palestinian amora. *Y. Yev.* 4:2 attributes this tradition to R. Zeira in the name of R. Huna.

61. Contrast, e.g., Gen. 2:19, where *vayitser* is written with only one *yod*. The double *yod* appears only in Gen. 2:7.

62. The text of the *Yerushalmi* is corrupt. See *P'nei Moshe* and *Korban HaEdah* ad loc. See Lieberman 1994, 76–77 (*Hellenism*), and 22–23 (*Greek*).

63. Theodor and Albeck 1965, 127. Alternatively: Seven, live; eight, go. I have translated according to Lieberman 1994, 77 (*Hellenism*). See Wasserstein 1985, 227–29, for a critique of Lieberman's reading. My own hesitation about Lieberman's translation is that it allows more flexibility concerning the eight-month child's survival than the rest of *Gen. Rab.* 14:2. For, if the seven-month child is *more likely* to survive than the eight-month child, it seems that it is possible, according to R. Abbahu, that an eight-month child can survive. (This is explicitly stated in the *Yerushalmi Yevamot* parallel, at least according to the printed versions, but given the manuscript variants in both *Genesis Rabbah* passages, it is reasonable to assume they exist for the *Yerushalmi* as well.) Lieberman signals his own addition in this translation, as he places in parenthesis the Greek word *mallon* (more than). One could fill in the gap in the language in other ways.

64. See Lieberman 1994, 77 (*Hellenism*), "R. Abbahu resorted here to the *notaricon*, paronomasia and the numerical value of letters, and combined them together for the purpose of investing letters of the Greek alphabet with mysterious significance." R. Abbahu is considered to be well-versed in Greek wisdom (Lieberman 1994, 22–24 [*Greek*]). See also Lachs 1970 and Levine 1975.

65. Lieberman 1994, in *Hellenism* (76), simply states that the interlocutors are non-Jews, but in *Greek* (22) he suggests that they are "probably Christians, with whom R. Abbahu had frequent discussions." I see nothing that firmly establishes that the questioners were Christian, but patristic authors also maintained the nonviability of eight-month children. See, e.g., Tertullian, *De anima*, chap. 37.

66. I have focused exclusively on traditions explicitly engaged with the question of the viability of seven- and nine-month children and the nonviability of eight-month children. A large number of sources primarily concerned with paternity mention seven- and nine-month children as well, without mentioning eight-month children, implying their nonviability. The distinction between the seven- and nine-month children already appears in tannaitic compilations and is then carried over into the amoraic compilations, including the *Bavli*, which has no parallel to *Gen. Rab.* 14:2 and 20:6. See, e.g., *m. Yev.* 5:2 and 12:6; *m. Bek.* 8:1; *t. Shab.* 16:4; *t. Yev.* 6:1 and 12:5, *t. Bek.* 6:2; *b. Yom.* 75a; *b. Yev.* 35b and 100a; and *b. Nid.* 8b. And see G. Kessler 2001, 346–66, for further discussion.

67. King 1998, 112, emphasis added.

68. Another coping mechanism for the death of a newborn might be found in the debate about whether it is considered *nefel,* and thus not viable, until thirty days after birth. See *b. Shab.* 135b–136a.

69. On the motif of the special status of seven-month children in comparative perspective, see Lieberman 1994, 76 n. 240 (*Hellenism*) and van der Horst 1978.

70. This tradition's lack of attribution of any role to menstrual blood in conception and nurturing the fetus, in contrast to Hippocratic, Aristotelian, and Galenic sources, is explored in the following chapter.

71. *Leviticus Rabbah* 14 is discussed at length in the following chapter. For other rabbinic sources about the "stirring up" or "raising up" of breast milk, see *t. Nid.* 2:1; *y. Nid.* 1:5(49b); *y. Sot.* 4:4(19c); *b. Nid.* 9a; and *b. Ket.* 60a. See also Rashi on *b. Ket.* 39a, s.v. "lest she have to wean." However, all of these traditions are concerned with the production of breast milk in a woman who is lactating and becomes pregnant. Except for *b. Nid.* 9a, none of the traditions explicitly mention that God transforms blood into milk. *B. Nid.* 9a attributes the transformation of blood into milk to God by interpreting Job 4:14, *Who can bring a clean thing from an unclean? Not one*, as "Who can bring a clean thing from an unclean, not God?" For secondary sources, see Preuss 1978, 404; Kottek 1980; Rosner 1977; and Gruber 1992. Despite the fact that rabbinic traditions demonstrate consonance with Greco-Roman sources on the connection between breast milk and blood, I have not found a tradition that suggests, like some Greco-Roman sources, any connection between semen and blood.

72. The other leading theory maintains that breast milk is produced from the woman's nutriment. See Dean-Jones 1994, 215–22. See also Buell 1999, 154–59. Hippocratic texts mention both theories, and although Aristotle primarily maintains the link between menstrual blood and milk, traces of the theory that milk comes from mother's nutriment also appear in Aristotle (Dean-Jones 1994, 218). Galen also maintains that breast milk was formed from menstrual blood (Kottek 1980, 8; and Preuss 1978, 404 n. 322). Herophilus maintained that menstrual blood was transformed into breast milk after birth (Von Staden 1989, 292). Soranus, albeit less explicitly, links menstrual blood and breast milk when he writes, "The uterus itself brings the seed to perfection, whereas the breasts prepare milk as food for the coming child; and menses occurring, the milk stops, whereas lactation occurring, menstruation appears no more" (*Gyn.* 1.15; Temkin 1991b, 14). Precisely when blood or nutriment gets changed into breast milk remains a matter of debate, which might also surface among the rabbinic sources mentioned above. Hippocratic works suggest a variety of times for the production of breast milk (Dean-Jones 1994, 215–22). Aristotle also offers different points at which menstrual blood becomes milk. He writes, "When [as soon as] the animal is pregnant milk is found, but at first—and then again later—it is unfit for use" (*History of Animals* 522a4; Barnes 1984, 828). Here it seems that milk is formed immediately upon conception. However, he also claims that menstrual blood was converted to breast milk after about a month of pregnancy. He writes, "After conception, and when the above-mentioned days are past [thirty days for female embryos and forty days for males], the discharge no longer takes its natural course but finds its way to the breasts and turns to milk" (583a32–34; Barnes 1984, 913–14).

73. Clement of Alexandria also adapts Greco-Roman notions about the production of breast milk and implicates God in the process (*Paid.* 1.39.3). See Buell 1999, 154–59. Buell, writing on a related passage in *Paidogogos*, points out, "that this portion of chapter six is not merely a discourse on physiology, but rather an inter-

pretation of spiritual matters in light of physiological and developmental concepts" (1999, 167).

74. Greco-Roman sources appeal to nature, precisely where R. Meir invokes God. For example, Aristotle writes, "Milk is formed in the females of all internally viviparous animals, becoming useful for the time of birth. For *nature* has made it for the sake of the nourishment of animals after birth (*Generation of Animals* 776a15–17; Barnes 1984, 1200). And, "As to man's growth, first within his mother's womb and afterward to old age, *the course of nature,* in so far as man is specially concerned, is after the following manner (*History of Animals* 581a8–10; Barnes 1984, 910). Herophilus also attributed the blood flowing up to the breasts "by natural course" (Von Staden 1989, 292). And see Soranus *Gyn.* 2.21 (Temkin 1991b, 89).

75. *Lev. Rab.* 14:2 asserts God's role in providing sustenance for Israel and the world.

76. That both God and the fetus occupy the focus of these traditions at the expense of the woman is discussed in the following chapter.

77. The *Yerushalmi* version maintains that Dinah is changed from male to female at the moment of birth, but *Genesis Rabbah* and the *Bavli* seem to open up the possibility that this change occurs after birth. The *Bavli,* however, then suggests that such a change occurs during the first forty days of gestation.

78. Preus explains that theories of generation arose in order to answer certain questions, for example, "Why do children usually resemble their parents, and sometimes fail to resemble one or both parents? What determines the sex of offspring?" He continues, "Many of the answers to questions about the source and nature of seed were developed as theories explaining some or all variations in resemblance and lack of resemblance to parents" (1977, 65). See also Boylan 1984 and Dean-Jones 1994, 178.

79. *MRI B'shalakh* 8 (Horovitz and Rabin 1970, 144; Lauterbach 1933–35, 2:65). The mention of "a drop of liquid," semen, being the primary human contribution to procreation is discussed in the following chapter.

80. *M. Ber.* 9:3, which most likely predates the tradition in the *Mekhilta,* implies that God determines the sex of the fetus when it characterizes a prayer about the fetus's sex being in vain.

81. I read the Hebrew word *ben* as here specifically referring to a son, instead of a child. The concreteness of the image being replicated suggests that the image maker's, and God's, rendering be presumed to be somewhat exact. For rabbinic traditions that interpret the biblical use of *banim* as "sons" specifically, and not "daughters," see *Sifre Deut. Ki Tetse* 43 and *b. Yev.* 77b, both interpreting Deut. 23:9. See also *b. Nid.* 70b–71a, where, in the context of answering the question of what men do so that they may have male children, Ps. 127:3, *Sons [banim] are an inheritance of the Lord,* is cited. See also *Num. Rab.* 3:8, which, although a much later compilation, explicitly interprets the mention of *banim* in Ps. 127:3 as "sons." The *Mekhilta* passage cites Ps. 127:3 a few lines above the cited passage.

82. The Castanata and Munich manuscripts add that God "created/formed the fetus in its mother's womb and he resembled the form of his father."

83. See, e.g., Rosner 1977; Kottek 1981, 305, citing *b. Ber.* 60a; van der Horst 1990, 300–301); and Levinson 2000b. See also Satlow 1994, 158–59. Cf. *b. Ber.* 60a, and

b. Nid. 25b, 28a, and 70b–71a. See Preuss 1978, 390–92, for additional citations. On rabbinic "eugenics" more broadly, see Satlow 1995, 303–13. Satlow includes a number of *Bavli* traditions on sex determination, provides citations of numerous additional sources, contextualizes these traditions among Roman sources in late antiquity, and discusses why these traditions, most of which are attributed to Palestinian sages, are unique to the *Bavli*.

84. The emission of seed (*mazria/mazraat*) is commonly understood as connoting orgasm. See, e.g., Rosner 1977, 173 and 175; and Levinson 2000b, 124. Perhaps this source provides evidence of rabbinic absorption of the link between pleasure, orgasm, and conception prevalent in antiquity. See Brown 1983 for Greco-Roman and Christian sources. However, the same words (*mazria* and *mazraat*) appear in another tradition in *b. Nid.* 31a, which maintains that the man "*mazria* the white" parts of the body and the woman "*mazraat* (the) red" parts of the body, and here it seems difficult to understand *mazria/mazraat* as connoting "orgasm."

85. Levinson (2000b, 124) uses *b. Nid.* 31a to frame his discussion about rabbinic cultural androgyny, which he sees as buttressed by the rabbinic adoption of "Hippocratic-Galenic two-seed embryology." While I am sympathetic to his overall desire to expose the ambiguities surrounding gender and identity in rabbinic sources, I think his grounding of this in the notion that the rabbis' adopted a two-seed embryology wherein both men and women produce male and female seed is somewhat premature. It requires that one imports the idea of men and women producing both male and female seed into traditions about sex determination, where no evidence is present in the texts. See also Koren 2004. These sources, especially when the "parallel" in *Lev. Rab.* 14:8 is included, say nothing about men and women producing both male and female seed. (*Lev. Rab.* 14:8 surprisingly says nothing explicit about seed whatsoever.) Instead, they seem to suggest that women produce male seed and men produce female seed, thus operating out of a more rigid two-sexed model than a more fluid androgynous model. I have not found Greco-Roman sources concerned with who emits seed first, which is different from who provides the strongest seed. Finally, Stol points out the difference between the *Bavli* sources on sex determination when viewed in context of Greco-Roman theories. He writes, "The deviating Jewish opinion derives from Leviticus 12:2, 'If a woman gives seed and bears a male child . . .'. Female seed engenders a boy. Clearly, the Word of God forced the Rabbis to reverse this accepted rule" (2000a, 8).

86. Satlow maintains that this tradition is attributed to Palestinian sages (1995, 304; and see 1994, 158–59). But Levinson examines manuscripts and suggests that the tradition is correctly attributed to Babylonian sages (2000b, 124 n. 32). Levinson grants that there are parallels in Palestinian sources at *Lev. Rab.* 14:8 and *Midrash Tanhuma* (*Tazria'* 3). However, *Midrash Tanhuma* (ca. eighth century CE) probably borrows from the *Bavli*, and *Lev. Rab.* 14:8 exhibits some significant differences. Most relevant, there is no mention of the woman or man emitting seed (*mazra'at/ mazria'*). (As seen in the following chapter, *Leviticus Rabbah* 14 almost in its entirety refuses to entertain the notion of a woman emitting seed, despite its basis in Lev. 12:2.) *Lev. Rab.* 14:8 simply states that the males always come from women and females always come from men and provides scripture, quite selectively, to prove this.

Lev. Rab. 14:8 does, however, record a parable: "[The process whereby the sex of the offspring is determined may be compared to] two who enter a bathhouse. The first one who sweats [*mazia'*], goes out first." Both Margulies (1993, 312) and Chanokh Zelman in his *Etz Yosef* appeal to the *Bavli* tradition about the emission of seed to explain this parable—but to different ends. According to Margulies, the one who emits seed first, forgoes his/her influence on the fetus's gender: if the man emits seed first, then the child will be born a girl; if the woman emits seed first, the child will be born a boy. But according to *Etz Yosef*, the one who emits first dictates the gender of the child, which is the "opposite" gender since males come from women and females come from men. In other words, if the man emits first, his influence, since he causes the birth of girls, will remain. And if a woman emits first, her influence, which causes the birth of boys, will remain. My point is not to decide the correct interpretation, but to point out the alternatives and their reliance on the *Bavli's* tradition, which seems especially methodologically problematic since no precise parallel exists in Palestinian sources.

87. See *y. Kel.* 8:3(31c), *Eccles. Rab.* 5:10, and *b. Nid.* 31a (the same page that seems to ignore God's role in sex determination). However, *b. Ber.* 60a and *b. Nid.* 70b–71a do implicate God in sex determination. Also worthy of note is that in contrast to almost all rabbinic traditions about procreation examined in the next chapter, here the woman and man are themselves portrayed as equal: both produce the other.

88. Certainly the fact that this tradition appears in the *Bavli* also contributes to its centrality, as if the *Bavli* represents all that "the rabbis" say on a given topic. Still, *b. Ber.* 60a and *b. Nid.* 70b–71a invoke God in sex determination, and they receive considerably less attention.

89. Satlow 1995, 313, speculates about the theology evident in *Yerushalmi* traditions, in contrast to *Bavli* traditions.

90. Margulies 1993, 310. Lev. 12:2 states in full, *When a woman emits seed and bears a male child: then shall she be unclean seven days; as in the days of her menstrual sickness* [*niddah*] *shall she be unclean.* Thus this passage is connected to the base verse of Lev. 12:2 and its mention of *niddah*, even though it ends with the citation of Lev. 12:3. Margulies points out that this *petihta*, and its concern for observing *niddah*, is a shift away from the point of this chapter, which focuses on the creation of the embryo and the care of the fetus. However, it clearly asserts that God *gives* the child/son to the parents. Furthermore, since 14:7 discusses the sex of the fetus, it provides a bridge with *Lev. Rab.* 14:8, also concerned with sex determination. Cf. *b. Shev.* 18b, where men are given male children as a reward for observing *niddah*. And cf. *b. Nid.* 70b–71a for God giving sons as a reward for sexual restraint and in answer to men's prayers.

91. This theory about sex determination seems open to the question posed in *b. Nid.* 71a, "Have not many done so, to no success?" Nevertheless, *Lev. Rab.* 14:7 seems content to (have God) explicitly praise those who observe *niddah* and implicitly blame those who do not. The assumption of the preference for male children is consistently maintained throughout *Leviticus Rabbah* 14 (see Chapter 5).

92. The translation follows Gordis 1951, 184 and 321–22, and Seow 1997, 336–37,

with some modification. Cf. *Gen. Rab.* 65:12. The *Bavli* traditions that mention the emission of seed and *Lev. Rab.* 14:8 also attach the notion that men produce female offspring and women produce male offspring to scripture.

93. Cf. *y. Ber.* 9:5(14a) and *b. Ber.* 60a. For a discussion of the differences between these traditions, see G. Kessler 2001.

94. Both the *Yerushalmi* and *Genesis Rabbah* traditions seize upon the fact that no time frame is given for the Mishnah's teaching that praying about the sex of the fetus is of no consequence—a wasted prayer. Instead of interpreting *m. Ber.* 9:3 to teach that such prayer is ineffective throughout pregnancy, the *Yerushalmi* suggests that this is so only once the woman has begun labor. *Genesis Rabbah* goes further, minimally maintaining that even at the moment of birth the sex can be changed. The amoraic traditions also change the Mishnah's concern about a man praying for a male child to women—either Rachel or Leah—praying for the birth of a girl, but in order that another male child will be born. For a discussion of this text in the context of rabbinic traditions about body malleability informed by queer theory, see G. Kessler 2007. There I also point out that one of the motivations for this midrash is to account for the peculiar fact that Dinah is the only named daughter whose birth story is recorded in the Torah.

95. *M. Ber.* 9:3 literally states that this is a "vain prayer," but the force of the phrase has a stronger connotation in that such a prayer takes God's name in vain. See Exod. 20:7. I thank Burton Visotzky for this insight and the translation.

96. Literally, "who sits on the birthing stool" (*mashber*). Preuss writes, "the expression 'to sit on the *mashber*' gradually came to be used for 'parturition,' so that the literal meaning of the phrase became forgotten" (1978, 396).

97. Vilna edition adds, "Just as this potter, after he makes a cruse, breaks it and makes another, so too I can do such, even on the birthing stool."

98. *Y. Ber.* 9:5(14a) states, "the essence of Dinah's conception was male."

99. The use of '*ahar* may also be being understood as '*aher*—masculine for "another." See *Midrash Tanhuma Vayyetze* 8, where it is pointed out that '*aher*, not '*aheret* (the feminine for "another") is used, thus intimating further that originally Dinah was male.

100. This is my suggested reading of the text. In Theodor's commentary (Theodor and Albeck 1965, 844–45), he cites parallels and earlier commentaries on the midrash, providing previous interpretations of the apparent textual problem. Having found none of the previous suggestions perfectly satisfactory, I am suggesting a new understanding of the text. I believe it to be the strongest reading because it makes sense of R. Yehudah's response to the objection raised against him, and because it follows the chronology (birth order) of the biblical text. Theodor cites that some commentators have understood the verse "May God grant me another son" to refer to Joseph, not Benjamin. Clearly, in the biblical text, the verse is referring to Benjamin. My suggested reading maintains the biblical birth order and does indeed allow that Rachel is praying for another son, Benjamin.

101. *Lev. Rab.* 14:8 and *Gen. Rab.* 72:6 (and parallels) again demonstrate that even though they both attribute sex determination to God, their depictions of God might differ. According to *Lev. Rab.* 14:8, God works from the attribute of judgment, but in *Gen. Rab.* 72:6, God works from the attribute of mercy.

102. *Gen. Rab.* 14:5 and *Lev. Rab.* 14:9 credit God with the creation of sinews, bones, tendons, and flesh, without any mention of the parents' contributions.

103. I read this tradition from the *Yerushalmi*, which appears embedded within a discussion of inherited traits of animals, as a rabbinic tradition concerned with generic heredity, not as a tradition about the creation of the embryo or a tradition about specific inherited traits. Commenting on Aristotle's theory of resemblance, Dean-Jones distinguishes between general and specific inherited traits: "The process described so far has explained how a 'generic' individual of a species could be reproduced; what has passed from father to embryo via the semen has been the form of the species. This does not explain what makes each individual unique in features, or how parents pass on to their children their own idiosyncratic characteristics which are not contained in the species form" (1994, 193). She also writes that Aristotle maintained "that we do not say a child resembles its parents in the materials of its body, its flesh and blood (the uniform parts, *ta homoiomere*) but in the arrangement of the flesh and blood, its face, hands, etc. (the nonuniform parts, *ta anomoiomere*)" (1994, 164). See also Balme 1990.

104. However, no close parallels for either *Lev. Rab.* 23:12 or *MRI B'shalakh* 8 appear in the *Bavli*.

105. *Lev. Rab.* 23:12 first assumes the facial features of the fetus as sculpted in the image of the father and then imagines that God can reshape the fetus in the image of the adulterer.

106. *Gen. Rab.* 85:5 mentions that one of the five sons of R. Yosi "had dark eyes, that resembled his mother's." I have found no other sources that mention facial features resembling the mother. *Gen. Rab.* 86:6, without specific mention of facial features, does assert that Joseph resembles his mother, Rachel. See Levinson 2000b, 135ff. However, *Gen. Rab.* 84:8 specifically states, "*Now Israel loved Joseph more than all his children, because he was a son of his old age* (Gen. 37:3). R. Judah said this means that his facial features resembled his."

107. This is supported in the next chapter. On Hippocratic theories of resemblance, see Dean-Jones 1994, 162–66.

108. On environment contributing to the fetus, see Preus 1977, 66; and Boylan 1984, 86. On Aristotle's theory of resemblance based on woman's contribution from blood, see Dean-Jones 1994. Aristotle also writes, "the offspring derive their nature from their mothers as plants do from the earth" (*Politics* 7.16, cited from Stol 2000b, 63). On patristic theories, especially about Jesus, see Harlow 1999. In Chapter 5, I include more discussion about the relationship between rabbinic and patristic theories of procreation.

109. Preuss, writing in 1911, already observed, "In all the foregoing, the only point is the psychic influence of the mother on the child at the moment of conception. The Talmud only rarely admits to such an influence on the pregnancy itself" (1978, 392). Preuss's only examples are the later expansion of *Lev. Rab.* 23:12 in *Num. Rab.* 9:1, where the woman's actions, not her physiology or appearance, have an impact on the fetus who nevertheless resembles not her but her husband or the adulterer, and *Num. Rab.* 9:5, about a female donkey who was cauterized and bore an offspring with a flame mark. The subject heading of this section in Preuss's work is "Psychic Maternal Influences on the Fetus," yet again revealing that the woman

contributes nothing material to the fetus. For a more recent analysis of maternal imagination, see Stol 2000b. In all of the instances of such "psychic influence" that I have found, the offspring does not physically resemble the mother, but the object/man whom she was imagining during intercourse. In *Gen. Rab.* 26:7, R. Berekiah interprets *When the sons of God came into the daughters of men and they gave birth to children for them* (Gen. 6:4) to mean, "A woman would go out into the market and see a young man and desire him, and she would go and have sex and bring forth a young man like him." See Stol, for an earlier, albeit more detailed, tradition about Gen. 6:4 in the *Testaments of the Twelve Patriarchs* (2000b, 60–61). *Gen. Rab.* 73:10, in the context of its interpretation of Jacob's flocks conceiving by the rods he places in the watering troughs (Gen. 30:37ff.), states that the offspring resembled the *rods*, not the mother. In late manuscripts of *Gen. Rab.* 73:10 the text adds, "*Ma'aseh*: A Cushite married a Cushite woman and he begat from her a white son. He took his son and came to Rabbi and said to him, 'Perhaps he is not my son.' Rabbi said to him, 'Do you have any pictures in your house?' He said, 'Yes.' Rabbi said, 'Are they black or white?' He said, 'White.' Rabbi said to him, 'From here was your white son.'" According to this tradition, the son resembles the pictures, not the woman. Cf. *Num. Rab.* 9:34. Stol 2000b, 59 cites a presumably well-known story in antiquity where Persinna, the black Ethiopian queen gave birth to a white *daughter* due to the picture of a white Andromeda in the bedroom. The rabbinic versions interestingly focus on the birth of a white son, not daughter, perhaps indicating that the pictures the woman sees during sexual intercourse are of men. *B. Bab. Metz.* 84a relates that R. Yohanan would sit by the gates of the *mikveh* so that women would see/meet him after they had immersed and they would have sons as beautiful and learned as he was. Again, the sons resemble R. Yohanan, not their mothers. In *b. Bek.* 6b–7a, the rabbis discuss firstlings that resemble their mothers, but here the resemblance is of species, not specific inherited traits. Cf. *t. Bek.* 1:5. See Satlow 1995, 310–12, for some parallels in Roman sources and insightful comments about the *Bavli*'s concern for men's thoughts and actions during intercourse, not women's. He writes, "This schema lessens the perceived female contribution to the fetus. This dialectic, I believe, underscores the androcentric nature of these texts" (312). I think his comments are also applicable to rabbinic traditions about maternal influence cited in this note.

110. Cf. Gen. 30:5 and 30:17.

111. This tradition previously mentioned Sarah being kept in Pharaoh and Avimelech's houses. Cf. *b. Bab. Metz.* 87a, where the features of Isaac's face were changed at his weaning banquet to resemble Abraham's, in order to dispel doubts of Abraham's paternity. Cf. *Mid. Tanhuma* (Buber), *Vayishlakh* 25.

112. The rabbis derive *ziv 'eykonin* (facial features) from *lizkunav* (his old age). Cf. *Gen. Rab.* 84:8.

113. The *Mekhilta* (*B'shalakh* 8) makes it clear that even though semen is necessary for procreation, God makes the son resemble his father.

114. The national concerns are already apparent in *Genesis Rabbah*, since Sarah might be pregnant by Avimelech. See Genesis 20.

115. In the *Tanhuma* tradition, this passage interprets Gen. 25:19, not Gen. 21:2. The *Tanhuma* continues to question the apparent superfluousness in Gen. 25:19,

"Why does scripture state both, *And these are the generations of Isaac, son of Abraham* and *Abraham begot Isaac* (Gen. 25:19)? If scripture states *Isaac son of Abraham*, don't I know that *Abraham begot Isaac*? And why does scripture state *Abraham begot Isaac*? Because all who saw Abraham were saying, 'Surely Abraham begot Isaac because the features of their faces were just like each other's.' Therefore scripture says, *Abraham begot Isaac*." Cf. *Mid. Tanhuma* (*Toldot* 6), where a similar tradition is stated about David's son with Avigail.

116. The part of the text not translated above reads:

What did the facial features of their fathers resemble? [Literally: What was the essence of their fathers like?] The greats of the families, as it is written concerning Reuben, *These are the families of the Reubenites* (Num. 26:7). [And as it is written concerning Shimeon], *These are the families of the Shimeonites* (Num. 26:14). R. Hoshaiah said, "Reuben, the Reubenite, Shimeon the Shimeonite." R. Merinos son of R. Hoshaiah, "This is also said concerning the Baronites, Savronites, Siborites." R. Huna in the name of R. Idi said, "the letter *hay* is at the beginning of the word and the letter *yod* is at its end. God [YH] testified on their behalf that they are the sons/children of their fathers."

117. The text does not say that the daughters are pregnant, but I suggest that it implies this based on their request for a signature and seal from their husbands, and the king's request that they produce such signs, which recalls Tamar's proof of pregnancy by Judah in Genesis 38.

118. Levinson (2000b, 124 n. 31) notes the "judaization" of rabbinic embryology.

119. S. Schwartz 2001, 162ff. Schwartz, in agreement with Hayes, does not see such accommodation as intentional. See Hayes 1997.

120. Berkowitz 2006. See also Boyarin 1999.

121. Berkowitz 2006, 162.

122. However, a *baraita* in the Babylonian Talmud (*b. Ket.* 30a, *b. Sot.* 8b, *b. Sanh.* 56a), as Berkowitz notes, maintains "that even though the four rabbinic executions are annulled, they are still in force through acts of God" (2006, 161).

123. As M. Stol writes, "Basic to all these descriptions of the prenatal development of man—whether Jewish or Muslim—is that God is the Creator steering the process in every stage" (2000a, 16).

124. As above, I stress the normativity of Rabbi, not his exceptionality in this tradition.

125. *Gen. Rab.* 34:10 cites two proof texts, but *b. Sanh.* 91b cites only one.

126. Interestingly, this text is itself a reversal of a more popular exchange between Rabbi and Antoninus where Antoninus learns from Rabbi. See Meir 1999 and Rubenstein 2002.

127. Seth Schwartz points out some of the difficulties in reading intent into rabbinic sources (2001, 164). For this reason, a discussion of rabbinic resistance does not frame this chapter but sits perhaps oddly at the end.

128. For rabbinic sources on idolatry that *function* as accommodation, see S. Schwartz 2001, 173.

129. On the "hidden transcript," see Scott 1990, 1–44. See also Boyarin 1999; 46ff.; and Berkowitz 2006, 154ff.

130. Most of the contemporary scholarship on rabbinic embryology emphasizes its consonance with Greco-Roman sources, often presented using the language of influence. For example: "The Talmud reflects the influence of Greek, Babylonian and Persian medicine" (Muntner 1977, 13); "There are very few original ideas in the Talmudic corpus on embryology, but it is obvious that the Sages were well aware of the Greek and Roman theories on embryology" (Kottek 1981, 314); "That there was indeed Greek influence on rabbinic embryology is proved beyond any doubt by several passages" (van der Horst 1990, 299); and "many comments dispersed throughout classical rabbinic literature clearly show traces of Aristotelian and Galenic influence" (Levinson 2000b, 123). However, the opposite position has been suggested by Solomon Kagan in *Jewish Medicine* (1952): "Dr. L. Kazenelson stated that the ancient Greek medicine had no influence upon the medical thoughts of the Talmudists during the stages of development of the Talmud, as there was at that time continuous warfare between Judaea and Greece, and no exchange of ideas or knowledge could filter through (cited from Newmyer 1985, 34–35). Satlow (1995, 313) briefly speculates that the lack of traditions about eugenics in the *Yerushalmi* might be due to theology.

131. For example, if ignorance or outright denial, one must read into these traditions a Greco-Roman context that is not evident in the text but supported by other traditions; if adaptation, one might expect, as possibly evident in the *Bavli*'s take on sex determination (or at least one of the *Bavli*'s takes) some mention of male and/or female seed.

132. In midrashic sources about embryology, the recognition of pregnancy is the only topic utterly devoid of any mention of God that I have found. I also remain unconvinced that on this topic midrashic traditions demonstrate consonance with Greco-Roman notions about this, as rabbinic sources place primacy on Gen. 38:24 to establish the recognition of pregnancy at three months.

133. Although I evoke the image of "God's womb" here, I do not think that these traditions overturn—though they do complicate and possibly subvert—masculine imagery of God in rabbinic sources. Verna Harrison (1990 and 1996) has argued for the transcendence of gender vis-à-vis God in Cappadocian authors, but I do not see that forefronted in rabbinic traditions about embryology. I see these traditions more in line with Buell's readings of maternal imagery of God in the writings of Clement of Alexandria (1999, 177–79)—despite the chronological proximity of most of these sources to the Cappadocians. Buell writes, "Clement transposes the key characteristics of a mother—conception, parturition, and lactation—to the divine realm; these maternal characteristics are then appropriated to a divine *father* figure" (1999, 178). On biblical traces of God's womb, see Trible 1978, 31–71.

Chapter 5

I owe the title of this chapter to Elizabeth Clark's references to Augustine's "theology of reproduction" in her article "Vitiated Seeds and Holy Vessels" (1988). See also E. Clark 2001.

1. *Gen. Rab.* 4:7.

2. *Lev. Rab.* 14:9. Cf. *Gen. Rab.* 14:5. And see Aristotle *Generation of Animals* 739b22 (Barnes 1984, 1148). Cf. Clement *Paid.* 1.48.1–2.

3. I focus on rabbinic theories of procreation, by which I specifically mean rabbinic traditions that explicitly describe the creation of the embryo and the care of the fetus—and set out to do so. Rabbinic theories of procreation surfacing in traditions that do not have as their main purpose an explicit interest in explaining the process of coming into being are of less concern, except insofar as they reveal that rabbinic traditions overwhelmingly set forth a "one-seed" theory of procreation, not a "two-seed" theory, as some scholars have suggested.

4. I provide a brief summary of biblical and Greco-Roman sources below, and I also make note of procreation theories in Second Temple Jewish writings.

5. God's involvement in the creation of the embryo also appears in patristic theories of procreation. See Buell 1999, 98–100; and E. Clark 1988 and 2001. See below.

6. Stephen Newmyer, in an article concerned with Greek influence on rabbinic sources in the larger area of medicine, writes, "To point to evidence of Rabbinic familiarity with Greek sources, however, is not to ignore the fundamental ideological differences which separated the two schools. For the Talmudists, disease and health are essentially religious categories, a position which finds scriptural authority in such passages as the Lord's pronouncement (Exod. 15:16), 'I am the Lord your healer'" (1985, 40). He continues, "Nothing could be further from the totally non-religious orientation of Hippocratic medicine" (ibid.). In contrast to this assertion about Hippocratic medicine, Newmyer casts Galen as a possible exception, writing, "For in as much as Galen was an ardent teleologist, seeing God behind all the workings of nature, his science may have been less obnoxious to the Rabbis than might otherwise have been the case" (ibid., 39). However, see Temkin 1991a for Hippocrates among the Christians. Finally, it seems probable that the distinction that I am suggesting between more scientific beliefs evident in Greco-Roman medical sources would not accurately portray everyone's beliefs about generation and that many people still ascribed importance to gods and goddesses of love and fertility. Some evidence for this surfaces in early Christian discourse against Eros, discussed in Pagels 1988, 69–76.

7. See *m. Avot* 3:15.

8. See also *b. Nid.* 30b–31b, which brings together rabbinic traditions about embryology and the creation of the embryo. I begin with *Leviticus Rabbah* 14 instead of the *Bavli* because my emphasis is on Palestinian traditions, its redaction date is set before that of the *Bavli*, and it contextualizes the traditions in *Bavli Niddah* within their broader rabbinic context.

9. Again, the only comparably extensive passage on the creation of the embryo, but less so regarding the care of the fetus, appears in *b. Nid.* 31a, which borrows a number of traditions "originally" appearing in *Leviticus Rabbah* 14, expands other traditions from additional Palestinian compilations, and contributes its own traditions not evident in extant Palestinian compilations. Still, I think that *Leviticus Rabbah* 14 is more extensive and, although this puts me in the middle of debates about the unity of individual chapters as a whole in *Leviticus Rabbah*, ultimately

unified. See below. *B. Nid.* 31a, in contrast, sets forth competing theories of procreation on the same page.

10. See *Mekhilta of R. Ishmael B'shalakh* 8 (Horovitz and Rabin 1970, 143–44); *Mekhilta of R. Shimeon ben Yohai B'shalakh* (Epstein and Melamed n.d., 93–94; Hoffman 1905, 67), and *b. Nid.* 31a.

11. Much of *Lev. Rab.* 14:2, 3, and 4 remains unparalleled in extant Palestinian sources.

12. See Visotzky 2003, 31–41, for the anthological nature of *Leviticus Rabbah*. However, despite some of the broad similarities between *Leviticus Rabbah* 14 and the *Mekhilta of Rabbi Ishmael* (*B'shalakh* 8), many of the embryological traditions in this chapter remain unparalleled in extant tannaitic and amoraic compilations of Palestinian provenance, but they are picked up especially in *Bavli Niddah,* and later in *Midrash Tanhuma.* The lack of parallels precisely of *Lev. Rab.* 14:2–14:6 challenges the notion of *Leviticus Rabbah* 14's anthological character (making no claims to other chapters or the document as a whole), since, stated simply, how does *Leviticus Rabbah* 14 gather materials heretofore unrecorded? One could posit the existence of a nonextant source or sources, as Visotzky does (e.g., 2003, 171 n. 106) but that remains an argument from silence and an assumption of sources that we cannot reproduce and therefore cannot prove. I can only stress that Lev. 12:2, and in particular the meaning of *tazria'* in the context of procreation theories, remains uninterpreted in tannaitic sources and earlier amoraic ones (*Yerushalmi, Genesis Rabbah, Pesikta de Rav Kahana,* and others). The nonembryological traditions in *Leviticus Rabbah* 14, however, have parallels, especially with *Genesis Rabbah,* and those traditions appear to have been placed in *Leviticus Rabbah* with little alteration (e.g., *Lev. Rab.* 14:1, which parallels *Gen. Rab.* 8:1, and *Lev. Rab.* 14:9, which parallels *Gen. Rab.* 14:5 with slight, albeit in my reading, significant modification).

13. Visotzky 2003, 7.

14. Neusner, though he champions the thematic unity and compositional integrity of *Leviticus Rabbah,* repeatedly neglects to connect almost all of the *petihtaot* to the base verse of Lev. 12:2 (1986b, 64 and 306–13). In my reading, the *petihtaot* repeatedly engage with Lev. 12:2, subverting, or at least interpreting away, even the possible biblical reference to female seed. The mention of male offspring in Lev. 12:2 also receives continual focus, and provides one of the reasons for the repeated statement "it is better if it is male" (see below).

15. Cf. *Gen. Rab.* 8:1. In its biblical context Ps. 139:5 is rendered *You have beset me behind and before,* using the Hebrew root ts.r.h.

16. Psalm 139, even if attributed to David, is used by the rabbis in a more general way. See, e.g., *Mekhilta of R. Ishmael* (*B'shalakh* 8); *Mekhilta of R. Shimeon ben Yohai* on Exod. 15:11; *t. Nid.* 4:10; *y. Nid.* 3:3(50d)); *Lev. Rab.* 14:8; and *b. Nid.* 25a and 31a.

17. Job 36:3 in its biblical context is rendered *I will fetch my knowledge from afar, and to my Maker I will ascribe righteousness.*

18. Cf. *Gen. Rab.* 63:5; 17:7 and *b. Sanh.* 39a.

19. See manuscript variants in Margulies 1993, 301–2, which I have incorporated into this translation.

20. Cf. *Eccles. Rab.* 5:11. In this parallel version, the text states that men deposit

a white drop with their wives. See also *Mekhilta of R. Ishmael B'shalakh* 8 (Horovitz and Rabin 1970, 144).

21. Cf. *b. Nid.* 30b. *Lev. Rab.* 31:8 states, "The Holy Blessed One said to the child, all nine months that you were in your mother's womb, who gave light to you, not I?" Cf. *Num. Rab.* 15:7.

22. The statement "and it is better if it is a male" is the repeated conclusion to all of the proems in *Leviticus Rabbah* 14.

23. In contrast to the traditions in *Lev. Rab.* 14:3, which I do see as gynophobic, I don't at this moment see the comparison here between the womb and prison as necessarily gynophobic, but it might be. *B. Nid.* 30b, in contrast, imagines the days in the womb as the happiest in a man's life.

24. Cf. *b. Nid.* 31a.

25. Literally, "so that it does not become a *shefir, shilya,* or *sandal*." See G. Kessler 2001.

26. Visotzky (2003, 23–40) notes some structural affinities between *Leviticus Rabbah* and Hellenistic writings. I set forth some preliminary comparisons between rabbinic traditions and patristic sources later in this chapter.

27. Dean-Jones 1994, 152–53. Dean-Jones notes that Galen was the exception. See Lloyd 1983, 109. Lloyd is quite certain that Galen does not attribute any role to menstrual blood in the fashioning of the embryo. However, Preus suggests that Galen remains undecided on the role of menstrual blood in generation: "He is not sure whether to follow Aristotle's theory that menstrual fluid is the female contribution to generation, or the theory that the fluid found in the vagina during excitation is a female semen, or the theory that there is some third sort of seed" (1977, 84). Buell writes, "Galen holds that women contribute both menstrual blood and seed to the event of conception" (1999, 23 n. 7). Nevertheless, Galen did maintain that menstrual blood was necessary for nutrition, as May writes, "Suffice it to say here that both semens have in his opinion both the material and efficient causes and that the *menstrual blood is merely nutritive*"(1968, 631–32 n. 24, my emphasis).

28. Dean-Jones 1994, 200. She further notes, "Soranus goes so far as to say that the menses derived their appellation of the 'monthly' [*epimanion*], from the fact that they became the food for the embryo, and a sailor's monthly rations were called [*epimania*], *Gyn.* 1.19" (1994, 200 n. 179).

29. Cf. *t. Nid.* 2:1; *y. Sot.* 4:4(19c); and *b. Ket.* 60b. Recall that *Lev. Rab.* 14:3 also refers to the womb as the place of shame and the breasts as a place of honor.

30. Contrast Philo's *Questions and Answers on Genesis* 3.47.

31. Galen, *On the Usefulness of the Parts of the Body*, book 14 (May 1968, 621). On Galen's distinction between Nature and nature, see Boylan 1984, 102. He points out, "What Galen meant by this was that Nature, not merely nature, was involved in generation."

32. King 1998, 33. I have not found any Palestinian rabbinic sources that indicate that the rabbis viewed the man as hotter and the woman as colder.

33. Hebrew: *me'eiha*, "womb" or "intestines."

34. Cf. *b. Bek.* 45a.

35. See Fonrobert 2000, 56–59; and Baker 2002, 34–76, esp. 48–59.

36. Fonrobert, interpreting *Lev. Rab.* 14:4's parallel in *b. Bek.* 45a, perceives the

house as inanimate, but Baker, using different sources that refer to "her house" or "his (the husband's) house," argues for the "animation and dynamism" present in the homology (e.g., 2002, 192 nn. 66 and 67). If *Lev. Rab.* 14:3 and 14:4 are linked, the pregnant woman as house is a precarious construct—one that needs God's constant supervision.

37. It is perhaps significant here that the text brings the metaphor of the woman as a house, but not as a field. See, however, *Lev. Rab.* 15:5.

38. Baker 2002, 57.

39. Or "afterbirth" (Hebrew, *shilya'*).

40. The text concludes, "*And here shall your proud waves be stayed* (38:11). R. Aibu said, [read] 'your proud filth.' Because this fetus goes forth full of filth and all types of smelly things, but everybody hugs him and kisses him. And it is better if it is a male. *When a woman conceives and bears a male* (Lev. 12:2)." I revisit this part of the passage below.

41. Hasan-Rokem 2003, 92.

42. Hebrew: *be'avon*. This statement means that the word "iniquity" is written with an "extra" *vav*.

43. Jesse, David's father. Cf. *b. Shab.* 55b.

44. See Visotzky 1995, 102 n. 30, for manuscript variants.

45. See Margulies's manuscript variants (1993, 308). See also Visotzky 1995, 104. For my purposes here, it is irrelevant whether or not David's parents engaged in coitus interruptus, as Visotkzy maintains, or merely turned away from each other *after* having had sex (Feldman 1995, 133 n. 3; Biale 1992, 44). The text, in either case, clearly asserts that God is credited with inserting the semen into the womb.

46. Margulies 1993, 308–9.

47. See Visotzky 1995, 101–5 and 2003, 165–67. On Ps. 51:7 see Feldman 1995, 83–90 and 98. And see Biale 1992, 44.

48. The Hebrew root *y.h.m.*, however, is itself a somewhat odd choice for Ps. 51:7, only meaning "conceive," or perhaps more accurately "become heated" (recall *Lev. Rab.* 14:3's image of the boiling womb) in Gen. 30:39 and 41 and 31:10 in the context of Jacob's flocks.

49. Visotzky (2003, 11–22) strongly cautions against thematic unity as an organizing principle of *Leviticus Rabbah,* instead favoring an anthological or encyclopedic organization. In contrast, Neusner (e.g., 1985a; 1986b) argues for such unity, although he repeatedly states that *Leviticus Rabbah* 14 seems to lack some crucial connecting points in his translation and brief explanations (1986b, 64 and 306–13). Whether or not *Leviticus Rabbah* as a whole sets forth such unity, I have found that the sections of this chapter are thematically linked enough to at least assume some sort of unity until proven otherwise. If one emphasizes Ps. 51:7, as Visotzky does, then such unity is somewhat challenged, but Ps. 27:10, in my reading, potently retains such unity. The chapter's unity could suggest some sort of redactional intent, but it could also signal the constraints set by the materials that a redactor/collector had at his disposal. (But see my remarks above about the unparalleled *petihtaot*.) For my purposes, which are to read *Leviticus Rabbah* 14 as a whole, the larger question about anthology or integrity is not at issue.

50. And this might be the stronger "anti-Christian" polemic, that God creates

David with Jesse's semen, not "immaculate seed." See Visotzky 1995 and 2003. The polemic, then, is more anti-*Christ*, than anti-Christian per se, especially in light of E. Clark's assertion that both Augustine and Julian, despite their differences, maintained that "God creates all humans from seed" (2001, 26).

51. This statement seems to be in agreement with the notion, prevalent in both the Hippocratic corpus and Aristotle's writings, that a woman is most fertile right after menses. See Dean-Jones 1994, 154, 170–72, and 186, for references. See also Rousselle 1988, 37: "There was no doubt in ancient times that the most fertile phase in the female cycle was that which immediately followed the menstrual period." She later writes, "It is astonishing that throughout the whole of antiquity no one realized that an error had been made in relation to women's fertile period. . . . But Soranus clearly stated that if a woman wanted to avoid pregnancy she must avoid intercourse in the days immediately following her period" (1988, 45).However, Margulies (1993, 308) interprets "after her menstrual period" as "after her immersion," presumably based on R. Yohanan's statement in *b. Nid.* 31b:

And R. Yitzhak said in the name of R. Ami (Asi), "A woman becomes pregnant only near her menstrual period, as it is said, *Behold, I was brought forth in iniquity* (Ps. 51:7)." But R. Yohanan said "[a woman becomes pregnant only] after her ritual immersion, as it is said, *And in cleansing [uvehet'] did my mother conceive me* (Ps. 51:7). What verse teaches that this *het'* means "cleansing"? *And he shall cleanse [vehite'] the house* (Lev. 14:52). And we translate, "And he shall cleanse the house." And if you want to, learn it from this verse, *You shall cleanse me (tehat'eni) with hyssop and I shall be pure* (Ps. 51: 9).

Even in the *Bavli* text, the most fertile period remains disputed. R. Yohanan's view is championed by modern interpreters for two reasons: first, it comes closer to contemporary understanding that conception often occurs at "mid-cycle." Second, it justifies the rabbinic addition of "white days"—additional days after menstruation and before immersion—that a woman must wait until she is sexually permitted to her husband. See Meacham 1999a, 28–32. Nonetheless, the tradition in *Leviticus Rabbah* explicitly states "after or near menstruation," with no mention of ritual immersion. The *Bavli* text supports that the simple reading of "after or near menstruation" is appropriate, for if "after immersion" were meant, there would be no reason for R. Yohanan's opinion to be stated. See Feldman 1995, 86–87 and 247.

52. Contrast, possibly, *Lev. Rab.* 14:9, discussed below. *Lev. Rab.* 14:5 appears exceptional in its explicit connection between menstruation and sin. See Fonrobert 2000 for a more comprehensive survey of menstrual (im)purity in rabbinic literature, which does not, however, include this text or a similar tradition in *b. Nid.* 31b. See also Klawans 2000, which discusses the rabbinic compartmentalization of ritual and moral impurity in tannaitic sources.

53. Dean-Jones writes that the most favorable time for conception "was just after menstruation when the womb would be empty and the seed would not be flushed out by the flow of blood" (1994, 170–71).

54. Margulies 1993, 309. Only secondarily can one inquire about this tradition's possible relation to "original sin" and its categorization as "anti-Christian polemic."

55. Margulies notes that the Oxford manuscript reads "embryo" (1993, 309).

56. See *b. Nid.* 9a.

57. Translated according to how it will be midrashically understood. The verse is usually translated, *You measure my rising up and lying down; You are acquainted with all my ways.* Cf. *b. Nid.* 31a. See also the interpretations of Num. 23:10 in *Gen. Rab.* 94:9 and *b. Nid.* 31a.

58. See Margulies's notes (1993, 309–10) on the peculiarity of the question "How does R. Yohanan interpret this word?" Some manuscripts attribute the next statement to R. Shimeon ben Lakish. I follow Margulies's text.

59. God is not specifically mentioned as the subject of this verb but God is clearly implied by the context, both that of the biblical verse, which speaks of God's "knowing"/"scattering," and the context provided from the previous sections of *Leviticus Rabbah*. The partial parallel to this tradition in *b. Nid.* 31a makes explicit God's involvement.

60. The relationship between this text and *y. Kel.* 8:3(31c), discussed below, should not be overlooked. Each of the three contributions that a man makes by way of his semen—the marrow, bones, and sinews—are here also attributed to the father. Thus in the end, God usurps the father's contributions to the embryo and it is God who ultimately "creates" the marrow, bones, and tendons. The Oxford manuscript does mention that a drop is for flesh (*basar*), which the "three partners" texts list among the mother's contributions.

61. See van der Horst 1990, 290ff.; Lloyd 1983; Dean-Jones 1994, 161ff.; Preus 1977, 70ff.; and Boylan 1984 and 1986. On pangenesis in rabbinic sources, see Kottek 1981, 304, and Preuss 1978, 387, both citing *b. Hull.* 69a. Preuss also notes a tradition in the *Bavli* that links semen and the brain (1978, 203).

62. Dean-Jones cites Aristotle: "Our own statement therefore must be the opposite of what the early people said. They said the semen is that which was drawn from the whole of the body; we are going to say the semen is that whose nature is to be distributed to the whole of the body" (1994, 194, quoting *Generation of Animals* 725a21–24).

63. See, e.g., van der Horst 1990, 293–94; Preus 1977, 78ff.; and Dean-Jones 1994, 60–61. See also Buell 1999, 154ff., which notes the transformation of blood into milk and semen in the writings of Clement.

64. *Lev. Rab.* 14:7 and 14:8 were discussed in the previous chapter. *Lev. Rab.* 14:8 includes women in its discussion about the sex of the offspring, but in contrast to the *Bavli* parallels, there is no explicit mention of the woman emitting seed. Furthermore, I maintain some distinction between rabbinic traditions about sex determination and the creation of the embryo. Rabbinic sources in general and *Lev. Rab.* 14:8 in particular grant women involvement in sex determination seen as a hereditary aspect, but this does not mean that they actively contribute to the creation of the embryo.

65. I have drawn from manuscript variants and later parallels for this puzzling passage. See Margulies's notes (1993, 316–17). Specifically, I have kept the reading preserved in the London manuscript, which provides Margulies's foundational text, reconstructed from his variants but not presented in his printed text. For example, I have translated that the menstrual blood goes forth "from its source" not "to its source" as Margulies suggests in his printed version.

66. Hebrew: *notsar,* "created"/"formed." Here the actual creation of the embryo is being discussed.

67. Cf. Aristotle, *Generation of Animals* 739b22 (Barnes 1984, 1148): "When the material secreted by the female in the uterus has been fixed by the semen of the male (this acts in the same way as rennet acts upon milk, for rennet is a kind of milk containing vital heat, which brings into one mass and fixes the similar material, and the relation of the semen to the menstrual blood is the same, milk and the menstrual blood being of the same nature)." See Dean-Jones 1994, 188, for problems with Aristotle's use of this analogy and his overall theory of generation.

68. See, e.g., Feldman 1995, 133; Kottek 1981, 300–304; and Biale 1992, 55–56. Cf. *Gen. Rab.* 14:5. At first glance, this tradition seems to have much in common with Aristotle's theory of generation, especially since it uses the metaphor of a curdling agent. However, it seems that this tradition is more in line with what eventually has come to be attributed to Aristotle, but is not, strictly speaking Aristotle's own theory. According to Aristotle, the woman's menstrual blood is indeed less active than the man's semen, but it is not totally passive in generation. See Dean-Jones 1994, 184–99. In *Lev. Rab.* 14:9 the woman's blood seems totally passive in the creation of the embryo—albeit moving and shaking. Furthermore, we do not know from this tradition if the blood continues to be useful during gestation, as it is in both Hippocratic sources and Aristotle's writings, but *Leviticus Rabbah* 14 does not suggest such contribution to fetal development elsewhere.

69. It should also be noted that Job 10:10–13 makes no mention of blood out of which the embryo is curdled.

70. The significance of this reading will become more apparent in the following sections of this chapter. However, since I return to it repeatedly, I thought it best mentioned in the text and not relegated to a footnote. My alternative understanding of *Lev. Rab.* 14:9 is in contrast to those proposed by Kottek (1981, 301) and Biale (1992, 55–56). Both Kottek's and Biale's works have their merits. Kottek translates the text, working from the standard (Vilna) edition, with its complexity intact. Although Biale does not contextualize *Lev. Rab.* 14:9 among other traditions in *Leviticus Rabbah* 14, he does situate it within the rabbinic discourse of *niddah*. However, he begins with the assumption that, "Following certain strands of ancient medicine, the rabbis held that menstrual blood is necessary for conception" (1992, 55). But the rest of *Leviticus Rabbah* 14 never explicitly suggests that blood contributes to the creation of the embryo; to the contrary, it resists or denies such a notion. (I find the appeal to menstrual blood in the creation of the embryo and the development of the fetus quite undersupported not only in *Leviticus Rabbah* 14, but in rabbinic literature in its entirety.) My claim is not that I have the right reading—this tradition is far too obscure to make any such claim for either reading—but that this alternative reading should be explored as a possibility. It has the distinct advantage of working within the evidence of *Leviticus Rabbah* 14. Nevertheless, I remain open to the possibility that *Leviticus Rabbah* 14 presents opposing interpretations, and I do not want to succumb to the disadvantageous strategy of imposing absolute consistency on the chapter, despite my claim for an uncanny degree of thematic unity. Finally, the *mashal* that follows this difficult statement could be seen as undercutting my alternative reading. I think that this can be explained by *Lev. Rab.*

14:9's drawing from *Gen. Rab.* 14:5, where the parallel tradition appears without this obscure statement. In other words, it appears that the redactor of *Leviticus Rabbah* added the statement about a woman's womb being full of blood, etc., thus altering it slightly to fit its context, but otherwise maintained the tradition as it was presented in *Gen. Rab.* 14:5.

71. The parallel in *Gen. Rab.* 14:5 cites Job 10:12 at the end of the passage.

72. M. Stol writes, "To put it in the words of a mother in the Book of Maccabees, reassuring her sons about the reality of a future Resurrection: 'I do not know how you came to be in my womb. It was not I who gave you spirit and life, nor did I determine the order of the elements of each of you. Surely, then, the Creator of the Universe, Who shaped man's coming into being and fathomed the fashioning of everything, with mercy will restore spirit and life to you' (2 Macc. 7:22–3). Indeed, God's ability to make man born is the guarantee that He equally has the power to resurrect him" (2000a, 16).

73. *Lev. Rab.* 14:1 and *Gen. Rab.* 8:1 both begin by reading Ps. 139:5 as alluding to this world and the next, a topic that returns in *Lev. Rab.* 14:9.

74. See Visotzky 2003, 20–22 and 24 n. 3, for a discussion of the "messianic peroration." Visotzky points out that a sufficient number of the chapters of *Leviticus Rabbah* lack a messianic flourish to doubt its centrality to the redaction of the document. Nevertheless, he lists chapter 14 as one of the chapters that does contain such a flourish, albeit a short one. I suggest that *Lev. Rab.* 14:9, with its concern about the future and the process of resurrection is a rather lengthy messianic peroration, which begins with the debate between Beit Hillel and Beit Shammai and then resumes with the end of the passage.

75. Some patristic sources use Isa. 66:7 to establish Mary's virginity *in partu*. See Hunter 2007, 174; and see Methodius's *Oration on Simeon and Anna*, though the authorship of this is disputed.

76. *Y. Kel.* 8:3(31c) is not about the creation of the embryo but about inherited traits. Furthermore, it does not use the language of "seeds." See below.

77. *Genesis Rabbah* records a number of traditions that remain content, like biblical sources, to attribute pregnancy only to God, leaving human contributions to inference. See below.

78. Contrast *b. Yev.* 98a, which mentions that twin brothers originate from one drop. See Meacham 1992. See Chapter 3 for discussion of *Gen. Rab.* 63:8.

79. The context of this text is that Reuben differs from Jacob even though he was his firstborn because Jacob did not have a nocturnal emission until he was eighty. However, as we've just seen, Jacob was also "the first drop." The text simultaneously seems to affirm both the differences and similarities between Jacob and Reuben.

80. Hebrew: *metipah kedusha*. For additional traditions that imply the role of male seed in procreation, without any mention of female seed, see *Gen. Rab.* 45:5 and *Gen. Rab.* 53:6. See also *y. Yev.* 9:3, which implies that offspring of an Amonite convert come from an "unfit drop"/*metipah pesulah*. See also *b. Avod. Zar.* 20a.

81. Cf. *Lev. Rab.* 18:1 and 27:9; *Eccles. Rab.* 12:1; and *b. Avod. Zar.* 20a. And see *Avot d'Rabbi Natan* 16. For a reading that explores the concept of "wasted seed" in rabbinic sources, see Satlow 1994.

82. *M. Avot*'s mention of seed as a "fetid drop" answers the question "From where do we come?" It does not answer the question "How do we come from a fetid drop?" In *Gen. Rab.* 63:8, R. Halfota answers the question "Why was Esau born first?" not "How did Esau come to be?" *Gen. Rab.* 99:6 addresses a question of scriptural exegesis, asking what it might mean that Reuben is called Jacob's "might and the beginning of his strength," and, finally, *Gen. Rab.* 46:2 answers why Abraham was circumcised at the age of ninety-nine.

83. This is not to claim that the rabbis never discuss procreation and pregnancy without mentioning God. In addition to the above traditions, see, e.g., *Gen. Rab.* 45:4, 51:9, 85:5, and 94:9. However, when the rabbis *theorize* procreation, when they imagine, reflect upon, and describe the process of coming into being, the creation of the embryo and the care of the fetus, they consistently invoke God.

84. Delaney points out that the meaning of the male role in procreation is not self-evident. She writes, "it may be (1) that in intercourse the male is thought to open the path for a fetus that comes by other means; (2) that intercourse stops menstruation, which allows for (1); or that the product of ejaculation (3) feeds the fetus or (4) contributes in some other way to its formation" (1991, 11).

85. *Mekhilta of R. Ishmael B'shalakh* 8 (Horovitz and Rabin 1970, 144). Cf. *Mekhilta of R. Shimeon ben Yohai*. Both *Mekhilta*s attach this tradition to Exod. 15:11, *Who is like you, God, among the gods, glorious in holiness, fearful in praises, doing wonders,* but *Mekhilta of R. Ishmael* places it under interpretations of "fearful in praises" and *Mekhilta of R. Shimeon ben Yohai* at "doing wonders." See Chapter 4 for further discussion of this tradition. *Midrash Tanhuma* (*Tazria'* 2) picks up these traditions in the context of interpreting Lev. 12:2. See *b. Nid.* 31a, where the motif of contrasting human and divine powers of procreation also appears. See also *b. Ber.* 10a and *b. Meg.* 14a.

86. I discuss rabbinic traditions that use agricultural imagery to describe procreation below.

87. Rabbinic traditions consistently maintain that God grants children, but I focus on traditions that more specifically suggest that God gives "conception," or pregnancy. For examples of the former, see *Mekhilta of R. Ishmael B'shalakh* 8 (Horovitz and Rabin 1970, 143), interpreting *Sons/children are an inheritance of the Lord* (Ps. 127:3); *Gen. Rab.* 53:8, 71:1, and 71:2; *Pesikta de Rav Kahana* 20:1; and *Ruth Rab.* 7:14.

88. Frymer-Kensky discusses Num. 5:28 in its biblical context, pointing out, "Conception is the reward for innocence, either in the sense that the woman is capable of bearing seed . . . or that she is being rewarded for her innocence. We cannot discard the further possibility that the waters themselves, coming from the sacred realm (holy water, with dust from the tabernacle floor) and bearing the name of God, *were believed to function as an impregnating force, and that the woman was believed to become pregnant as a direct result of this trial*" (1999b, 467, emphasis added). She also writes, "There is no explicit statement about 'divine conception' in the Old Testament. It appears, however, in post-biblical literature. . . . It is possible that this idea, which is known from other Near Eastern religions, was not considered impossible in Israel, and that a reflection of this idea is seen in the 'conception' of the innocent woman" (1999b, 473). It also seems possible that *Gen. Rab.* 53:6, if not Gen. 21:1–2 and similar biblical verses, at least point to the idea of "divine conception."

89. See also *Pesikta Rabbati* 42:2: "Sarah said, *Behold, God has prevented me from giving birth* (Gen. 16:2). The Holy Blessed One said [to Sarah], 'You have benefitted yourself. By your life, you said, *God has prevented me from giving birth,* in the same language, I will visit you [with pregnancy]' . . . as scripture states, *And God visited Sarah . . . and she became pregnant and gave birth* (Gen. 21:1–2)." Buell writes about Clement's mention of "angels who assist at procreation," explaining, "Clement locates the cause of barrenness in neither human partner but in the absence of angelic intervention, and the source of desire for intercourse to angels. This etiology emphatically underscores a view of procreation as a suprahuman endeavor" (1999, 25–26).

90. The midrash that immediately follows, interpreting Gen. 21:2 does mention male seed, "this teaches that she did not steal seed from another." But this interpretation seeks to understand the mention of "to Abraham" (which should be redundant) in Gen. 21:2, and perhaps also indicates the rabbis anxiety about Abraham's advanced age at the time of Isaac's conception. See Chapter 4 for further discussion. I see the two traditions not as mutually exclusive or even necessarily contradictory, but as a point of productive tension in rabbinic theorizing of procreation, which, consistent with *Leviticus Rabbah* 14, brings together male seed and God. For my purposes here, I let the first statement attributed to R. Yehudah stand on its own, teaching that God in God's glory alone gave Sarah pregnancy, which is supported by the later text in *Pesikta Rabbati,* cited in the previous note, and by the later parallel version of this text in *Midrash Sekhel Tov,* cited in Theodor's notes (Theodor and Albeck 1965, 560).

91. See Chapter 4 for further discussion of this tradition. Other rabbinic traditions use the Hebrew root *p.k.d.,* which in this context means "to be visited so as to conceive," and I think even when God is not explicitly mentioned, God's role is implied because of the allusion to Gen. 21:1 and 1 Sam. 2:21. See, e.g., *Sifre Numbers, Naso*; and *Gen. Rab.* 53:6, 53:8, 56:2, 60:13, 71:1–2, 72:6, and 73:1.

92. Contrast *y. Kel.* 8:3(31c), *b. Nid.* 31a, and *Eccles. Rab.* 5:10, discussed below.

93. *Gen. Rab.* 73:4. Cf. *b. Tan.* 2a; *b. Sanh.* 113a; and *Deut. Rab.* 7:6. See also *b. Bek.* 45a.

94. See also *Mekhilta of R. Ishmael* (*B'shalakh* 8) Horovitz (1970: 143–44); and *Mekhilta of R. Shimeon bar Yohai* (*B'shalakh* 8).

95. See Delaney 1986, 1991, 8–16, and 1998a, 137–39; E. Martin 1991; and Franklin 1997, 17–72 and 187–90.

96. Cf. *Gen. Rab.* 87:14 and *b. Hull.* 79a for more on mules' ears.

97. Menstrual blood is implied because, to state the obvious, men also bleed.

98. Later manuscripts of *Leviticus Rabbah* apparently append the statement "The man emits the white and the woman emits the red, and from their the embryo is formed/created." See Margulies's variants (1993, 314).

99. Hebrew: *b'adam.* The context within which this tradition appears in the *Bavli* indicates that the creation of the embryo is meant. *Eccles. Rab.* 5:10 reads, "At the time the embryo (*valad*) is formed/created (*notsar*) in its mother's womb, there are three partners in him/it."

100. Just before this tradition, the *Bavli* also mentions that sexual intercourse

is permitted during the last trimester of pregnancy, because from it, the fetus is made white (*meluvan*).

101. Others translate (not incorrectly) as "brain matter." The "marrow that is in his head" is unique to the *Bavli*.

102. The printed version of *Bavli Niddah* does not include blood as one of the contributions from the mother. However, Vatican MS 111 and Munich MS 95 both include blood. Also lacking in the printed version is God's contribution of the *nefesh*. *Gen. Rab.* 14:9 discusses five names for "breath of life." It states, "*Nefesh*: this is the blood, [as it is said], *For the blood is the life* [*nefesh*] (Deut. 12:23)," making it interesting that both the blood and the *nefesh* are not mentioned here.

103. Cf. *Lev. Rab.* 23:12, discussed in Chapter 4.

104. The phrase "our rabbis taught" indicates that the *Bavli* presents this tradition as a *baraita*, a tannaitic statement not found in the Mishnah. However, *Sifra Qedoshim* 1:7 (Weiss 1862, 86d), which is the only extant tannaitic parallel, simply states, in the context of why one should honor one's parents and God, "the three of them are partners in him." Cf. *Mekhilta of R. Ishmael Bahodesh* 8 (Horovitz and Rabin 1970, 231) for a tannaitic parallel that does not mention that the three of them are partners in him. Cf. *y. Kid.* 1:7(61b) and *b. Kid.* 30b.

105. Palestinian traditions hardly use either word at all; the *Bavli* uses the words only in the context of procreation, most of which occur in the oft-cited tradition about sex determination (see Chapter 4 for citations). *Eccles. Rab.* 5:10 presents an even more expanded version of the "three partners" tradition. However, the dating of *Ecclesiastes Rabbah* is disputed, being possibly as late as the eighth century CE or, according to Hirshman, redacted during the sixth or seventh century (Strack and Stemberger 1996, 318). Regardless of the dating of the document, parallels between the *Bavli* and *Ecclesiastes Rabbah*, which is what we have in 5:10, are, according to Strack and Stemberger (1996, 317), later additions. Even if *Ecclesiastes Rabbah*'s borrowing of *Bavli* material is not adopted as an overarching principle, *Eccles. Rab.* 5:10 is best seen as drawing from *b. Nid.* 31a because the language used is consistent with the *Bavli* and is lacking in all of Palestinian rabbinic literature.

106. Note that the *Bavli* does not explicitly cite Lev. 12:2 in connection with this passage, but only cites that verse when it discusses sex determination.

107. The mention of a woman "emitting first," also appearing first in the *Bavli*, is concerned with sex determination, which I consider distinct from the creation of the embryo. Whether the "three partners" tradition should be understood as setting forth a notion of female seed is discussed below.

108. One other statement on *b. Nid.* 31a might suggest that both men and women "seed" the embryo, but it is less explicit: "If a man puts different seeds in a bed each grows in the manner of its own particular species, but the Holy Blessed One creates the embryo in the woman's womb in such a manner that all grow into one and the same kind." One could read into the second part of this passage mention of "two seeds," but I don't think the comparison needs to work quite that closely. Urbach points out that "the analogy seeks to emphasize the difference between man the sower and the Holy One, blessed be He, who forms a figure [the embryo]" (1987, 233–34). This tradition is attributed to the Palestinian tanna R. Yosi the Galilean, but I have not found a parallel in Palestinian sources.

109. See *b. Nid.* 16b, where the angel appointed over conception delivers the "drop" before God and God decrees what will be of this drop: rich or poor, strong or weak, wise or foolish, and so on. And see *b. Yev.* 78a, *b. Sot.* 27a, and *b. Sanh.* 36b, which distinguish between offspring from a "fit" and "unfit" drop. See also *b. Yev.* 98a and *b. Nid.* 27a. And see *b. Nid.* 9a, which states that "although semen is impure, the man created from it is pure." In some medieval versions of the tradition about the angel appointed over conception that delivers the drop to God (*b. Nid.* 16b), the "drop" is a mixture of two seeds (e.g., *Seder Yetsirat Ha-Valad*, Jellinek 1967, 1:156, constrast ibid., 1:153, and *Mid. Tanhuma* [*Pekudei* 3]) but I do not find this supported in the *Bavli*. See Meacham 1992, 145.

110. See, e.g., Feldman 1995, 132; Kottek 1981, 301–4; van der Horst 1991; Satlow 1994, 158–59; and Boyarin 1997b, 9. Most of these authors examine other rabbinic traditions about the creation of the embryo, mentioning *Lev. Rab.* 14:9 (similarly decontextualized) and other traditions in the *Bavli*, but except for the often-cited *Bavli* tradition about sex determination, which also appears in *b. Nid.* 31a, the other traditions about the creation of the embryo in *b. Nid.* 31a have not been considered.

111. It also has much in common with *Mekhilta of Rabbi Ishmael* (*B'shalakh* 8) in that it consistently contrasts humanity and God's powers to (pro)create.

112. Though it does not suggest the other option presented in *Lev. Rab.* 14:6, that all the semen is used. The *Bavli* also only explicitly invokes God in David's being "winnowed" from the finest part of "the drop," perhaps bringing together what appear as separate traditions in *Lev. Rab.* 14:5 and 14:6. But God's involvement is implied via Ps. 139:3.

113. Cf. *Lev. Rab.* 14:3. The *Bavli* cites this as an interpretation of Job 9:10, *Who does great things past finding out and wonders without number?*

114. See also *b. Meg.* 14a, "There is no artist/creator [*tsayyar*] like our God. A person creates a shape on the side of a wall but cannot imbue it with *ruah* and *neshamah,* innards or intestines. But the Holy Blessed One creates a shape within a shape and places in it *ruah* and *neshamah,* innards and intestines." Cf. *b. Ber.* 10a.

115. See Satlow 1994, 159; and Boyarin 1997b, 9. Feldman (1995, 132–33), Kottek (1981, 300–304), and van der Horst (1990, 300–301) acknowledge that this is not the only theory of procreation presented in rabbinic sources.

116. This is also accurate for the "three partners" tradition in *y. Kel.* 8:3(31c).

117. See *Lev. Rab.* 23:12. In the previous chapter I noted that *Bavli* traditions reflect more of an openness to human influence in sex determination, and the same could be said of the "three partners" tradition. This is not surprising since these two traditions have much in common, and I tend to think that the "three partners" tradition is influenced by the one about sex determination—not the other way around.

118. See also *Mekhilta of Rabbi Ishmael* (*B'shalakh* 8), discussed above.

119. Hoffman 1996, 172; and Boyarin 1997a, 65.

120. Levinson 2000b, 124 n. 31. See also Urbach 1975, 218. Boyarin (1997b, 9) also considers God's roles.

121. All the more the rabbis do not represent contemporary feminist beliefs about gender and reproduction.

122. Boylan (1984) mentions a third theory of generation in antiquity, which he calls the "furrowed field theory." This theory seems, in pre-Socratic writers, to attribute *all* "relevant causes for generation" to the male or the "most important elements" of generation to the male (Boylan 1984, 85). This is how some post-Aristotelian authors understand Aristotle's own "one-seed" theory, but it need not be the only way that Aristotle's theory of generation is understood. In this context, I consider the "furrowed field theory" as a one-seed theory.

123. This summary is by no means exhaustive, and by necessity a number of nuances and details are obscured. I focus on theories as articulated in the Hippocratic corpus, Aristotle, and Galen. For theories of the pre-Socratic writers, see, for example, Needham 1934, 27–31; Preus 1977; Lloyd 1983, 87–88; Boylan 1984; Dean-Jones 1994, 148–52. For scholarship on Greco-Roman theories of generation, see, for example, Needham 1934; Preus 1977; Horowitz 1976; Lonie 1981; Lloyd 1983; Boylan 1984 and 1986; R. Smith 1988; Hanson 1992; Dean-Jones 1994; Harlow 1999; and Buell 1999, 21–31. Additional references may be found in each of these sources. For scholarship on rabbinic theories of procreation, see, e.g., Feldman 1995, 132–40; Kottek 1981, 300–304; van der Horst 1990; Levinson 2000b, 120–25; and Stol 2000a, 5–16. Pieter van der Horst offers the most comprehensive comparison of Greco-Roman, rabbinic, and New Testament theories. See also Satlow 1994, 157–59, and Boyarin 1997b, 9, for brief remarks.

124. For the equality, or exactness of the two seeds, see Boylan 1984, 52; and Lloyd 1983, 92.

125. See Lloyd 1983, 88–94, for differences between this view as set forth in the Hippocratic embryological treatises and the treatise *On Regimen*. However, Lloyd concludes, "Both treatises maintain that there is, overall, not just a general similarity, but a precise equality in the contributions of each of the two parents" (92).

126. Aristotle appears to maintain that women also produce seed in some of his writings, especially in *History of Animals*, book 10. However, it remains unclear whether this section is a later interpolation or an earlier work of Aristotle that preserved his own earlier opinion. See Dean-Jones 1994, 14–15. She places *History of Animals* 10 within the Hippocratic corpus. On the complexities of Aristotle's theory, see also Boylan 1984 and 1986 and Preus 1977.

127. On Galen's syncretism, see Preus 1977; Lloyd 1983; Boylan 1984 and 1986; Cadden 1993; and Singer 2001.

128. Lloyd 1983, 110.

129. Boylan 1986, 59. However, Galen does not think that menstrual blood in and of itself contributes to the creation of the embryo, but rather it supplies nutriment (May 1968, 632 n. 24; Lloyd 1983 109). Preus (1977, 84) writes, "The second book of *On Seed* examines the female seed, and here Galen has problems which he does not fully resolve. He is not sure whether to follow Aristotle's theory that menstrual fluid is the female contribution to generation, or the theory that the fluid found in the vagina during excitation is a female semen, or the theory that there is some third sort of seed." Preus points out, "But the theory that the ovaries produce the female seed, which is impelled to the womb at the time of copulation—as it were, a female ejaculation—is not consonant with the theory that the menstrual fluid is the female seed."

130. It is not clear to me whether this view, which eclipses all contributions of the woman—even lesser ones—should be seen as taking Aristotle's one-seed theory to its "logical" extreme, or if it is a return to, or merely continuation of, pre-Socratic theories where the woman is the passive "woman/field" planted by the man/seed. See Preus 1977 and Boylan 1984.

131. See Noonan 1965, 89, for a brief overview and his connection of this extreme one-seed theory (= "furrowed field theory"?) to the Stoics and Soranus. See also Harlow 1998, 160: "This meant [for Soranus] that female seed could not be useful in the reproductive process and that, as in Aristotle's theory, the male seed must be the author of generation. Soranus is hazy as to any female contribution other than providing a vessel and nourishment for the foetus. In some cases he implies that menstrual blood is analogous to male semen and in others plays down its role, going so far as to argue that it might be harmful to health."

132. See Lloyd 1983, 86–94; and Dean-Jones 1994.

133. Dean-Jones 1994, 178. Although Lloyd frames his discussion about "two-seed" theories of generation as alternative theories that challenge the notion of utter subordination of women in Greco-Roman culture, he too reiterates that the proponents of such a theory were not motivated by primarily ideological concerns (1983, 94 and 107). Rabbinic traditions examined in the previous chapter did not expound upon children resembling their mothers.

134. See above for my alternative reading of *Lev. Rab.* 14:9. And see further, below.

135. See van der Horst 1990, 300–301, for the mixture of Aristotelian and Hippocratic theories in the "three partners" tradition. See note 129 on Galen's confusion about women's contribution.

136. See note 131 above. Soranus is still three to four centuries removed from most of the rabbinic traditions examined here, if dated according to the redaction of compilations. On the difficulty in fixing Aristotle's theory about the male contribution only to "efficient cause," however, see Boylan 1984.

137. See Chapter 4. Buell (1999, 172–77) discusses Clement's writings about the production of semen from blood.

138. Situating rabbinic traditions among Greco-Roman medical theories, assuming they represent Greco-Roman culture as a whole, forecloses upon the possibility that people continued to believe in the usefulness or necessity of gods and goddesses in procreation. If, in nonelite, nonmedical discourse, people still maintained a belief in and worshipped such deities, the distinction that I am suggesting does not speak for the cultures "at large." I have, however, maintained and perhaps further perpetuated a methodological flaw in my own reliance on so-called medical sources *alone* for rabbinic context. Perhaps others, more qualified than I, will be able to further situate rabbinic traditions about procreation among Greco-Roman nonmedical sources.

139. See also Eccles. 11:5 and Job 31:15. That God fashions the embryo in the womb is also expressed in Isa. 44:2 and 24 and 49:5; and Jer. 1:5.

140. See Satlow 1994, 157. See Frymer-Kensky 1999a, 295 and 301, on the general lack of information about sex and sexuality in the Hebrew Bible.

141. Milgrom (1991, 743–44) and Meacham (1999a, 25–28) suggest that Leviticus 12 and 15 contain evidence of a "two-seed" theory of conception. See below.

142. Perhaps in keeping with its ancient Near Eastern context, the more common way to frame this topic is to refer to the biblical God's roles in fertility. See, e.g., Frymer-Kensky 1992.

143. In the Hebrew Bible, barrenness is always connected to women's infertility. See *b. Yev.* 64a for rabbinic traditions about the barrenness of the patriarchs, and see *Num. Rab.* 10:5. On the motif of barrenness in the Hebrew Bible, see Callaway 1986 and Frymer-Kensky 1992, who also cites ancient Near Eastern traditions.

144. 1 Sam. 1:5 states that God closed Hannah's womb. 1 Sam. 2:20 states that "God visited Hannah." Sarah, Rebekah, Rachel, and Manoah's wife are all called barren (*'aqarah*). None of the verses listed above explicitly mentions that the husband "went into her," and only 1 Sam. 1:19 states that Elkanah "knew his wife."

145. *B. Bab. Kam.* 92a extends this to include even the hens in his household, which did not lay eggs.

146. See Pardes 1992, 39–59. Cf. Gen. 4:25.

147. There are some exceptions, for example, Gen. 16:4, where Abram "goes into Hagar and she becomes pregnant." Yet according to *Gen. Rab.* 45:5, God is responsible for Hagar's pregnancy. Nor is God invoked when Lot's daughters "lay with their father" (Gen. 19:32ff.) or when David "lay with" Batsheva (2 Sam. 11:4 and 12:24) or when Tamar becomes pregnant (Gen. 38:18). Genealogies in the Hebrew Bible do not mention God. However, they are concerned with lineage/heredity, not theorizing procreation. This does not mean that they do not have the cumulative effect of erasing women, by and large, from genealogy, and thus possibly setting forth a procreation theory that totally excludes women.

148. Gen. 38:8–9 comes closest. There, *zera'* ("offspring" or "seed") is clearly linked to pregnancy, but the phrase *shikhvat zera'* is not used. Furthermore, the verse states *Onan veshihet artsah*, which is usually understood as "Onan spilled/wasted his seed/semen on the ground." See *Gen. Rab.* 85:5 and cf. *Gen. Rab.* 26:4. However, "his seed/semen" is read into the verse. This may be a correct interpretation, but it is significant that it relies on filling in a textual lack. Cf. Gen. 6:12, where the verse makes the lack in Gen. 38:9 all the more apparent: *For all flesh had corrupted (hishhit) its way (darko) upon the earth*. Stol writes, "In Hebrew, the word 'seed' (*zera'*) is primarily the seed of plants, particularly of cultivated crops sown by the farmer. It can also stand for 'offspring,' but it seldom denotes the semen of man. A notable exception in which *zera'* means 'semen' occurs in Genesis 38:9 when Onan spills his 'seed' on the ground. Another can be found in the laws of purity (Leviticus 15:16). Very often, 'seed' in the Hebrew Bible stands for 'offspring'" (2000a, 4). In fact, Lev. 15:16 uses *shikhvat zera'*, not *zera'*, and it seems plausible that the use of *zera'* in Gen. 38:9 could mean "offspring " in both occurrences. Stol further writes, "The Akkadian word for seed (*zeru*) hardly ever means 'semen'" (ibid). Robert Alter, in contrast, translates biblical uses of *zera'* as seed, explaining, "this is thought of both figuratively and in the most concretely physical way" (1983, 6). However, when the same word is used attached to women, Alter translates as "offspring"; for example, he translates Gen. 24:60, "may your offspring take the gates of its foes" (1983, 54). See also Gen. 3:15 and 4:25 and 16:10.

149. In the Bible, semen and menstrual blood, along with other bodily discharges from men and women, are linked only in the context of impurity (Leviticus

15). See Eilberg-Schwartz 1990, 177–94. One may read into Leviticus 15 a concern about fluids that are involved in procreation, but they are not explicitly named as such in the text. See Meacham 1999a, 25–28, for such an interpretation.

150. Although the grammatically active attribution of woman's seed in Lev. 12:2 has vexed interpreters for generations, the active grammatical structure of *vatahar vateled* has received little notice. Translating *vatahar* as "conceives" further eclipses such action since conception is still commonly thought to be passive. See E. Martin 1991.

151. I rely on van der Horst (1990) and Satlow (1994, 156–58) for sources, leaving open the possibility that other sources attribute the creation of the embryo to male seed and God. For example, Philo, interpreting Exod. 21:22–25, writes, "But if the child which was conceived had assumed a distinct shape in all its parts, having received all its proper connective and distinctive qualities, he shall die; for such a creature as that is a man, whom he has slain while still in the workshop of nature [God], who had not thought it as yet a proper time to produce him to the light, but had kept him like a statue lying in a sculptor's workshop, requiring nothing more than to be realeased and sent out into the world" (*De specialibus legibus* III.108–9). On Philo's conflation of nature and God, see Buell 1999, 100 n. 9.

152. Satlow 1994, 157–58; van der Horst 1990, 297–99. For a discussion about Greco-Roman procreation theories in the context of "gnostic" sources, see R. Smith 1988.

153. Van der Horst 1990, 298. He also cites 1 Enoch 5:14 (van der Horst 1990, 297).

154. Ibid., 298, citing *Quaestiones ad Genesim* 3.47, the context of which is about why men are circumcised. Van der Horst also cites *On the Creation of the World* 132, "(The menstural blood) too is said by physical scientists to be the bodily substance of embryos" (298). See also Buell 1999, 24 n. 7. Satlow's point is that despite the primacy given to semen in Philo's theories, it remains of "low order," according to *On the Creation of the World* 67 (1994, 158).

155. See van der Horst 1990, Satlow 1994, and Boyarin 1997b, 9.

156. Recall that according to *Lev. Rab.* 14:3 God raises the blood to the breasts, away from the fetus, throughout pregnancy. *Lev. Rab.* 14:3 also records a tradition that again suggests that God protects the fetus in not allowing it to be pushed out when the mother eats. *Lev. Rab.* 14:8, however, states that the fetus eats what its mother eats and drinks what its mother drinks, but it does not explain how the nutriment is passed on to the fetus. In contrast to the lack of mention of blood as important during gestation, *b. Nid.* 31a maintains that sexual intercourse is beneficial to both the fetus and the woman during the last three months of pregnancy because it "whitens" and "strengthens" the fetus. Cf. *Num. Rab.* 10:4.

157. I return to this below.

158. E. Clark 1988, 376, citing *Contra Julian* 6.59(19).

159. For patristic sources on the conception of Jesus, see Harlow 1999. See also E. Clark 1988 and 2001. These traditions are beyond the scope of the present study; my mention of Jesus is confined to the possible engagement *Lev. Rab.* 14:5 suggests with such patristic theories.

160. Buell's work on Clement (1999) and E. Clark's on Augustine (1986, 1988 and 2001) have greatly informed my own research.

161. The differences between rabbinic and patristic attitudes about procreation, sexuality, and marriage are not absolute. Here I refer to what is commonly understood as an overall positive rabbinic valuation of marriage and procreation and a more negative view attributed to patristic authors, especially Augustine despite his more moderate stand when viewed in context. For an exploration of the differences among rabbinic sources about marriage along geographical (and to some extent chronological lines), see Boyarin 1993; see also Gafni 1989. For discussions of more renunciative rabbinic traditions, see Fraade 1986; Biale 1992, 33–59; and Boyarin 1993. For patristic advocates of marriage and procreation, see Hunter 1987, 1989, and 2007. For a detailed examination of Jewish and Christian attitudes about sexuality and procreation as it pertains to the specific exegesis of Gen. 1:28, see J. Cohen 1989. See Pagels 1989 for an overview of Christian interpretations of Genesis 1–3.

162. See Buell 1999, 22–27, for Clement's eclectic use of procreation theories.

163. Clement *Strom.* 6.147.4, cited from Buell 1999, 100.

164. Translated according to Buell 1999, 100 n. 10.

165. Buell translates part of this passage toward the end of her more general explanation of gender hierarchy in Clement's use of the seed/soil imagery, writing, "According to this image, the process of procreation consists of the unilateral activity of the man, the farmer, who sows seed into a 'living field,' the woman. The male and female roles are radically asymmetrical. Not only does the man play the active role in this model, but he also offers the essence of new life: '[seed] contains the principle of creation and has assembled in it the ideas of nature . . .' (*Paid.* 2.83.3)" (1999, 38).

166. Pagels 1989, 27. Buell points out that Philo, who shares Clement's procreative imagery of farming (e.g., *Who Is the Heir* 115), "frequently uses the terms *nature* and *God* interchangeably" (1999, 100 n. 9).

167. *Paid.* 2.93, emphasis added.

168. Cf. *b. Yev.* 34b. See also *t. Nid.* 2:7. See Labovitz 2002, 171ff., for additional sources and an extended discussion of rabbinic sources that link women and land by virtue of their ownership and productivity. See also *Gen. Rab.* 84:4–5, which uses agricultural imagery to describe Er and Onan's nonprocreative intercourse. See Satlow 1994, 152–53.

169. Theodor and Albeck 1965, 1253. See Labovitz 2002, 178.

170. Cf. *Gen. Rab.* 85:5 and *b. Shab.* 118b. See Labovitz 2002, 178–79. The phrase "by way of a sheet" might come to teach of R. Halfota's potency, or that he is simply doing his obligation and thus not supposed to feel pleasure, but perhaps the text invokes some of the miraculousness of conception here, thus implicating God in these "plantings."

171. See also *Gen. Rab.* 72:6.

172. If one brings together the excerpts from Clement cited above from *Strom.* 6.147.4 and *Paid.* 2.83, Clement also allocates the (pro)creative process primarily to God. See also Philo: "What of the first beginnings of plants? Do they consist in the depositing of the seed in farming, or are they the invisible works of nature? What of the generation of men and other animals? Are not the parents as it were accessories,

while nature is the original, the earliest and the real cause?" (*Who Is the Heir* 115, cited in Buell 1999, 100 n. 9).

173. See Frymer-Kensky 1992, 88ff. She writes, "Agricultural fertility is a matter of vital concern to the peoples of the ancient world, who cannot take fertility for granted and believe that fertility is fragile." She continues, "But the ancient farmers were also very aware that sometimes you could put a seed in the ground and it wouldn't grow. The ground might be too saline, or the birds might eat the seed, or locusts might devour the growing plants. . . . There are so many reasons that a seed might not grow that it is a miracle every time it really does so" (91). And she succinctly points out, "Like the other Near Eastern peoples, Israel was concerned with fertility. . . . God must be the only power who brings fertility, and God alone must be enough" (92). See also Biale 1992, 23–28.

174. *Gen. Rab.* 73:4 and parallels, cited above. The parallel at *b. Tan.* 2b, recorded in the name of R. Yohanan, states, "In the west (Palestine) they said also the key to sustenance, as it is written, *You open your hand* (Ps. 145:6). Why didn't R. Yohanan also [attribute this key to God]? He would say, If you have rain, you have sustenance." Again, Frymer-Kensky writes, "To the Bible, God's fertility-bringing power lies in God's power over rain" (1992, 92).

175. The text states "kings," but I have rendered it in the singular according to the rest of the passage.

176. This text reads the Hebrew *vayetar* ("entreat"; "pray") as related to *hatar* ("digging," or "making an opening"). This is made explicit in some manuscripts, stating, "In the west they call digging, entreating." Cf. *b. Yev.* 64a.

177. Cf. *Lev. Rab.* 14:2, "R. Levi said, it is customary in this world that when one deposits an ounce of silver with his friend in secret and the friend returns to him a litra of gold in public, will he not praise him? So too men deposit to the Holy Blessed One a white drop in secret and the Holy Blessed One returns to them complete and beautiful living beings in public." It might be possible to understand R. Levi's final statement in *Gen. Rab.* 63:5 as a further comment on God fashioning the womb from digging within, since the text previously credits God with fashioning Rebekah's womb. However, since *Lev. Rab.* 14:2, also attributed to R. Levi, mentions that the litra of gold provided by God is the child, it seems more likely that here too the "gold" alludes to the embryo, not the womb. This reading also takes into account the last part of Gen. 25:21, *and Rebekah his wife conceived*.

178. Again, see *b. Ber.* 10a and *b. Meg.* 14a.

179. *Lev. Rab.* 14:6, discussed above, uses agricultural imagery to describe God's distribution of semen.

180. E. Clark 1988, 371.

181. Ibid., 369.

182. E. Clark 2001, 19. See also Brown 1983 and Pagels 1989.

183. Clark 2001, 26.

184. Ibid.

185. *Leviticus Rabbah*'s redaction date in the first half of the fifth century does not preclude that many traditions contained within it are much earlier. However, the interpretations of Lev. 12:2, *When a woman* tazria' *and gives birth to a male*,

which is the base verse of *Leviticus Rabbah* 14, that have to do specifically with the issue of seed first appear in, and appear unique to, *Leviticus Rabbah*. In other words, no Palestinian compilation prior to *Leviticus Rabbah,* nor for that matter contemporaneous with it, worry over the possible mention of woman's seed in Lev. 12:2, suggesting that *Leviticus Rabbah* 14 is not best characterized as strictly biblically or exegetically motivated.

186. However, Visotzky points out, "By the fifth century original sin had finally replaced free will in doctrinal discussion. This was fueled by the Pelagian controversy in which the British free will advocate found his views on Adam and Eve attacked by none less than Augustine and Jerome. Since Pelagius had visited Palestine and Jerome lived there, and since the bishop of Hippo's letters and writings were widely circulated in Palestine, it may be surmised that even Jews had heard of the controversy regarding free will and original sin" (1995, 102). And see Visotzky (forthcoming) for a more detailed exploration of rabbinic and Pelagian sources and methodological considerations about the difficulties of establishing an exegetical encounter on linguistic terms, or because of the "language barrier."

187. E. Clark notes that in *De nuptiis* 2.26(13) "Augustine mentions in passing that reproduction occurs through "the commingling of seminal elements of the two sexes in the womb" (2001, 37 n. 112).

188. Julian appeals to Heb. 11:11 in *Opus imperfectum* 3.85.3–4, but he apparently understands the verse to refer to Sarah conceiving through faith, not emitting seed. E. Clark writes, "Strictly speaking, Julian probably accepted the same medical theory as Augustine that deemed male seed largely responsible for the creation of a child. (His claim that children are born *de vi seminum* is meant to challenge Augustine's view that sin is transmitted through the reproductive act, not to stand as a biological statement about the relative contributions of male and female)" (1988, 386).

189. See E. Clark 1988, 386ff., and 2001, 18–19 and36ff.

190. *Opus imperfectum* 3.85.4 (Teske, 1999a 325). Cf. *Opus* 2.56, 2.83, 3.88.3–4, and 2.179. See E. Clark 1988, 387.

191. Part of Julian's attack on Augustine is the former's seeming location of the transmission of original sin with men in particular. See E. Clark 1988, 376 and 387.

192. Ibid., 376, citing *Contra Julian* 4.12(2), 5.34(8), and 6.59(19).

193. *Lev. Rab.* 14:6, discussed above, does not present a theory about the origins of male seed, but imagines that God either distills the seed or distributes it to various body parts. I think it possible that one of the reasons that this tradition does not consider where semen originates in the body—as Greco-Roman authors did—implies that the rabbis, like Augustine, would have imagined God creating the seed.

194. Augustine's separation of the creation of the embryo from lust would seem, at first, to be at odds with much of rabbinic literature, *Leviticus Rabbah* 14 included. However, *Leviticus Rabbah* 14 mentions "lust" only once, in 14:5, where it is at odds with the creation of the embryo (David). See below.

195. E. Clark points out that Julian's statements about procreation are also informed by theology and refers to them as well as "bio-theology" (1988, 375).

196. My emphasis on theology is not meant to dismiss the ways ancient biology also reflects shared rabbinic and patristic (and Hellenistic) assumptions about

gender hierarchies. However, I see theology as the primary motivating factor and the construction of gender as a predictable corollary.

197. This seems accurate for Clement as well, but Buell's (1999) detailed analysis of Clement suggests that his rhetoric of procreation also, and perhaps more primarily, serves to delineate proper lineage and authority amid competing Christian claims.

198. E. Clark 2001, 24. See also E. Clark 1988, 373–74.

199. For patristic debates about the relative goods or ills of marriage, and so on, see, e.g., Brown 1988, Pagels 1989, and Hunter 1987, 1989, 1993, and 2007. See also J. Cohen 1989, 221–70. The question of "anti-Christian polemic" in *Leviticus Rabbah* has been addressed by Visotzky (1995, 93–105, and 2003, 161–72) and Neusner (e.g., 1986b, 94–105, and 1986c, 67–87), to differing conclusions. Visotzky is on the whole quite skeptical of anti-Christian polemic in *Leviticus Rabbah,* though he presents *Lev. Rab.* 14:5 as an almost certain anti-Christian polemic. In contrast to both Visotzky and Neusner, I limit my own engagement with the question of anti-Christian polemic in *Leviticus Rabbah* to chapter 14 of the compilation. Furthermore, I explore if the chapter's only relationship with Christian notions about procreation is best characterized as of the "anti" variety.

200. See Biale 1992, 44; and Visotzky 1995, 101–5 and 2003, 165–67. Visotzky provides a compelling line of transmission for *Lev. Rab.* 14:5's engagement with original sin, briefly noting the possible inroads through the Pelagian controversy, and then focusing on Syriac and Greek fathers (1995, 102–4). Visotzky's argument could be further supported by Origen's comments on Mary's unique conception of Jesus in *Hom. Lev.* 8:2(6), where he interprets Lev. 12:2 writing, "Therefore, let these words be for us a confirmation of what we observed that the Lawgiver did not add to Scripture superfluously, 'If a woman receives seed and bears a son,' but that there is a mystical exception, which separated Mary alone from the rest of women whose birth was not by the conception of seed but by the presence 'of the Holy Spirit and the power of the Most High' (Lk. 1:35)" (trans. Barkley 1990, 155). Later in the same homily (8:3[5]; Barkley 1990, 157), Origen cites Ps. 51:7 (LXX Ps. 50:5). See Roll 2003 for a discussion of Origen's homily in the context of the "churching of women" after childbirth in early Christianity.

201. Feldman 1995, 98, cautions, "Lest one be guilty of the heresy that even legitimate sexual activity is somehow sinful when it lacks procreative intent, a standard commentary elucidates the above Midrash." Heresy or not, the text seems to suggest a connection between iniquity and nonprocreative sexual activity and Feldman's and previous commentators' attempts to dissuade one of this possibility do as much to establish it as anything else. See Biale 1992, 246 n. 59, for a similar point.

202. Note that Psalm 51 is about David's iniquity in that he has intercourse with Batsheva, presumably simply to satisfy his own needs, that is, without any intention of procreation.

203. Ps. 51:4 parallels verse 51:7, stating, *Wash me from my iniquity and cleanse me from my sin.*

204. Visotzky 1995, 105, emphasis added. Visotzky (forthcoming) revisits the question of original sin and the Pelagian controversy in rabbinic sources.

205. Visotzky 1995, 104.

206. The difference between David and both Jesus and *'adam* is that God creates David (and all embryos/Israel) with semen.

207. Biale 1992; Boyarin 1993. See also the important contribution of Fraade (1986), whose methodological insights into the very discourse about asceticism are quite profound.

208. Biale writes, "The midrashic reading of the Song certainly did not efface the eroticism of the text, but neither could it embrace it fully on the human plane" (1992, 59).

209. Biale 1992, 58; see also 34–35.

210. Boyarin 1993, 61 and 75. These quotes are from *Carnal Israel*'s second chapter, but see also chap. 4.

211. I focus on *Leviticus Rabbah* 14 in the following pages, but most of what I suggest about *Leviticus Rabbah* 14 also applies to rabbinic traditions about the creation of the embryo more generally.

212. Boyarin 1993, e.g., 107.

213. E. Clark writes, "Against the Manichean belief that a human birth would have 'confined' Jesus to the womb, Augustine constantly affirms that God is everywhere and cannot be subjected to 'confinement'" (1986, 394).

214. See my comments about *Lev. Rab.* 14:7's use of Eccles. 11:5 in the previous chapter, which admit, in the context of sex determination, to human lack of understanding. Cf. *Gen. Rab.* 65:12.

215. *Leviticus Rabbah* 14 then echoes biblical sources on a profound level. See above where in a number of biblical sources, while sexual intercourse is implied but God's granting of pregnancy explicit, the text does not mention sexual intercourse.

216. I have found it particularly striking, and no less significant, that, in contrast to Richard Smith's opening to his article about "gnostic" theories of generation (1988, 345, where he writes, "This is an essay about the vagina, the womb, and blood; it is also about the penis, the testicles, and semen. It is about sexual intercourse, embryology, and birth," *Leviticus Rabbah* 14 is far less about these things than God.

217. The majority of both parties maintained that the primary, most godly, purpose of sex was procreation and both constructed marriage as the proper outlet for sexuality.

218. *Lev. Rab.* 14:2, imagines men depositing a "white drop," which God has given to them, back to God, and God delivers to them beautiful children. The parallel in *Eccles. Rab.* 5:11, however, mentions that men deposit the white drop *with their wives*. See also *Mekhilta of R. Ishmael B'shalakh* 8 (Horovitz and Rabin 1970, 144).

219. See Klawans 2000. Particularly interesting in this context is Klawans's explanation of both moral and ritual impurity as "two *distinct but analogous perceptions of contagion*" (158 and 38).

220. See Leviticus 15 and Lev. 18:19 and 20:18, which seem to ascribe moral impurity to those who bring such substances together. See Klawans 2000, 40, 105, and 107. Perhaps biblical prohibitions of sex with a menstruant contribute to the rabbinic hesitation, in my readings, to fully promote Greco-Roman theories about the comingling of these two bodily substances in the creation of the embryo. Even in the "three partners" tradition in the *Bavli*, semen and blood are not explicitly said to commingle. In the *Yerushalmi*'s version, which lacks much specificity (see

above), the tradition appears in tractate *Kelayim*, about forbidden mixtures. The first mention of blood and semen mixing is in the medieval text (ca. eleventh century) *Yetsirat Ha-Valad* (Jellinek 1967, 155).

221. The postpartum woman is ritually impure (see Lev. 12:2–6), but this is not transmitted to the newborn.

222. Possibly R. Abbahu, see Margulies's notes ad loc. (1993, 307).

223. Margulies (1993, 307) suggests that the appearance of the word "iniquity" is possibly a scribal error brought about by *Lev. Rab.* 14:5's mention of Ps. 51:7, directly following.

224. For the possible transmission of birth impurity to midwives and the woman's husband in early Christian and patristic sources, see Roll 2003, 118–20.

225. I have not found a parallel in Palestinian compilations.

226. The exegesis of Job 14:4 is attributed to R. Ilai, most likely the third-generation amora, not the contemporary of R. Meir.

227. This is not meant to critique Lieberman's work, but to suggest that to continue in the tradition of my teacher's teacher entails examining rabbinic theories of procreation in ways that explore Greco-Roman, Christian, and broader rabbinic contexts, to name just a fraction of the scope of Lieberman's work. My point is that previous scholarship on rabbinic theories of procreation have had the more limited goal of explaining rabbinic traditions primarily in light of Greco-Roman medical theories.

228. See Delaney 1986 and 1991.

229. The context of this midrash is the construction of the *mishkan*, which is equated with the creation of the world and the creation of humanity. Just as the embryo develops from the navel, the world develops from the "founding stone," just below the *mishkan*.

Epilogue

1. See especially Duden 1993 and Michaels 1999.

2. See, e.g., Petchesky 1987, Stabile 1992, Duden 1993, Berlant 1997, and Hartouni 1997. And see Haraway 1988.

3. Petchesky 1987, 268.

4. Ibid., 267–68.

5. These years are marked by the appearance of Lennart Nilsson's images of fetuses in two issues of *Life* magazine.

6. Duden 1993, 12 (original emphasis) and 17. See Michaels 1999 for a critique of some elements of Duden's work.

7. Hartouni 1997, 13.

8. See Fonrobert 2000 for "ruptures" in rabbinic discussions about menstruation based on the rabbinic gender trouble that emerges from a consideration of women's bodily sensation. I do not foreclose the possibility of such a rehabilitative reading on traditions about pregnancy, but I remain skeptical of it.

9. I have come to see contemporary disputes about abortion in the United

States as about far more than the fate of fetuses or the unborn; they are about the constructions of gender, power, religion, and nationality.

10. Ginsburg 1998, 104.

11. I had been advised, at numerous times during this project, not to use the word "theology" because it is a Christian term and Jews don't do theology. I have chosen to use the term "theology"—with the understanding that what the rabbis do not engage in is "systematic" or "dogmatic" theology—as a convenient shorthand for rabbinic constructions or depictions of God, despite the fact that it too does not appear in rabbinic sources. In contrast to the terms "Jewishness" and "Judaism," which have a viable alternative within the sources, "(rabbinic) Israel," I have found no alternative to "theology" in rabbinic sources.

12. See, e.g., S. Stern 1994, 10–11 and 222–23; S. Cohen 1999; Baker 2005; Satlow 2005; and Goodblatt 2006. See also R. Kraemer 1989 and 1991 for epigraphic evidence.

13. S. Cohen 1999, 5.

14. The problems that surface when one uses the word "Judaism" (and "Christianity") for late antique sources have been eloquently articulated by others. See, e.g., Boyarin 2003, 67–74; and Lieu 2002, 226–31, and 2004, 1–26. I am suggesting that reference to "rabbinic Israel" be seen as a viable alternative when referring to rabbinic sources, which do not figure prominently in Lieu's work (see 2004, 23 n. 61) but are central to Boyarin.

15. For more on the importance of language in the context of rabbinics scholarship, see Boyarin 2003 and 2004.

16. See Boyarin 2003.

17. Baker 2005, 114.

18. Yuval 2006, 23.

19. It also points to a difference between Second Temple sources and rabbinic ones. However, the focus on the occurrence of the terms "Jews/Judeans" and "Jewishness" in nonrabbinic Jewish sources might occlude the extent to which they also use the term "Israel." For a recent examination of the terms "Jews" and "Judaism" in postbiblical sources, see Mason 2007. This article was brought to my attention when this book was at its final stages, and it is therefore not fully integrated here.

20. Boyarin notes that Frend posited, "After circa A.D. 100 there was less of a tendency for Christians to claim to be Israel and more of a tendency to contrast Christianity and Judaism as separate religions" (2003, 72 n. 25). If Frend is correct, then it seems difficult to maintain that rabbinic sources, which are all redacted post-100 CE, would be reacting to Christians. But see Boyarin 1999, 134 n. 12. And see Lieu 2002 for the problems of imposing the terms "Christian" and "Christianity" on traditions known as "early Christian" literature.

21. Neusner (1989) often refers to "an Israel."

22. See, e.g., S. Cohen 1983, 1990, and 1999; Hayes 2002; Neusner 1995; Porton 1994; and Schiffman 1985. Here is not the place to engage with the details of each of these scholars' interpretations, but it is important to note that rabbinic traditions about converts are open to multiple and often conflicting readings. Thus Hayes, at the conclusion of her study, writes, "For the rabbis, genealogy and biological filiation were not dispensed with, but they were overcome. Although native descent

continued to guarantee membership in the community of Israel, it was not viewed as a sine qua non because the rabbis recognized the power of halakhic (legal) conversion to alter biological fact" (2002, 194). She also writes, "Increasingly in rabbinic texts, genealogical concerns are secondary to moral-religious concerns as the rabbis distanced themselves from Ezran [holy seed] rhetoric and ideology" (2002, 194). Shaye Cohen, in contrast, asserts, "Israel is primarily a descent group that one joins at birth" (2005, 103). However, see S. Cohen 1983, 1990, and 1999 for more nuanced readings. Cohen often makes note of *b. Yev.* 47b, which declares that a convert is "like an Israelite in all respects," but he also draws attention to other rabbinic sources that conflict with this one. Thus he writes, "a convert is not an Israelite, but he is a Jew" (1983, 33; but see 1999, 160). Although I understand the distinction between Israelite and Jew that Cohen makes, at least regarding rabbinic sources this strikes me as problematic. Hayes's statement that "the term 'Israel' is an elastic one, embracing the foreign-born Jew, as well as the native-born Jew" (2002, 191) is a compelling alternative view.

23. I have been tempted to pursue how such "innateness" might in and of itself be seen as a response to Christianity and a further distancing between "Jews being born" and "Christians being made" (see note 26 below). However, I have not done so because this would contribute to what I am arguing against here, namely, seeing rabbinic sources as that responsive to Christian interpretations. Furthermore, it seems like the very distinction between "being made" and "being born" has to be rethought or at least nuanced in the wake of Buell 2005 and Lieu 2004 and, I hope, my own project.

24. Hayes 2002, 197.

25. Rabbinic traditions concerning "matrilineal descent" do not explicitly answer what constitutes Israel but what constitutes, or does not constitute, valid *kiddushin*.

26. S. Cohen 2005, 103. Cohen contrasts this with Tertullian's statement, "Christians are made, not born" (102). Himmelfarb, however, writes, "Of course, by some point in Christian history, perhaps late in the fourth century, being a Christian was in fact largely a matter of birth," but she quickly qualifies, "the idea of Christianity as an identity that transcended birth was enshrined in the New Testament and other works from the early period" (2006, 176). Limberis (2000, 377) also points to a difference between "second-generation Christians born into a Christian home" and "those people newly converted to Christianity."

27. Hayes 2002, 197.

28. See, e.g., *y. Bik.* 1:4(64a). And see Levinson 2000a, 345–46; S. Cohen 1990 and 1999; and Hayes 2002. If one emphasizes the malleability of genealogy in such passages, as Hayes does, and highlights the centrality of practices and beliefs in rabbinic narratives about fetuses, as I have done, then in many ways, the fetus and the convert, initially set up as quite different, tell a very similar story of what it means to be Israel.

29. Jakobovits 1959, 183: "Similarly inconclusive are the Talmudic statements attributing personal functions and discernment to embryos—such as their participation in the Song of Moses and in the acceptance of the divine law, their maledic-

tion of sinners, the dispute of Rebekkah's twin sons within her womb, and David's composition of Psalms before his birth."

30. Preuss 1978, 384 (first published in 1911). See Aptowitzer 1924; Aptowitzer does attempt, in his inquiry into the status of the embryo, to bring aggadic and halakhic sources together.

31. See, e.g., Romney-Wegner 1990; Boyarin 1993; Peskowitz 1997; Ilan 1997; Hauptman 1998; Hasan-Rokem 2000 and 2003; Fonrobert 2000; and Baskin 2002.

32. I have applied Tropper's (2004) insights into *m. Avot* and the ways in which its succession lists and those of early Christian sources adapt Greco-Roman writings both structurally and topically. Although Tropper points out differences between the rabbinic and Christian sources, and surely there are differences between rabbinic and patristic uses of embryology as well as similarities, he has suggested that both are drawing from Greco-Roman models, not that one is directly borrowing from or reacting to the other. Tropper's focus on a third-century text, in contrast to my own focus on later rabbinic sources dated to the time after the Christianization of Rome, could be questioned. However, the stance I have taken in this book, born out of my readings of this specific topic, has encouraged me to be more reluctant to read too much of a Christian impact on even these later sources. Visotzky (2003) also contextualizes the fifth-century compilation *Leviticus Rabbah* among Hellenistic literary forms.

33. Recently, Himmelfarb has emphasized, based on liturgical texts, the importance of ancestral merit for rabbinic Israel (2006, 177–81). The medieval tradition about fetuses serving as guarantors, and already the amoraic versions that have children serve as guarantors, that Israel will keep the Torah precisely because the patriarchs lack such merit is a powerful countertradition. I also suggest that rabbinic traditions about embryology and theories of procreation insist that all Israel is created and cared for by God, thus bridging a potential gap between biblical and rabbinic Israel.

34. See S. Cohen 1984 and D. Stern 1996. I take the notion of canonized dissent from Boyarin (1993, e.g., 28–29). Boyarin subsequently sees this as a more unique contribution of the *Bavli* (2004), but see Fraade 2007.

35. *Lev. Rab.* 14:8; *b. Nid.* 30b.

References

Primary Sources

Albeck, Ch., ed. 1952–59. *Mishnah*. 6 vols. Tel Aviv: Dvir; Jerusalem: Bialik Institute.
Buber, Solomon, ed. 1964. *Midrasch Tanhuma*. 2 vols. Reprint. Jerusalem.
Epstein, J. N., and E. Z. Melamed, eds. N.d. *Mekhilta D'Rabbi Shimon B. Yohai*. Reprint. Jerusalem: Hillel Press.
Finkelstein, Louis, ed. 1969. *Sifre on Deuteronomy*. Reprint. New York: Jewish Theological Seminary.
Friedmann, Meir, ed. 1969. *Tanna debe Eliyahu* (*Seder Eliyahu Rabbah* and *Seder Eliyahu Zuta*). Jerusalem: Wahrmann Books. Originally published in Vienna, 1902–4.
Hoffmann, David Z. 1905. *Mechilta de-Rabbi Simon ben Jochai*. Frankfurt am Main: J. Kauffmann.
Horovitz, H. S., ed. 1992. *Sifre Numbers*. Reprint. Jerusalem: Shalem.
Horovitz, H. S., and I. A. Rabin, eds. 1970. *Mekhilta D'Rabbi Ishmael*. Reprint. Jerusalem: Wahrmann.
Jellinek, A., ed. 1967. *Beit HaMidrash*. Jerusalem: Wahrmann.
Jones, W. H. S., trans. 1995. "Nutriment." In Hippocrates, vol. 1: *Ancient Medicine. Airs, Waters, Places. Epidemics 1 and 3. The Oath. Precepts. Nutriment*. Loeb Classical Library.
Lauterbach, Jacob, ed. 1933–35. *Mekhilta of Rabbi Ishmael: A Critical Edition on the Basis of MSS and Early Editions with an English Translation, Introduction and Notes*. 3 vols. Philadelphia: JPS.
Lieberman, Saul, ed. 1964. *Midrash Debarim Rabbah*. Jerusalem: Wahrmann.
Mandelbaum, B., ed. 1962. *Pesikta de Rav Kahana: According to an Oxford Manuscript with Variants, Commentary and Introduction*. 2 vols. New York: Jewish Theological Seminary.
Margulies, M., ed. 1993. *Midrash Wayyikra Rabbah: A Critical Edition Based on Manuscripts and Geniza Fragments with Variants and Notes*. 2 vols. New York and Jerusalem: Jewish Theological Seminary.
Midrash Tanhuma. 1969. Reprint. Jerusalem: Levin-Epstein.
Pirkei Rabbi Eliezer. 1973. Reprint. Jerusalem: Eshkol.
Schechter, S., ed. 1888. *Avot D'Rabbi Nathan*. Frankfurt: J. Kauffmann.
Talmud Yerushalmi. 1523. Venice edition. Reprint, Leipzig, 1925.
Theodor, J., and Ch. Albeck, eds. 1965. *Midrash Bereshit Rabba: Critical Edition with Notes and Commentary*. 3 vols. 2nd ed. Jerusalem: Wahrmann.

Weiss, I. H., ed. 1862. *Sifra.* Reprint, New York: Om Publishing, 1947.
Zuckermandel, M. S., ed. 1970. *Tosephta.* Jerusalem: Wahrmann.

Secondary Sources

Aaron, David H. 1995. "Imagery of the Divine and the Human: On the Mythology of Genesis Rabba 8:1." *Journal of Jewish Thought and Philosophy* 5:1–62.
Addelson, Kathryn Pyne. 1999. "The Emergence of the Fetus." In *Fetal Subjects, Feminist Positions,* ed. Lynn M. Morgan and Meredith W. Michaels. Philadelphia: University of Pennsylvania Press.
Adler, Rachel. 1977. "A Mother in Israel: Aspects of the Mother-Role in Jewish Myth." In *Beyond Androcentrism: New Essays on Women and Religion,* ed. Rita M. Gross. American Academy of Religion Aids for the Study of Religion 6. Missoula, Mont.: Scholars Press.
Aitken, Ellen. Forthcoming. "The Leaping Child: Imagining the Unborn in Early Christian Literature. In *Imagining the Fetus: The Unborn in Myth, Religion, and Culture.* Oxford: Oxford University Press.
Alexander, Philip. 1992. " 'The Parting of the Ways' from the Perspective of Rabbinic Judaism." In *Jews and Christians: The Parting of the Ways, A.D. 70 to 135,* ed. James D.G. Dunn. Tübingen: J.C.B. Mohr (Paul Siebeck).
Alter, Robert. 1983. *The Art of Biblical Narrative.* New York: Basic.
Aptowitzer, V. 1924. "Observations on the Criminal Law of the Jews." *Jewish Quarterly Review* 15: 55–118.
———. 1942. "Emdat Ha-Ubar B'Dinei Onshin Shel Yisrael." *Sinai* 6: 26–50.
Asad, Talal. 1993. *Genealogies of Religion: Discipline and Reasons of Power in Christianity and Islam.* Baltimore: Johns Hopkins University Press.
Auge, Francoise Heritier. 1989. "Semen and Blood: Some Ancient Theories Concerning Their Genesis and Relationship." In *Zone: Fragments for a History of the Human Body: Part Three,* ed. Michel Feher. Cambridge, Mass.: MIT Press.
Bacher, W. 1898. "Meir et Cleopatre." *Revue des Etudes Juives* 5.
Baker, Cynthia M. 2002. *Rebuilding the House of Israel: Architectures of Gender in Jewish Antiquity.* Stanford, Calif.: Stanford University Press.
———. 2005. "When Jews Were Women." *History of Religions* 45 (22): 114–34.
Bakhos, Carol. 2006. *Ishmael on the Border: Rabbinic Portrayals of the First Arab.* Albany: State University of New York Press.
———. 2007. "Figuring (out) Esau: The Rabbis and Their Others," *Journal of Jewish Studies* 58 (2): 250–62.
Balme, David M. 1987. "Aristotle's Biology Was Not Essentialist." In *Philosophical Issues in Aristotle's Biology,* ed. Allan Gotthelf and James G. Lennox. Cambridge: Cambridge University Press.
———. 1990. "Human Is Generated by Human." In *The Human Embryo: Aristotle and the Arabic and European Traditions,* ed. G. R. Dunstan. Exeter: University of Exeter Press.

Barkley, Gary Wayne, trans. 1990. *Origen: Homilies on Leviticus 1–16*. Fathers of the Church: A New Translation. Washington, D.C.: Catholic University of America Press.

Barnes, Jonathan, ed. 1984. *The Complete Works of Aristotle*. Vol. 1. Princeton, N.J.: Princeton University Press.

Baskin, Judith. 1983. *Pharoah's Counsellors: Job, Jethro, and Balaam in Rabbinic and Patristic Tradition*. Chico, Calif.: Scholars Press.

———. 1985. "Rabbinic and Patristic Exegetical Contacts in Late Antiquity: A Bibliographical Reappraisal." In *Approaches to Ancient Judaism*, vol. 5, *Studies in Judaism and Its Greco-Roman Context*, ed. William Scott Green. Atlanta, Ga.: Scholars Press.

———. 1989. "Rabbinic Reflections on the Barren Wife." *Harvard Theological Review* 82 (1): 101–14.

———. 1997. "Rabbinic Judaism and the Creation of Woman." In *Judaism Since Gender*, ed. Miriam Peskowitz and Laura Levitt. New York: Routledge.

———. 2002. *Midrashic Women: Formations of the Feminine in Rabbinic Literature*. Hanover, N.H.: University Press of New England for Brandeis University Press.

Berkowitz, Beth. 2002. "Decapitation and the Discourse of Antisyncretism in the Babylonian Talmud." *Journal of the American Academy of Religion* 70 (4): 743–69.

———. 2006. *Execution and Invention: Death Penalty Discourse in Early Rabbinic and Christian Cultures*. Oxford: Oxford University Press.

Berlant, Lauren. 1997. *The Queen of America Goes to Washington City: Essays on Sex and Citizenship*. Durham, N.C.: Duke University Press.

Bettenson, Henry. 1956. *The Early Christian Fathers: A Selection from the Writings of the Fathers from St. Clement of Rome to St. Athanasius*. New York: Oxford University Press.

———. 1970. *The Later Christian Fathers: A Selection from the Writings of the Fathers from St. Cyril of Jerusalem to St. Leo the Great*. New York: Oxford University Press.

Biale, David. 1992. *Eros and the Jews: From Biblical Israel to Contemporary America*. New York: Basic Books.

Blowers, Paul M. 1988. "Origen, the Rabbis, and the Bible: Toward a Picture of Judaism and Christianity in Third-Century Caesarea." In *Origen of Alexandria: His World and His Legacy*, ed. Charles Kannengiesser and William L. Petersen. Notre Dame, Ind.: University of Notre Dame Press.

Bokser, Baruch. 1987. "Todos and Rabbinic Authority in Rome." In *Religion, Literature, and Society in Ancient Israel, Formative Christianity and Judaism*, ed. Jacob Neusner et al. Lanham, Md.: University Press of America.

Boyarin, Daniel. 1990. *Intertextuality and the Reading of Midrash*. Bloomington: Indiana University Press.

———. 1992. "'This We Know to Be the Carnal Israel': Circumcision and the Erotic Life of God and Israel." *Critical Inquiry* 18 (Spring): 474–505.

———. 1993. *Carnal Israel: Reading Sex in Talmudic Culture*. Berkeley: University of California Press.

———. 1994. *A Radical Jew: Paul and the Politics of Identity.* Berkeley: University of California Press.
———. 1997a. "Jewish Studies as Teratology: The Rabbis as Monsters." *Jewish Quarterly Review* 88: 57–66.
———. 1997b. *Unheroic Conduct: The Rise of Heterosexuality and the Invention of the Jewish Man.* Berkeley: University of California Press.
———. 1998. "Gender." In *Critical Terms for Religious Studies*, ed. Mark C. Taylor. Chicago: University of Chicago Press.
———. 1999. *Dying for God: Martyrdom and the Making of Christianity and Judaism.* Figurae: Reading Medieval Culture. Stanford, Calif.: Stanford University Press.
———. 2001. "Justin Martyr Invents Judaism." *Church History* 70: 427–61.
———. 2003. "Semantic Differences; or, 'Judaism'/'Christianity.'" In *The Ways That Never Parted*, ed. Adam H. Becker and Annette Yoshiko Reed. Tübingen: B. Mohr (Paul Siebeck).
———. 2004. *Border Lines: The Partition of Judaeo-Christianity.* Divinations: Rereading Late Ancient Religion. Philadelphia: University of Pennsylvania Press.
———. Forthcoming. "Rethinking Jewish Christianity: An Argument for Dismantling a Dubious Category (to Which Is Appended a Correction of My *Border Lines*)." *Jewish Quarterly Review.*
Boylan, Michael. 1984. "The Galenic and Hippocratic Challenges to Aristotle's Conception Theory." *Journal of the History of Biology* 15: 89–118.
1986. "Galen's Conception Theory." *Journal of the History of Biology* 19: 47–77.
Brett, Mark G. 1996. *Ethnicity and the Bible.* Leiden: E. J. Brill.
Bronner, Leila L. 1994. *From Eve to Esther: Rabbinic Reconstructions of Biblical Women.* Louisville, Ky.: Westminster John Knox Press.
Brooks, Roger. 1988. "Straw Dogs and Scholarly Ecumenism: The Appropriate Jewish Background for the Study of Origen." In *Origen of Alexandria: His World and His Legacy*, ed. Charles Kannengiesser and William L. Petersen. Notre Dame, Ind.: University of Notre Dame Press.
Brown, Peter. 1969. *Augustine of Hippo: A Biography.* Berkeley: University of California Press.
———. 1983. "Sexuality and Society in the Fifth Century A.D.: Augustine and Julian of Eclanum." In *Tria corda: Scritti in onore di Arnaldo Momigliano*, ed. E. Gabba. Biblioteca di Athenaeum 1. Como: New Press.
———. 1988. *The Body and Society: Men, Women and Sexual Renunciation in Early Christianity.* Lectures on the History of Religions, vol. 13. New York: Columbia University Press.
Buell, Denise Kimber. 1999. *Making Christians: Clement of Alexandria and the Rhetoric of Legitimacy.* Princeton, N.J.: Princeton University Press.
———. 2000. "Ethnicity and Religion in Mediterranean Antiquity and Beyond." *Religious Studies Review* 26: 243–49.
———. 2001. "Rethinking the Relevance of Race for Early Christian Self-Definition." *Harvard Theological Review* 94: 449–76.

———. 2002. "Race and Universalism in Early Christianity." *Journal of Early Christian Studies* 10 (4): 429–68.

———. 2005. *Why This New Race? Ethnic Reasoning in Early Christianity*. New York: Columbia University Press.

Buell, Denise Kimber, and Caroline Johnson Hodge. 2004. "The Politics of Interpretation: The Rhetoric of Race and Ethnicity in Paul." *Journal of Biblical Literature* 123: 235–52.

Burns, J. Patout. 1998. "Traducianism." In *Encyclopedia of Early Christianity*, ed. Everett Ferguson. New York: Garland Publishing.

Burrus, Virginia. 2000. *"Begotten, Not Made": Conceiving Manhood in Late Antiquity*. Stanford, Calif.: Stanford University Press.

Butler, Judith. 1990. *Gender Trouble: Feminism and the Subversion of Identity*. New York: Routledge.

Butterworth, G. W. 1973. *Origen: On First Principles*. Gloucester, Mass.: Peter Smith.

Cadden, Joan. 1993. *Meanings of Sex Difference in the Middle Ages: Medicine, Science, and Culture*. Cambridge: Cambridge University Press.

Cahill, Lisa Sowle, and Margaret A. Farley, eds. 1995. *Embodiment, Morality, and Medicine*. Boston: Kluwer Academic Publishers.

Callaway, Mary. 1986. *Sing, O Barren One: A Study in Comparative Midrash*. SBL Dissertation Series 91. Atlanta: Scholars Press.

Casper, Monica J. 1999. "Operation to the Rescue: Feminist Encounters with Fetal Surgery." In *Fetal Subjects, Feminist Positions*, ed. Lynn M. Morgan and Meredith W. Michaels. Philadelphia: University of Pennsylvania Press.

Chadwick, H. 1966. *Early Christian Thought and the Classical Tradition: Studies in Justin, Clement, and Origen*. Oxford: Oxford University Press.

Cixous, Helene. 1993. "The Laugh of the Medusa." In *Feminisms: An Anthology of Literary Theory and Criticism*, ed. Robyn Warhol and Diane Herndl. New Brunswick, N.J.: Rutgers University Press.

Clark, Elizabeth A. 1986. *Ascetic Piety and Women's Faith: Essays on Late Antique Christianity*. Studies in Women and Religion 20. Lewiston, N.Y.: Edwin Mellen Press.

———. 1988. "Vitiated Seeds and Holy Vessels: Augustine's Manichean Past." In *Images of the Feminine in Gnosticism*, ed. Karen King. Philadelphia: Fortress Press.

———. 1999. "Origenist Controversy." In *Augustine Through the Ages: An Encyclopedia*, ed. A. Fitzgerald. Grand Rapids, Mich.: Eerdmans.

———. 2001. "Generation, Degeneration, Regeneration: Original Sin and the Conception of Jesus in the Polemic between Augustine and Julian of Eclanum." In *Generation and Degeneration: Tropes of Reproduction in Literature and History from Antiquity to Early Modern Europe*, ed. Valeria Finucci and Kevin Brownlee. Durham, N.C.: Duke University Press.

Clark, Gillian. 1998. "Bodies and Blood: Late Antique Debate on Martyrdom, Virginity and Resurrection." In *Changing Bodies, Changing Meanings*, ed. David Montserrat. London: Routledge.

Clements, Ruth. 2005. "Origen's Readings of Romans in *Peri Archon*: (Re)Constructing Paul." In *Early Patristic Readings of Romans*, ed. Kathy L. Gaca and L. L. Welborn. New York: T & T Clark International.

Cohen, Aryeh. 1998. *Rereading Talmud: Gender, Law and the Poetics of Sugyot*. Atlanta: Scholars Press.

Cohen, Boaz. 1966. *Jewish and Roman Law: A Comparative Study*. New York: Jewish Theological Seminary.

Cohen, Gerson D. 1991. "Esau as Symbol in Early Medieval Thought." In *Studies in the Variety of Rabbinic Cultures*. Philadelphia: JPS.

Cohen, Jeremy. 1989. *Be Fertile and Increase, Fill the Earth and Master It: The Ancient and Medieval Career of a Biblical Text*. Ithaca, N.Y.: Cornell University Press.

Cohen, Shaye J. D. 1983. "Conversion to Judaism in Historical Perspective: From Biblical Israel to Post-biblical Judaism." *Conservative Judaism* 36 (4): 31–45.

———. 1984. "The Significance of Yavneh," *Hebrew Union College Annual* 55: 27–53

———. 1990. "The Rabbinic Conversion Ceremony," *Journal of Jewish Studies* 41: 177–203

———. 1997. "Why Aren't Jewish Women Circumcised?" *Gender & History* 9 (3): 560–78.

———. 1998. "The Conversion of Antoninus." In *The Talmud Yerushalmi and Graeco-Roman Culture*, ed. Peter Schäfer. Tübingen: Mohr Siebeck.

———. 1999. *The Beginnings of Jewishness: Boundaries, Varieties, Uncertainties*. Berkeley: University of California Press.

———. 2005. *Why Aren't Jewish Women Circumcised? Gender and Covenant in Judaism*. Berkeley: University of California Press.

Collins, John J. 1985. "A Symbol of Otherness: Circumcision and Salvation in the First Century." In *"To See Ourselves as Others See Us": Christians, Jews, "Others" in Late Antiquity*, ed. Jacob Neusner and Ernest Frerichs. Chico, Calif.: Scholars Press.

Connery, John. 1977. *Abortion: The Development of the Roman Catholic Perspective*. Chicago: Loyola University Press.

Crego, Paul. 1996. "Theodoret of Kyros on the Relationship of the Body and the Soul Before Birth." *Greek Orthodox Theological Review* 41 (1): 19–37.

Danielou, Jean. 1955. *Origen*. Trans. Walter Mitchell. New York: Sheed and Ward.

Dean-Jones, Lesley. 1991. "The Cultural Construct of the Female Body in Classical Greek Science." In *Women's History and Ancient History*, ed. Sarah B. Pomeroy. Chapel Hill: University of North Carolina Press.

———. 1994. *Women's Bodies in Classical Greek Science*. Oxford: Oxford University Press.

Delaney, Carol. 1986. "The Meaning of Paternity and the Virgin Birth Debate." *Man: Journal of the Royal Anthropological Society* 21 (3): 494–512.

———. 1991. *The Seed and the Soil: Gender and Cosmology in Turkish Village Society*. Berkeley: University of California Press.

———. 1998a. "Abraham and the Seeds of Patriarchy." In *Genesis*, vol. 2 of *The Feminist Companion to the Bible* (2nd ser.), ed. Athalya Brenner. Sheffield: Sheffield Academic Press.

———. 1998b. *Abraham on Trial: The Social Legacy of Biblical Myth.* Princeton, N.J.: Princeton University Press.

de Lange, N. 1976. *Origen and the Jews: Studies in Jewish-Christian Relations in Third-Century Palestine.* Cambridge: Cambridge University Press.

Doelger, Franz. 1934. "Das Lebensrecht des ungeborenen Kindes und die Fruchtabtreibung in der Bewertung der heidnischen und christlichen Antike." In *Antike und Christentum,* 4:1–60. Münster: Aschendorffsche Verlagsbuchhandlung.

duBois, Page. 1988. *Sowing the Body: Psychoanalysis and Ancient Representations of Women.* Chicago: University of Chicago Press.

Duden, Barbara. 1993. *Disembodying Women: Perspectives on Pregnancy and the Unborn.* Trans. Lee Hoinacki. Cambridge, Mass.: Harvard University Press.

———. 1999. "The Fetus on the 'Farther Shore': Toward a History of the Unborn." In *Fetal Subjects, Feminist Positions,* ed. Lynn M. Morgan and Meredith W. Michaels. Philadelphia: University of Pennsylvania Press.

Dunn, Geoffrey. 1998. "Tertullian and Rebekah: A Re-Reading of an 'Anti-Jewish' Argument in Early Christian Literature." *Vigiliae Christianae* 52 (2): 119–45.

Dunn, James D. G. 1999. "Was Judaism Particularist or Universalist?" In *Judaism in Late Antiquity,* part 3, *Where We Stand: Issues and Debates in Ancient Judaism,* ed. Jacob Neusner and Alan J. Avery-Peck, 2:57–73. Leiden: Brill.

Eilberg-Schwartz, Howard. 1990. *The Savage in Judaism: An Anthropology of Israelite Religion and Ancient Judaism.* Bloomington: Indiana University Press.

———. 1994. *God's Phallus and Other Problems for Men and Monotheism.* Boston: Beacon Press.

Feldman, David. 1995. *Marital Relations, Birth Control, and Abortion in Jewish Law.* Reprint. New York: Schocken Books.

Fischel, Henry A. 1977. *Essays in Greco-Roman and Related Talmudic Literature.* New York: Ktav.

Fishbane, Michael. 1985. *Biblical Interpretation in Ancient Israel.* Oxford: Clarendon Press.

Fitzgerald, Allan D., ed. 1999. *Augustine Through the Ages: An Encyclopedia.* Grand Rapids, Mich.: Eerdmans.

Fonrobert, Charlotte. 1996. "Women's Bodies, Women's Blood: The Politics of Gender in Rabbinic Literature." Ph.D. diss., University of California.

———. 2000. *Menstrual Purity: Rabbinic and Christian Reconstructions of Biblical Gender.* Stanford, Calif.: Stanford University Press.

———. 2001. "When Women Walk in the Way of Their Fathers: On Gendering the Rabbinic Claim for Authority." *Journal for the History of Sexuality* 10 (3–4): 398–415.

Foucault, Michel. 1990. *The History of Sexuality.* Vol. 1, *An Introduction.* Trans. Robert Hurley. New York: Vintage Books.

Fox, Edward, trans. 1995. *The Five Books of Moses: Genesis, Exodus, Leviticus, Numbers, Deuteronomy.* New York: Schocken Books.

Fraade, Steven. 1986. "Ascetical Aspects of Ancient Judaism." In *Jewish Spirituality: From the Bible Through the Middle Ages,* ed. Arthur Green, New York: Crossroad Press.

———. 1987a. "Interpreting Midrash 1: Midrash and the History of Judaism." *Prooftexts* 7 (2): 179–94.

———. 1987b. "Interpreting Midrash 2: Midrash and Its Literary Contexts." *Prooftexts* 7 (3): 284–300.

———. 1991. *From Tradition to Commentary: Torah and Its Interpretation in the Midrash Sifre to Deuteronomy*. Jewish Hermeneutics, Mysticism, and Religion Series. Albany: State University of New York Press, 1991.

———. 1994. "Navigating the Anomalous: Non-Jews at the Intersection of Early Rabbinic Law and Narrative." In *The Other in Jewish Thought and History: Constructions of Jewish Culture and Identity*, ed. Laurence J. Silberstein and Robert L. Cohn. New York: New York University Press.

———. 2007. "Rabbinic Polysemy and Pluralism Revisited: Between Praxis and Thematization." *AJS Review* 31 (1): 1–40.

Fraenkel, Yonah. 1981. *Iyunim ha-Olamo ha-Ruhani shel Sipur ha-Agadah*. Tel Aviv: HaKibbutz ha-Meuhad.

———. 1991. *Darkhei ha-Agadah ve-ha-Midrash*. Givatayim, Israel: Yad la-Talmud.

Franklin, Sarah. 1997. *Embodied Progress: A Cultural Account of Assisted Conception*. London: Routledge.

———. 1999. "Dead Embryos: Feminism in Suspension." In *Fetal Subjects, Feminist Positions*, ed. Lynn M. Morgan and Meredith W. Michaels. Philadelphia: University of Pennsylvania Press.

Frend, W. H. C. "A Note on Tertullian and the Jews." *Studia Patristica X* (= *Texte und Untersuchungen*, no. 107, Berlin): 291–96.

Frymer-Kensky, Tikva. 1989. "Law and Philosophy: The Case of Sex in the Bible." *Semeia* 45.

———. 1992. *In the Wake of the Goddesses: Women, Culture, and the Transformation of Pagan Myth*. New York: Free Press.

———. 1999a. "Law and Philosophy: The Case of Sex in the Bible." Reprinted in *Women in the Hebrew Bible: A Reader*, ed. Alice Bach. New York: Routledge.

———. 1999b. "The Strange Case of the Suspected Sotah (Numbers V 11–31)." In *Women in the Hebrew Bible: A Reader*, ed. Alice Bach. New York: Routledge.

Gaca, Kathy L. 2003. *The Making of Fornication: Eros, Ethics, and Political Reform in Greek Philosophy and Early Christianity*. Berkeley: University of California Press.

Gafni, Isaiah M. 1989. "The Institution of Marriage in Rabbinic Times." In *The Jewish Family: Metaphor and Memory*, ed. David Kraemer. Oxford: Oxford University Press.

Gager, John. 2002. *Reinventing Paul*. Oxford: Oxford University Press.

Gasking, Elizabeth. 1967. *Investigations into Generation: 1651–1828*. Baltimore: Johns Hopkins University Press.

Geller, Mark J. 2000. "An Akkadian Vademecum in the Babylonian Talmud." In *From Athens to Jerusalem: Medicine in Hellenized Jewish Lore and in Early Christian Literature*, ed. Samuel Kottek and Manfred Horstmanshoff. Rotterdam: Erasmus.

Ginsburg, Faye. 1998. *Contested Lives: The Abortion Debate in an American Community*. Reprint. Berkeley: University of California Press.

Ginzberg, Louis. 1922. "Some Observations on the Attitude of the Synagogue Towards the Apocalyptic and Eschatological Writings." *Journal of Biblical Literature* 41: 115–36.

———. 1947. *The Legends of the Jews*. 6 vols. 1925. Reprint. Philadelphia: JPS.

———. 1955. "An Introduction to the Palestinian Talmud." In *On Jewish Law and Lore*. Philadelphia: JPS of America.

Glare, P. G. W., ed. 1973. *Oxford Latin Dictionary*. Oxford: Clarendon Press.

Goldberg, Abraham. 1994. "The Palestinian Talmud." In *Essential Papers on the Talmud*, ed. Michael Chernick. New York: New York University Press.

Goldenberg, Robert. 1994. "Did the Amoraim See Christianity as Something New?" In *Pursuing the Text: Studies in Honor of Ben Zion Wacholder on the Occasion of His Seventieth Birthday*. Journal for the Study of the Old Testament Supplement Series 184. Sheffield: Sheffield Academic Press.

———. 1998. *The Nations That Know Thee Not: Ancient Jewish Attitudes Toward Other Religions*. New York: New York University Press.

Goldin, Judah. 1988. *Studies in Midrash and Related Literature*. Philadelphia: JPS.

———. 1990. *The Song at the Sea: Being a Commentary on a Commentary in Two Parts*. Reprint. Philadelphia: JPS.

Goodblatt, David. 1994. *The Monarchic Principle: Studies in Jewish Self-Government in Antiquity*. Tübingen: Mohr.

———. 2006. *Elements of Ancient Jewish Nationalism*. Cambridge: Cambridge University Press.

Gorday, Peter. 1983. *Principles of Patristic Exegesis: Romans 9–11 in Origen, John Chrysostom, and Augustine*. New York: Edwin Mellen Press.

Gordis, Robert. 1951. *Koheleth: The Man and His World*. New York: Jewish Theological Seminary.

Gorman, Michael J. 1998. *Abortion and the Early Church: Christian, Jewish and Pagan Attitudes in the Greco-Roman World*. Reprint. Eugene, Ore.: Wipf and Stock.

Gray, Alyssa. 2003. "A Contribution to the Study of Martyrdom and Identity in the Palestinian Talmud." *Journal of Jewish Studies* 54 (2): 242–72.

———. 2005a. "The Power Conferred by Distance from Power: Redaction and Meaning in b. AZ 10a–11a." In *Creation and Composition: The Contribution of the Bavli Redactors (Stammaim) to the Aggadah*, ed. Jeffrey L. Rubenstein. Tübingen: Mohr Siebeck.

———. 2005b. *A Talmud in Exile: The Influence of Yerushalmi Avodah Zarah on the Formation of Bavli Avodah Zarah*. Providence, R.I.: Brown Judaic Studies.

Green, Monica. 1985. "The Transmission of Ancient Theories of Female Physiology and Disease through the Early Middle Ages." Ph.D. diss., Princeton University.

Green, William Scott. 1978. "What's in a Name? The Problematic of Rabbinic Biography." In *Approaches to Ancient Judaism: Theory and Practice*, 1:77–96. Brown Judaic Studies, no. 1. Missoula, Mont.: Scholars Press.

———. 1979. "Palestinian Holy Men: Charismatic Leadership and Rabbinic Tradition." *Aufstieg und Niedergang Der Romischen Welt* 19 (2): 619–47.

———. 1985. "Otherness Within: Towards a Theory of Difference in Rabbinic Judaism." In *"To See Ourselves as Others See Us": Christians, Jews, "Others" in*

Late Antiquity, ed. Jacob Neusner and Ernest S. Frerichs, 49–70. Chico, Calif.: Scholars Press.

Gruber, Mayer. 1992. *The Motherhood of God and Other Studies.* Atlanta: Scholars Press.

Gruen, Erich. 1998. *Heritage and Hellenism: The Reinvention of Jewish Tradition.* Berkeley: University of California Press.

Hall, Jonathan M. 1997. *Ethnic Identity in Greek Antiquity.* Cambridge: Cambridge University Press.

Hanson, Ann Ellis. 1990. "The Medical Writers' Woman." In *Before Sexuality: The Construction of Erotic Experience in the Ancient Greek World*, ed. David M. Halperin, John J. Winkler, and Froma I. Zeitlin. Princeton, N.J.: Princeton University Press.

———. 1991. "Continuity and Change: Three Case Studies in Hippocratic Gynecological Therapy and Theory." In *Women's History and Ancient History*, ed. Sarah B. Pomeroy. Chapel Hill: University of North Carolina Press.

———. 1992. "Conception, Gestation, and the Origin of Female Nature in the *Corpus Hippocraticum*." *Helios* 19 (1–2): 31–71.

Hamell, Patrick J. 1968. *Handbook of Patrology.* Staten Island, N.Y.: Alba House.

Haraway, Donna J. 1988. "Situated Knowledges: The Science Question in Feminism and the Privilege of Partial Perspective." *Feminist Studies* 14: 3.

———. 1997. *Modest_Witness@Second_Millennium.FemaleMan©_Meets_Onco Mouse™: Feminism and Technoscience.* New York: Routledge.

Hardacre, Helen. 1997. *Marketing the Menacing Fetus in Japan.* Berkeley: University of California Press.

Harlow, Mary. 1999. "In the Name of the Father: Procreation, Paternity and Patriarchy." In *Thinking Men: Masculinity and Its Self-Representation in the Classical Tradition*, ed. L. Foxhall and J. Salmon. London: Routledge.

Harrison, Verna. 1990. "Male and Female in Cappadocian Theology." *Journal of Theological Studies* 41: 441–71.

———. 1995. "The Allegorization of Gender: Plato and Philo on Spiritual Childbearing." In *Asceticism*, ed. Vincent Wimbush and R. Valantasis. Oxford: Oxford University Press.

———. 1996. "Gender, Generation and Virginity in Cappadocian Theology." *Journal of Theological Studies* 47: 38–68.

Hartouni, Valerie. 1997. *Cultural Conceptions: On Reproductive Technologies and the Remaking of Life.* Minneapolis: University of Minnesota Press.

Hasan-Rokem, Galit. 1998. "Narratives in Dialogue: A Folk Literary Perspective on Interreligious Contacts in the Holy Land in Rabbinic Literature of Late Antiquity." In *Sharing the Sacred: Religious Contacts and Conflicts in the Holy Land*, ed. Arieh Kofsky and Guy G. Stroumsa. Jerusalem: Yad Izhak Ben Zvi.

———. 2000. *The Web of Life: Folklore and Midrash in Rabbinic Literature.* Trans. Batya Stein. Stanford, Calif.: Stanford University Press, 2000.

———. 2003. *Tales of the Neighborhood: Jewish Narrative Dialogues in Late Antiquity.* Berkeley: University of California Press.

Hauptman, Judith. 1998. *Rereading the Rabbis: A Woman's Voice.* Boulder, Colo.: Westview Press.

Hayes, Christine. 1997. *Between the Babylonian and Palestinian Talmuds: Accounting for Halakhic Difference in Selected Sugyot from Tractate Avodah Zarah.* Oxford: Oxford University Press.

———. 1998. "Displaced Self-Perceptions: The Deployment of Minim and Romans in Bavli Sanhedrin 90b–91a." In *Religious and Ethnic Communities in Later Roman Palestine,* ed. Hayim Lapin. Potomac: University Press of Maryland.

———. 2002. *Gentile Impurities and Jewish Identities: Intermarriage and Conversion from the Bible to the Talmud.* Oxford: Oxford University Press.

———. 2007. "Rabbis and Their Jewish and Gentile Others." In *The Cambridge Companion to the Talmud and Rabbinic Literature,* ed. Martin Jaffee and Charlotte Fonrobert. Cambridge: Cambridge University Press.

Heine, Ronald E., trans. 1982. *Origen: Homilies on Genesis and Exodus.* Fathers of the Church: A New Translation. Washington, D.C.: Catholic University of America Press.

Heinemann, Joseph. 1971a. "The Proem in the Aggadic Midrashim—A Form-Critical Study." In *Scripta Heirosolymitana,* vol. 22, *Studies in Aggadah and Folk-Literature,* ed. J. Heinemann and D. Noy. Jerusalem: Magnes Press.

———. 1971b. "Profile of a Midrash." *Journal of the American Academy of Religion* 39: 141–50.

Herford, R. 1975. *Christianity in the Talmud and Midrash.* New York: Ktav.

Herr, Moshe D. 1971. "Dialogues Between Sages and Roman Dignitaries." In *Scripta Heirosolymitana,* vol. 22, *Studies in Aggadah and Folk-Literature,* ed. J. Heinemann and D. Noy. Jerusalem: Magnes Press.

———. 1972. "Persecution and Martyrdom in Hadrianic Days." In *Scripta Hierosolymitana,* vol. 23, ed. David Aheri and Israel Shatzman. Jerusalem: Magnes Press.

Hezser, Catherine. 1997. *The Social Structure of the Rabbinic Movement in Roman Palestine.* Tübingen: Mohr Siebeck.

Himmelfarb, Martha. 2006. *A Kingdom of Priests: Ancestry and Merit in Ancient Judaism.* Philadelphia: University of Pennsylvania Press.

Hirsch, W. 1947. *Rabbinic Psychology: Beliefs About the Soul in Rabbinic Literature of the Talmudic Period.* London: Edward Goldston.

Hirshman, Marc. 1996. *A Rivalry of Genius: Jewish and Christian Biblical Interpretation in Late Antiquity.* Trans. Batya Stein. New York: State University of New York.

———. 1999. *Torah for All the World's People* [in Hebrew]. Tel Aviv: Hakibbutz Hameuchad.

———. 2000. "Rabbinic Universalism in the Second and Third Centuries." *Harvard Theological Review* 93 (2): 101–15.

Hodge, Caroline Johnson. 2007. *If Sons, Then Heirs: A Study of Kinship and Ethnicity in the Letters of Paul.* Oxford: Oxford University Press.

Hoffman, Lawrence. 1996. *Covenant of Blood: Circumcision and Gender in Rabbinic Judaism.* Chicago: University of Chicago Press.

Horowitz, Maryanne Cline. 1976. "Aristotle and Women." *Journal of the History of Biology* 9: 186–213.

———. 1979. "The Image of God in Man—Is Woman Included?" *Harvard Theological Review* 72: 175–206.

Hunter, David G. 1987. "Resistance to the Virginal Ideal in Late Fourth Century Rome: The Case of Jovinian." *Theological Studies* 48: 45–64.

———. 1989. "On the Sin of Adam and Eve: A Little-Known Defense of Marriage and Childbearing by Ambrosiaster." *Harvard Theological Review* 82: 283–99.

———. 1992. "The Paradise of Patriarchy: Ambrosiaster on Woman as (Not) God's Image." *Journal of Theological Studies* 43: 447–69.

———. 1993. "Helvidius, Jovinian, and the Virginity of Mary in Late Fourth-Century Rome." *Journal of Early Christian Studies* 1: 47–71.

———. 2007. *Marriage, Celibacy, and Heresy in Ancient Christianity: The Jovinianist Controversy.* Oxford: Oxford University Press.

Huser, Roger John. 1942. *Crime of Abortion in Canon Law: An Historical Synopsis and Commentary.* Washington, D.C.: Catholic University Press.

Idel, Moshe. 1990. *The Golem: Jewish Magical and Mystical Traditions on the Artificial Anthropoid.* New York: State University of New York Press.

Ilan, Tal. 1997. *Mine and Yours Are Hers: Retrieving Women's History from Rabbinic Literature.* Leiden: Brill.

———. 1999. *Integrating Women into Second Temple History.* Tübingen: Mohr Siebeck.

Jakobovits, Immanuel. 1959. *Jewish Medical Ethics: A Comparative and Historical Study of the Jewish Religious Attitude to Medicine and Its Practice.* New York: Philosophical Library.

———. 1979. "Jewish Views on Abortion." In *Jewish Bioethics*, ed. Fred Rosner and J. David Bleich. New York: Sanhedrin Press.

Jastrow, Marcus. 1992. *A Dictionary of the Targumim, the Talmud Babli and Yerushalmi, and the Midrashic Literature.* Reprint. New York: Judaica Press.

Jones, W. H. S., trans. 1995. *Hippocrates.* Vol. 1: *Ancient Medicine. Airs, Waters, Places. Epidemics 1 & 3. The Oath. Precepts. Nutriment.* Loeb Classical Library. Cambridge, Mass. Harvard University Press.

Jouanna, Jacques. 1999. *Hippocrates.* Trans. M. B. DeBevoise. Baltimore: Johns Hopkins University Press.

Kadushin, Max. 1969. *A Conceptual Approach to the Mekilta.* New York: Jewish Theological Seminary.

Kalimi, I. 2002. "'He Was Born Circumcised': Some Midrashic Sources, Their Concept, Roots and Presumably Historical Context." *Zeitschrift für die Neutestamentliche Wissenschaft und die Kunde der Alteren Kirche* 93 (1–2): 1–12.

Kalmin, Richard.1990. "The Talmudic Story: Aggada as History." In *Proceedings of the Tenth World Congress of Jewish Studies.* Jerusalem: World Union of Jewish Studies.

———. 1991. "The Modern Study of Ancient Rabbinic Literature: Yonah Fraenkel's *Darkhei ha'aggadah vehamidrash.*" *Prooftexts* 14: 189–204.

———. 1999. *The Sage in Jewish Society of Late Antiquity.* London: Routledge.

———. 2003. "Rabbinic Traditions About Roman Persecutions of the Jews: A Reconsideration." *Journal of Jewish Studies* 54 (1): 21–50.

Kaminsky, Joel. 2007. *Yet I Loved Jacob: Reclaiming the Biblical Concept of Election.* Nashville: Abingdon Press.

Kapparis, Konstantinos. 2002. *Abortion in the Ancient World*. London: Duckworth.
Keller, Eve. 2000. "Embryonic Individuals: The Rhetoric of Seventeenth-Century Embryology and the Construction of Early-Modern Identity." *Eighteenth-Century Studies* 33 (3): 321–48.
Kelly, J. N. D. 1960. *Early Christian Doctrines*. New York: Harper.
Kessler, Edward. 2004. *Bound by the Bible: Jews, Christians, and the Sacrifice of Isaac*. Cambridge: Cambridge University Press.
Kessler, Gwynn. 2001. "The God of Small Things: The Fetus and Its Development in Palestinian Aggadic Literature." Ph.D. diss., Jewish Theological Seminary.
———. 2007. "Bodies in Motion: Preliminary Notes on Queer Theory and Rabbinic Literature." In *Mapping Gender in Ancient Religious Discourses,* ed. Todd Penner and Caroline V. Stichele. Biblical Interpretation Series 84. Leiden: E. J. Brill.
Kimelman, Reuven. 1980. "Rabbi Yohanan and Origen on the Song of Songs: A Third-Century Jewish-Christian Disputation." *Harvard Theological Review* 73 (3–4): 567–95.
———. 1981. "*Birkat Ha-Minim* and the Lack of Evidence for an Anti-Christian Jewish Prayer in Late Antiquity." In *Jewish and Christian Self-Definition*, vol. 2, ed. E. P. Sanders. Philadelphia: Fortress Press.
King, Helen. 1998. *Hippocrates' Woman: Reading the Female Body in Ancient Greece*. London: Routledge.
Klawans, Jonathan. 2000. *Impurity and Sin in Ancient Judaism*. Oxford: Oxford University Press.
Klein, Michele. 1998. *A Time to Be Born: Customs and Folklore of Jewish Birth*. Philadelphia: JPS.
Kohut, Alexander, ed. 1969. *Sefer Arukh HaShalem*. Reprint. Tel Aviv: Shiloh Press.
Koren, Sharon Faye. 2004. "Kabbalistic Physiology: Isaac the Blind, Nahmanides, and Moses de Lean on Menstruation." *AJS Review* 28 (2): 317–39.
Kottek, Samuel. 1980. "Breast-feeding in Ancient Jewish Sources, Historical and Legal Aspects. In *Human Milk: Its Biological and Social Value,* ed. S. Freier and A. I. Eidelman. Amsterdam-Oxford-Princeton: Elsevier.
1981. "Embryology in Talmudic and Midrashic Literature." *Journal of the History of Biology* 14 (2): 299–315.
———. 1996–97. "Alexandrian Medicine in the Talmudic Corpus." *Korot* 12: 80–89.
Kottek, Samuel, and G. Baader. 2000. "Talmudic and Greco-Roman Data on Pregnancy: A Renewed Examination." In *From Athens to Jerusalem: Medicine in Hellenized Jewish Lore and in Early Christian Literature,* ed. Samuel Kottek and Manfred Horstmanshoff. Rotterdam: Erasmus.
Kraemer, David. 1986. "A Developmental Perspective on the Laws of *Niddah*." *Conservative Judaism* 8: 26–33.
———. 1989. "On the Reliability of Attributions in the Babylonian Talmud." *Hebrew Union College Annual* 60: 175–90.
———. 1990. *The Mind of the Talmud: An Intellectual History of the Bavli*. Oxford: Oxford University Press.
———. 1999. "Rabbinic Sources for Historical Study." In *Judaism in Late Antiquity*,

part 3, *Where We Stand: Issues and Debates in Ancient Judaism*, vol. 1, ed. Jacob Neusner and Alan J. Avery-Peck. Leiden: Brill.

Kraemer, Ross S. 1989. "On the Meaning of the Term 'Jew' in Greco-Roman Inscriptions." *Harvard Theological Review* 82 (1): 35–53.

———. 1991. "Jewish Tuna and Christian Fish: Identifying Religious Affiliation in Epigraphic Sources." *Harvard Theological Review* 84 (2): 141–62.

———. 1993. "Jewish Mothers and Daughters in the Greco-Roman World." In *The Jewish Family in Antiquity*, ed. Shaye J. D. Cohen. Atlanta: Scholars Press.

Labovitz, Gail. 2002. "My Wife I Called 'My House': Marriage, Metaphor and Discourses of Gender in Rabbinic Literature." Ph.D. diss., Jewish Theological Seminary.

Lachs, S. T. 1969–70. "Rabbi Abbahu and the Minim." *Jewish Quarterly Review* 60: 197–212.

LaFleur, William. 1994. *Liquid Life: Abortion and Buddhism in Japan*. Princeton, N.J.: Princeton University Press.

Langston, Scott M. 2006. *Exodus Through the Centuries*. Malden, Mass.: Blackwell Publishing.

Lapin, Hayim, ed. 1998. *Religious and Ethnic Communities in Later Roman Palestine*. Studies and Texts in Jewish History and Culture. Potomac: University Press of Maryland.

Laqueur, Thomas. 1990. *Making Sex: Body and Gender from the Greeks to Freud*. Cambridge, Mass.: Harvard University Press.

Latour, Bruno. 1986. "Visualization and Cognition: Thinking with Eyes and Hands." *Knowledge and Society: Studies in the Sociology of Culture Past and Present* 6: 1–40.

Lauterbach, Jacob Z. 1970. *Studies in Jewish Law, Custom and Folklore*. New York: Ktav.

Lefkowitz, Mary R., and Maureen B. Fant. 1992. *Women's Life in Greece and Rome: A Source Book in Translation*. 2nd ed. Baltimore: Johns Hopkins University Press.

Levenson, Jon D. 1996. "The Universal Horizon of Biblical Particularism." In *Ethnicity and the Bible*, ed. Mark Brett. Leiden: Brill.

Levine, Baruch. 1989. *The JPS Torah Commentary: Leviticus*. Philadelphia: JPS.

Levine, Lee. 1975a. *Caesarea Under Roman Rule*. Leiden: Brill.

———. 1975b. "Rabbi Abbahu of Caesarea." In *Christianity, Judaism and Other Greco-Roman Cults: Studies for Morton Smith at Sixty*, ed. Jacob Neusner. Leiden: Brill.

———. 1989. *The Rabbinic Class of Roman Palestine in Late Antiquity*. New York: Jewish Theological Seminary.

———. 1998. *Judaism and Hellenism in Antiquity: Conflict or Confluence?* Seattle: University of Washington Press.

Levinson, Joshua. 2000a. "Bodies and Bo(a)rders: Emerging Fictions of Identity in Late Antiquity." *Harvard Theological Review* 93: 343–72.

———. 2000b. "Cultural Androgyny in Rabbinic Literature." In *From Athens to Jerusalem: Medicine in Hellenized Jewish Lore and in Early Christian Literature*, ed. Samuel Kottek and Manfred Horstmanshoff. Rotterdam: Erasmus.

Lewis, Charlton and Charles Short, eds. 1962. *A Latin Dictionary.* Oxford: Clarendon Press.
Lieberman, Saul. 1937–39. *Tosefet Rishonim* [in Hebrew]. 3 vols. New York: Jewish Theological Seminary.
———. 1949. "Response." *Proceedings of the Rabbinical Assembly* 12: 272–89.
———. 1955–58. *Tosefta Ki-fshutah: A Comprehensive Commentary on the Tosefta* [in Hebrew]. 10 vols. New York: Jewish Theological Seminary.
———. 1974. *Texts and Studies.* New York: Ktav.
———. 1994. *Greek in Jewish Palestine; Hellenism in Jewish Palestine.* Reprint. New York: Jewish Theological Seminary.
Lieu, Judith. 1994. "Circumcision, Women and Salvation." *New Testament Studies* 40: 358–70.
———. 2002. *Neither Jew nor Greek? Constructing Early Christianity.* London: T & T Clark.
———. 2004. *Christian Identity in the Jewish and Graeco-Roman World.* Oxford: Oxford University Press.
Limberis, Vasiliki. 2000. "'Religion' as the Cipher for Identity: The Cases of Emperor Julian, Libanius, and Gregory Nazianzus." *Harvard Theological Review* 93 (4): 373–400.
Lloyd, G. R. E. 1983. *Science, Folklore and Ideology.* Cambridge: Cambridge University Press.
Longrigg, James. 1998. *Greek Medicine from the Heroic to the Hellenistic Age: A Source Book.* New York: Routledge.
Lonie, Iain M. 1981. *The Hippocratic Treatises "On Generation," "On The Nature of the Child," "Diseases IV."* Berlin: Walter de Gruyter.
Macmullen, Ramsay. 1997. *Christianity and Paganism in the Fourth to Eighth Centuries.* New Haven, Conn.: Yale University Press.
Malkin, Irad, 2001. "Introduction." In *Ancient Perceptions of Greek Ethnicity*, ed. Irad Malkin. Center for Hellenic Studies Colloquia 5. Cambridge, Mass.: Harvard University Press.
Marmorstein, A. "Quelques problèmes de l'ancienne apologétique juive." *Revue des Etudes Juives* 68: 161–73.
———. 1935. "Judaism and Christianity in the Middle of the Third Century." *Hebrew Union College Annual* 10:225–63.
Martin, Dale. 1995. *The Corinthian Body.* New Haven, Conn.: Yale University Press.
Martin, Emily. 1991. "The Egg and the Sperm: How Science Has Constructed a Romance Based on Stereotypical Male-Female Roles." *Signs: Journal of Women in Culture and Society* 6 (31): 485–501.
Mason, Steve. 2007. "Jews, Judaeans, Judaizing, Judaism: Problems of Categorization in Ancient History." *Journal for the Study of Judaism* 38 (4–5): 457–512.
Mazusawa, Tomoko. 2007. *The Invention of World Religions.* Chicago: University of Chicago Press.
May, Margaret Tallmadge, trans. 1968. *Galen: On the Usefulness of the Parts of the Body.* Ithaca, N.Y.: Cornell University Press.

Meacham, Tirzah. 1992. "Fetal Death in the Palestinian Talmud: Death in the Chamber." In *Death and Taxes in the Ancient Near East*, ed. Sara E. Orel. Lewiston, N.Y.: Edwin Mellen Press.

———. 1999a. "An Abbreviated History of the Development of the Jewish Menstrual Laws." In *Women and Water: Menstruation in Jewish Life and Law*, ed. Rahel R. Wasserfall. Hanover, N.H.: Brandeis University Press.

———. 1999b. "Appendix B: Retroactive and Internal Impurity and the Varieties of Blood." In *Women and Water: Menstruation in Jewish Life and Law*, ed. Rahel R. Wasserfall. Hanover, N.H.: Brandeis University Press.

———. 1999c. "Tosefta as Template: Yerushalmi Niddah." In *Introducing Tosefta: Textual, Intratextual and Intertextual Studies*, ed. Harry Fox and Tirzah Meacham. New York: Ktav.

Meir, Ofra. 1993. *The Poetics of Rabbinic Stories* [in Hebrew]. Tel Aviv: Sifriat Poalim.

———. 1999. *Rabbi Judah the Patriarch: Palestinian and Babylonian Portrait of a Leader* [in Hebrew]. Tel Aviv: Hakibbutz Hameuchad.

Michaels, Meredith. 1999. "Fetal Galaxies: Some Questions About What We See." In *Fetal Subjects, Feminist Positions*, ed. Lynn M. Morgan and Meredith W. Michaels. Philadelphia: University of Pennsylvania Press.

Milgrom, Jacob. 1991. *Leviticus 1–16: A New Translation with Introduction and Commentary*. Anchor Bible. New York: Doubleday.

Moore, Keith L. 1988. *The Developing Human: Clinically Oriented Embryology*. 4th ed. Philadelphia: W. B. Saunders Company.

Moreshet, M. 1974. "Ha-Baraitot Ha-Ivriyot Ba-Bavli Uvi-Yrushalmi." In E. Y. Kutscher, *Sefer Zikaron Le-Hanokh Yalon*. Ramat Gan: Bar-Ilan University.

Morgan, Lynn. 1997. "Imagining the Unborn in the Ecuadoran Andes." *Feminist Studies* 23 (2): 323–50.

———. 1999. "Materializing the Fetal Body, or What Are Those Corpses Doing in Biology's Basement?" In *Fetal Subjects, Feminist Positions*, ed. Lynn M. Morgan and Meredith W. Michaels. Philadelphia: University of Pennsylvania Press.

———. 2003. "Embryo Tales." In *Remaking Life and Death: Toward an Anthropology of the Biosciences*, ed. Sarah Franklin and Margaret Lock. Santa Fe, N.Mex.: School of American Research Press.

Morgan, Lynn M., and Meredith W. Michaels, eds. 1999. *Fetal Subjects, Feminist Positions*. Philadelphia: University of Pennsylvania Press.

Morsink, Johannes. 1979. "Was Aristotle's Biology Sexist?" *Journal of the History of Biology* 12: 83–112.

Muntner, Suessman. 1977. "Medicine in Ancient Israel," In *Medicine in the Bible and Talmud*, ed. Fred Rosner. New York: Ktav.

Needham, Joseph. 1934. *A History of Embryology*. London: Cambridge University Press.

Nelson, W. David. 2006. *Mekhilta De-Rabbi Shimon Bar Yohai: Translated into English, with Critical Introduction and Annotation*. Philadelphia: Jewish Publication Society.

Neusner, Jacob. 1971. *Aphrahat and Judaism: The Christian-Jewish Argument in Fourth Century Iran.* Leiden: Brill.

———. 1980. "The Use of Later Rabbinic Evidence for the Study of Paul." In *Approaches to Ancient Judaism*, vol. 2, ed. William Scott Green. Chico, Calif.: Scholars Press.

———. 1982. *Judaism: The Evidence of the Mishnah.* Chicago: University of Chicago Press.

———. 1985a. *The Integrity of Leviticus Rabbah.* Chico, Calif.: Scholars Press.

———. 1985b. "Stable Symbols in a Shifting Society: The Delusion of the Monolithic Gentile in Documents of Late Fourth-Century Judaism." In *"To See Ourselves as Others See Us": Christian, Jews, "Others" in Late Antiquity*, ed. Jacob Neusner and Ernest S. Frerichs. Chico, Calif.: Scholars Press.

———. 1986a. *From Enemy to Sibling: Rome and Israel in the First Century of Western Civilization.* Ben Zion Bokser Memorial Lecture. New York: Queens College of the City University of New York.

———. 1986b. *Judaism and Scripture: The Evidence of Leviticus Rabbah.* Chicago: University of Chicago Press.

———. 1986c. *Judaism in the Matrix of Christianity.* Philadelphia: Fortress Press.

———. 1987a. *Judaism and Christianity in the Age of Constantine: History, Messiah, Israel, and the Initial Confrontation.* Chicago Studies in the History of Judaism. Chicago: University of Chicago Press.

———. 1987b. *What Is Midrash?* Philadelphia: Fortress Press, 1987.

———. 1989. *Judaism and Its Social Metaphors.* Cambridge: Cambridge University Press.

———. 1994. "The Talmud of the Land of Israel and the Mishnah." Reprinted in *Essential Papers on the Talmud*, ed. Michael Chernick. New York: New York University Press.

———. 1995. "Was Rabbinic Judaism Really 'Ethnic'?" *Catholic Bible Quarterly* 57: 281–305.

Neusner, Jacob, and Ernest S. Frerichs, eds. 1985. *"To See Ourselves as Others See Us": Christian, Jews, "Others" in Late Antiquity.* Chico, Calif.: Scholars Press.

Newman, Karen. 1996. *Fetal Positions: Individualism, Science, Visuality.* Stanford, Calif.: Stanford University Press.

Newmyer, Stephen. 1985. "Talmudic Medicine and Greek Sources." *Korot* 9: 34–57.

———. 1988. "Antoninus and Rabbi on the Soul: Stoic Elements of a Puzzling Encounter." *Korot* 9: 108–23.

———. 1993. "Asaph the Jew and Greco-Roman Pharmaceutics." In *Studies in Ancient Medicine*, vol. 7, ed. John Scarborough. New York: Brill.

Niehoff, Maren. 2005. "*Creatio ex Nihilo* Theology in *Genesis Rabbah* in Light of Christian Exegesis." *Harvard Theological Review* 99 (1): 37–64.

Noonan, John T., Jr. 1965. *Contraception: A History of Its Treatment by the Catholic Theologians and Canonists.* Cambridge, Mass.: Harvard University Press.

———. 1970. "An Almost Absolute Value in History." In *The Morality of Abortion: Legal and Historical Perspectives*, ed. J. T. Noonan Jr. Cambridge, Mass.: Harvard University Press.

Norris, Richard. 1998. "Soul." In *Encyclopedia of Early Christianity*, ed. Everett Ferguson. New York: Garland.

Nutton, Vivian. 1996. "Galen." In *The Oxford Classical Dictionary*, ed. S. Hornblower and A. Spawforth. Oxford: Oxford University Press.

O'Connell, Robert J. 1987. *The Origin of the Soul in St. Augustine's Later Works*. New York: Fordham University Press.

Pagels, Elaine. 1988. "'Freedom from Necessity': Philosophic and Personal Dimensions of Christian Conversion." In *Genesis 1–3 in the History of Exegesis: Intrigue in the Garden*, ed. Gregory Allen Robbins. Studies in Women and Religion 27. Lewiston, N.Y.: Edwin Mellen Press.

———. 1989. *Adam, Eve, and the Serpent*. New York: Vintage Books.

Pardes, Ilana. 1992. *Countertraditions in the Bible: A Feminist Approach*. Cambridge, Mass.: Harvard University Press.

———. 2000. *The Biography of Ancient Israel: National Narratives in the Bible*. Berkeley: University of California Press.

Peskowitz, Miriam. 1997. *Spinning Fantasies: Rabbis, Gender, and History*. Berkeley: University of California Press.

Peskowitz, Miriam, and Laura Levitt. 1997. *Judaism Since Gender*. New York: Routledge.

Petchesky, Rosalind. 1987. "Fetal Images: The Power of Visual Culture in the Politics of Reproduction." *Feminist Studies* 13 (2): 263–92.

Porton, Gary. 1988. *Goyim: Gentiles and Israelites in Mishnah-Tosefta*. Atlanta: Scholars Press.

———. 1994. *The Stranger within Your Gates: Converts and Conversion in Rabbinic Literature*. Chicago: University of Chicago Press.

———. 1999. "Who Was a Jew?" In *Judaism in Late Antiquity*, part 3, *Where We Stand: Issues and Debates in Ancient Judaism*, vol. 2, ed. Jacob Neusner and Alan J. Avery-Peck. Leiden: Brill.

Preus, Anthony. 1977. "Galen's Criticism of Aristotle's Conception Theory." *Journal of the History of Biology* 10 (1): 65–85.

Preuss, Julius. 1978. *Biblical and Talmudic Medicine*. Trans. Fred Rosner. New York: Sandhedrin Press. Originally published as *Biblisch-talmudische Medizin: Beitrage zur Geschichte der Heilkunde und der Kultur ueberhaupt* (Berlin: S. Karger, 1911).

Rabinowitz, Z. M. 1965. *Halakha and Aggada in the Liturgical Poetry of Yannai: The Sources, Language and Period of the Payyetan*. Tel Aviv: Z. M. Rabinowitz.

Rapp, Rayna. 1999. *Testing Women, Testing the Fetus: The Social Impact of Amniocentesis in America*. New York: Routledge.

Riddle, John M. 1997. *Contraception and Abortion from the Ancient World to the Renaissance*. Cambridge, Mass.: Harvard University Press.

———. 1997. *Eve's Herbs: A History of Contraception and Abortion in the West*. Cambridge, Mass.: Harvard University Press.

Robbins, Gregory Allen, ed. 1988. *Genesis 1–3 in the History of Exegesis: Intrigue in the Garden*. Studies in Women and Religion 27. Lewiston, N.Y.: Edwin Mellen Press.

Robinson, James M., ed. 1990. *The Nag Hammadi Library in English*. Rev. ed. San Francisco: HarperCollins.
Rokeah, David. 1998. *Justin Martyr and the Jews* [in Hebrew]. Jerusalem: Merkaz Dinur.
Roll, Susan K. 2003. "The Old Rite of the Churching of Women after Childbirth." In *Wholly Woman, Holy Blood: A Feminist Critique of Purity and Impurity*, ed. Kristen De Troyer, Judith A. Herbert, Judith Ann Johnson, and Anne-Marie Korte. Harrisburg, Pa.: Trinity Press International.
Romney-Wegner, Judith. 1990. *Chattel or Person? The Status of Women in Time and Torah*. Hoboken, N.J.: Ktav.
Rosner, Fred. 1977. "Sex Determination as Described in the Talmud." In *Medicine in the Bible and Talmud: Selections from Classical Jewish Sources*. New York: Yeshiva University Press.
———. 1979. *Jewish Bioethics*. New York: Sanhedrin Press.
Rothman, Barbara Katz. 1986. *The Tentative Pregnancy: Prenatal Diagnosis and the Future of Motherhood*. New York: Viking.
Rousselle, Aline. 1988. *Porneia: On Desire and the Body in Antiquity*. Trans. Felicia Pheasant. Oxford: Blackwell.
Rubenstein, Jeffrey. 1998. "Elisha ben Abuya: Torah and the Sinful Sage." *Journal of Jewish Thought and Philosophy* 7: 141–222.
———. 1999. *Talmudic Stories: Narrative Art, Composition, and Culture*. Baltimore: Johns Hopkins University Press.
———. 2002. *Rabbinic Stories: Stories from the Major Works of Classical Rabbinic Literature Produced between 200 and 600 C.E.* New York: Paulist Press.
———. 2003. *The Culture of the Babylonian Talmud*. Baltimore: Johns Hopkins University Press.
———. 2007. "Social and Institutional Settings of Rabbinic Literature. In *The Cambridge Companion to the Talmud and Rabbinic Literature*, ed. Charlotte Elisheva Fonrobert and Martin S. Jaffee. Cambridge: Cambridge University Press.
Rubin, Nissan. 1988. "Body and Soul in Talmudic and Mishnaic Sources." *Korot* 9: 151–64.
Ruether, Rosemary Radford. 1991. "The *Adversus Judaeos* Tradition in the Church Fathers: The Exegesis of Christian Anti-Judaism." In *Essential Papers on Judaism and Christianity in Conflict: From Late Antiquity to the Reformation*, ed. Jeremy Cohen. New York: New York University Press.
Saldarini, Anthony. 1998. "The Social World of Christian Jews and Jewish Christians." In *Religious and Ethnic Communities in Later Roman Palestine*, ed. Hayim Lapin. Potomac: University Press of Maryland.
Sanders, E. P. 1977. *Paul and Palestinian Judaism*. London: SCM.
———. 1980. "Puzzling Out Rabbinic Judaism." In *Approaches to Ancient Judaism*, vol. 2, ed. William Scott Green. Chico, Calif.: Scholars Press.
Sanders, E. P., et al., eds. 1981. *Jewish and Christian Self-Definition*. Vol. 2, *Aspects of Judaism in the Greco-Roman World*. London: SCM.
Sandmel, Samuel. 1962. "Parallelomania." *Journal of Biblical Literature* 81: 1–13.

Sarason, Richard. 1982. "The Petihtot in Leviticus Rabbah: 'Oral Homilies' or Redactional Constructions." *Journal of Jewish Studies* 33: 557–67.
Sasson, Vanessa. 2007. *The Birth of Moses and the Buddha: A Paradigm for the Contemporary Study of Religions.* Sheffield: Phoenix Press Ltd.
Satlow, Michael. 1994. "'Wasted Seed': The History of a Rabbinic Idea." *Hebrew Union College Annual* 65: 157–60.
———. 1995. *Tasting the Dish: Rabbinic Rhetorics of Sexuality.* Brown Judaic Studies. Atlanta: Scholars Press.
———. 2005. "A History of the Jews or Judaism? On Seth Schwartz's *Imperialism and Jewish Society, 200 B.C.E. to 640 C.E.*" *Jewish Quarterly Review* 96 (1): 151–62.
Schäfer, Peter. 1990. "Hadrian's Policy in Judaea and the Bar Kokhba Revolt: A Reassessent." In *A Tribute to Geza Vermes: Essays on Jewish and Christian Literature and History,* ed. Philip R. Davies and Richard T. White. Sheffield: Journal for the Study of the Old Testament Press.
———. 1997. *Judeophobia: Attitudes Toward the Jews in the Ancient World.* Cambridge, Mass.: Harvard University Press.
Schechter, Solomon. 1910. *Some Aspects of Rabbinic Theology.* New York: Macmillan.
Scheck, Thomas P., trans. 2002. *Origen: Commentary on the Epistle to the Romans, Books 6–10.* Fathers of the Church: A New Translation. Washington, D.C.: Catholic University of America Press.
Schiff, Daniel. 2002. *Abortion in Judaism.* Cambridge: Cambridge University Press.
Schiffman, Lawrence H. 1985. *Who Was a Jew? Rabbinic and Halakhic Perspectives on the Jewish-Christian Schism.* Hoboken, N.J.: Ktav.
———. 2003. "The Concept of Covenant in the Qumran Scrolls and Rabbinic Literature." In *The Idea of Biblical Interpretation: Essays in Honor of James L. Kugel,* ed. Hindy Najman and Judith H. Newman. Leiden: Brill.
Schultz, Jennifer. 2003. "Doctors, Philosophers, and Christian Fathers on Menstural Blood." In *Wholly Woman, Holy Blood: A Feminist Critique of Purity and Impurity,* ed. Kristen De Troyer, Judith A. Herbert, Judith Ann Johnson, and Anne-Marie Korte. Harrisburg, Pa.: Trinity Press International, 2003.
Schwartz, Regina. 1997. *The Curse of Cain: The Violent Legacy of Monotheism.* Chicago: University of Chicago Press.
Schwartz, Seth. 2001. *Imperialism and Jewish Society, 200 B.C.E. to 640 C.E.* Princeton, N.J.: Princeton University Press.
Scott, James C. 1990. *Domination and the Arts of Resistance: Hidden Transcripts.* New Haven, Conn.: Yale University Press.
Segal, Alan. 1977. *Two Powers in Heaven: Early Rabbinic Reports about Christianity and Gnosticism.* Leiden: Brill.
———. 1985. "Covenant in Rabbinic Literature." *Studies in Religion/Sciences Religieuses* 14: 53–62.
———. 1986. *Rebecca's Children: Judaism and Christianity in the Roman World.* Cambridge, Mass.: Harvard University Press.

Seow, C. L. 1997. *The Anchor Bible Ecclesiastes: A New Translation with Introduction and Commentary*. New York: Doubleday.
Simon, Marcel. 1937. "Melchisédech dans la polémique entre juifs et chrétiens et dans la légende." *Revue d'histoire et de philosophie religieuses* 17: 58–93.
———. 1986. *Verus Israel: A Study of the Relations Between Christians and Jews in the Roman Empire (135–425)*. Littman Library of Jewish Civilization. Oxford: Oxford University Press. Original French edition was published in 1948.
Singer, Peter N., trans. 2001. *Galen: Selected Works*. Oxford: Oxford University Press.
Smith, Anthony D. 1986. *The Ethnic Origins of Nations*. Oxford: Blackwell.
Smith, Jonathan Z. 1982. *Imagining Religion: From Babylon to Jonestown*. Chicago: University of Chicago Press.
———. 1985. "What a Difference a Difference Makes." In *"To See Ourselves as Others See Us": Christians, Jews, "Others," in Late Antiquity*, ed. Jacob Neusner and Ernest S. Frerichs. Chico, Calif.: Scholars Press.
———. 1996. "A Matter of Class: Taxonomies of Religion." *Harvard Theological Review* 89: 387–403.
———. 1998. "Religion, Religions, Religious." In *Critical Terms for Religious Studies*, ed. Mark C. Taylor. Chicago: University of Chicago Press.
Smith, Richard. 1988. "Sex Education in Gnostic Schools." In *Images of the Feminine in Gnosticism*, ed. Karen King. Philadelphia: Fortress Press
Smith, William Robertson. 1927. *Lectures on the Religion of the Semites: The Fundamental Institutions*. Ed. Stanley A. Cook. London: A. & C. Black.
Souter, Alexander, ed. 1949. *A Glossary of Later Latin to 600 A.D.* Oxford: Clarendon Press.
Stabile, Carol. 1992. "Shooting the Mother: Fetal Photography and the Politics of Disappearance." *Camera Obscura: A Journal of Feminism and Film* 28. Special issue: *Imaging Technologies, Inscribing Science*, ed. Paula Treichler and Lisa Cartwright.
Stern, David. 1988. "Midrash and Indeterminacy." *Critical Inquiry* 15: 132–61.
———. 1991. *Parables in Midrash: Narrative and Exegesis in Rabbinic Literature*. Cambridge, Mass.: Harvard University Press.
———. 1996. *Midrash and Theory: Ancient Jewish Exegesis and Contemporary Literary Studies*. Evanston, Ill.: Northwestern University Press.
Stern, Sacha. 1994. *Jewish Identity in Early Rabbinic Writings*. New York: Brill.
Stol, M. 2000a. *Birth in Babylonia and the Bile: Its Mediterranean Setting*. Groningen: Styx.
———. 2000b. "Maternal Imagination During Pregnancy in Babylonia." In *From Athens to Jerusalem: Medicine in Hellenized Jewish Lore and in Early Christian Literature*, ed. Samuel Kottek and Manfred Horstmanshoff. Rotterdam: Erasmus.
Stormer, Nathan. 2000. "Prenatal Space." *Signs* 26 (1): 109–44.
Stowers, Stanley. 1994. *A Rereading of Romans: Justice, Jews, and Gentiles*. New Haven, Conn.: Yale University Press.
Strack, H. L., and G. Stemberger. 1996. *Introduction to the Talmud and Midrash*. Trans. Markus Bockmuehl. 2nd printing. Minneapolis: Fortress Press.

Temkin, Owsei. 1991a. *Hippocrates in a World of Pagans and Christians*. Baltimore: Johns Hopkins University Press.

———, trans. 1991b. *Soranus' Gynecology*. Reprint, Baltimore: Johns Hopkins University Press. Originally published in 1956.

Tertullian. "A Treatise on the Soul" (*De anima*). In *Ante-Nicene Fathers*, vol. 3, ed. Alexander Roberts and James Donaldson.

Teske, Roland, trans. 1999a. Augustine. *Answer to the Pelagians III. Unfinished Work in Answer to Julian*. Hyde Park, N.Y.: New City Press.

Teske, Roland J. 1999b. "Soul." In *Augustine Through the Ages: An Encyclopedia*, ed. A. Fitzgerald. Grand Rapids, Mich.: Eerdmans.

Trachtenberg, Joshua. 2004. *Jewish Magic and Superstition: A Study in Folk Religion*. Reprint. Philadelphia: University of Pennsylvania Press.

Trible, Phyllis. 1978. *God and the Rhetoric of Sexuality*. Philadelphia: Fortress Press.

Trigg, Joseph Wilson. 1983. *Origen: The Bible and Philosophy in the Third Century Church*. Atlanta: John Knox Press.

Tropper, Amram. 2004. *Wisdom, Politics, and Historiography: Tractate Avot in the Contet of the Graeco-Roman Near East*. Oxford: Oxford University Press.

Urbach, E. E. 1971. "The Homiletical Interpretations of the Sages and the Exposition of Origen on Canticles, and the Jewish-Christian Disputation." In *Scripta Heirosolymitana: Studies in Aggadah and Folk-Literature*, vol. 22, ed. J. Heinemann and D. Noy. Jerusalem: Magnes Press.

———. 1987. *The Sages: Their Concepts and Beliefs*. Trans. Israel Abrahams. Cambridge, Mass.: Harvard University Press.

Van der Horst, Pieter Willem. 1978. "Seven Months' Children in Jewish and Christian Literature from Antiquity." *Ephemerides Theologicae Louanienses* 54: 346–60.

———. 1990. "Sarah's Seminal Emission: Hebrews 11:11 in the Light of Ancient Embryology." In *Greeks, Romans, and Christians: Essays in Honor of Abraham J. Malherbe*, ed. David L. Balch, Everett Ferguson, and Wayne A. Meeks. Minneapolis: Fortress.

Veltri, Guiseppe. 1998. "On the Influence of 'Greek Wisdom': Theoretical and Empirical Sciences in Rabbinic Judaism." *Jewish Studies Quarterly* 5: 300–317.

Vermes, Geza. 1982. "Jewish Literature and New Testament Exegesis: Reflections on Methodology." *Journal of Jewish Studies* 31: 361–76.

Veyne, Paul. 1988. *Did the Greeks Believe in Their Myths? An Essay on the Constitutive Imagination*. Trans. Paula Wissing. Chicago: University of Chicago Press.

Visotzky, Burton. 1995. *Fathers of the World*. Tübingen: J. C. B. Mohr.

———. 1999. "The Priest's Daughter and the Thief in the Orchard: The Soul of Midrash Leviticus Rabbah." In *Putting Body and Soul Together: Essays in Honor of Robin Scroggs*, ed. Virginia Wiles, Alexandra Brown, and Graydon F. Snyder. Valley Forge, Pa.: Trinity Press International.

———. 2003. *Golden Bells and Pomegranates*. Tübingen: Mohr Siebeck.

———. 2006. "Midrash, Christian Exegesis, and Hellenistic Hermeneutic." In *Current Trends in the Study of Midrash*, ed. Carol Bakhos. Leiden: Brill.

———. 2007. "*Midrash Aggadah: Al Kama Mi'Ekronot Ha'Arikhah shel Vayikra Rabbah*" [Hebrew]. In *Higgayon LaYona: HeBetim Hadashim BiHeker Sifrut

HaMidrash: MaAggadah VeHaPiyyut [New Directions in the Study of Midrash Aggadah: Jonah Fraenkel Volume], ed. Levinson, Elbaum and Hasan-Rokem. Jerusalem: Magnes Press.

———. 2008. "Goys 'Я'n't Us: Rabbinic Anti-Gentile Polemic in Yerushalmi Berachot 9:1." In *Heresy and Identity in Late Antiquity*, ed. Eduard Iricinschi and Holger Zellentin, 299–313. Tübingen: Mohr Siebeck.

———. Forthcoming. "Will and Grace: Aspects of Judaising in Pelagianism in Light of Rabbinic and Patristic Exegeses of Genesis)." In *The Exegetical Encounter Between Jews and Christians in Late Antiquity: Conference at University of Cambridge; 24–28 June, 2007, Proceedings*, ed. Edward Kessler. Leiden: Brill.

Von Balthasar, Hans Urs, ed. 1984. *Origen: Spirit and Fire: A Thematic Anthology of His Writings*. Trans. Robert J. Daly. Washington, D.C.: Catholic University of America Press.

Von Staden, Heinrich. 1989. *Herophilos: The Art of Medicine in Early Alexandria*. Cambridge: Cambridge University Press.

Wallach, L. 1941. "The Colloquy of Marcus Aurelius with the Patriarch Judah I." *Jewish Quarterly Review* 31: 259–86.

Wasserstein, A. 1985. "Normal and Abnormal Gestation Periods in Humans: A Survey of Ancient Opinion (Greek, Roman and Rabbinic)." *Korot* 9: 221–29.

Weitzman, Steve. 2005. *Surviving Sacrilege: Cultural Persistence in Jewish Antiquity*. Cambridge, Mass.: Harvard University Press.

Wolfson, Elliot. 1987. "Circumcision and the Divine Name: A Study in the Transmission of Esoteric Doctrine." *Jewish Quarterly Review* 78 (1–2): 77–112.

Yuval, Israel Jacob. 2000. *Shene goyim be-vitnekh: Yehudim ve-Notsrim, dimuyim hadadiyim*. Tel Aviv: Am Oved.

———. 2006. *Two Nations in Your Womb: Perceptions of Jews and Christians in Late Antiquity and the Middle Ages*. Berkeley: University of California Press.

Name and Subject Index

Abba bar Kahana, R., 93, 95
Abbahu, R., 57, 75, 85, 171n64
abortion, 18, 19, 128–29, 145n110
Abraham, 103, 189n82, 190n90
'adam, 10, 37, 74, 91–92, 101, 139n44, 140n46, 149n31
adultery, 69–70, 71, 166–67n31, 177n109
affiliation, narrative of, 12, 141–42n63
agricultural fertility, 118, 198n173
Aitken, Ellen, 147n138, 147n139
Alter, Robert, 195n148
"And the elder shall serve the younger" (Gen. 25:23), 56–57, 60, 61
Antoninus-Rabbi tradition, on occurrence of ensoulment, 65, 68, 76, 85, 86, 156n37, 165n19
Aristotle, 110, 177n102, 177n103, 183n27, 187n67, 187n68, 193n122
Augustine, 119–20, 197n161

Baker, Cynthia, 95, 97, 130, 131, 183–84n36
Bakhos, Carol, 59
barrenness, 112, 118, 190n89, 195n143
Barth, Frederik, 8
Bavli (Babylonian Talmud): circumcision in, 40; ensoulment in, 68–69, 166n27; gematria used in, 74; on order of fetal development, 168n41; rabbinization of fetus in, 41, 151n50; on sex determination of fetus, 78–79, 174–75n86; theory of female seed, 106–7; Torah study in, 35, 40, 41–42, 150n39
ben Lakish, Shimeon, R. (Reish Lakish), 49, 99, 100, 118
Berkowitz, Beth, 4, 85–86, 179n122
Bhabha, Homi, 86
Biale, David, 122, 187n70
bishop of Hippo and Julian of Eclanum, 119
Boyarin, Daniel: on defining religion, 141n53; dialectics of desire, 122; on erasure of Esau, 8, 160n81; on Gen. 25:23, 56, 155n31; on identities of Judaism and Christianity, 62; on Jewish identity, 203n20; on Judaism as Hellenistic religion, 162n1; on rabbinic ambivalence about sex, 122, 123; on "three partners" tradition, 108
Boylan, Michael, 193n22
breast milk, 73, 76–77, 124, 172n71, 172n72, 172–73n73
Brown, Peter, 122
Buell, Denise, 12, 139n38, 172–73n73, 180n133, 190n89

capital punishment, 85–86
Christianity: Church relations with Synagogue, 37, 47, 53, 54, 56, 57; Esau as Christian Rome, 59–60, 61; Jesus, 121–22, 147n138; Mary, virginity of, 188n75; original sin, 98, 119, 121–22, 199n184, 199n186, 200n200; Paul's letter to the Romans on prenatal Jacob and Esau, 51–55. *See also* Origen
Christian Rome, Esau as, 27, 47, 50, 59, 153n2
Church, Jacob as symbolic of, 37, 47, 53, 54, 56, 57
circumcision: Esau as uncircumcised, 51, 155n27, 161n93; Isaac's birth and, 103; Jacob as born circumcised, 50, 154n10, 161n93; in Talmud, 40
Clark, Elizabeth, 116, 119, 120, 199n188, 199n195
Clement of Alexandria, 116–17, 180n133, 190n89, 197n165
Cohen, Gerson, 53, 55, 157n41, 157n44
Cohen, Shaye, 131, 152n71, 203–4n22, 204n26
conception: angel appointed over, 192n109; barrenness, 112, 118, 190n89, 195n143; conditions for, 104, 185n53, 189n88; menstrual blood in, 187n67, 187n68, 187n70; optimal time for, 185n51, 185n53
converts and conversion, 4, 132, 140n49, 203n22, 204n22
crossing of the sea: as baptism, 43, 149n23; as birth, 43; as Creation, 43; fetuses singing at the, 7, 24, 26, 30, 32, 36–37

232 Name and Subject Index

curdling agent, metaphor of, 100, 101, 102, 187n67, 187n68

David (biblical figure): conception of, 97–98, 121, 184n45, 184–85n50, 192n112; Psalms attributed to, 122, 151–52n53
Dean-Jones, Lesley, 94, 110, 146n124, 177n103
Decalogue, 42–43, 44, 153n72
Delaney, Carol, 22, 189n84
Dinah (biblical figure), 9, 77, 79, 80, 173n77, 176n94
Duden, Barbara, 15–18, 20, 127, 128, 143n81

eight-month child, viability of, 73, 74–76, 170n58, 171n63, 171n65
embryos: components of (sinews, bones, marrow), 101–2, 104, 106, 108; facial features of, 69–70, 166–167n31; formation of, 163n12; gestation periods for, 68–76, 166n27, 167n33, 167n38, 167–68n39, 169n49, 170n54, 170n58, 171n63, 171n65, 183n21; male origin of, 98–100; order of formation, 72; personhood of, 143n81; subjectivity of, 143n81; *tazria'*, 35, 97, 104, 198–199n185; use of term, 15–17, 144n97; visualizations of, 16–17, 20, 143n81, 144n91. *See also* fetal formation and development
emissions (*mazra'at 'odem, mazria' haloven*), 106-7, 191n105, 191n106
ensoulment: biblical proof texts for, 68, 164n13; compared with giving of Torah, 68–70, 71, 166n27, 167n33, 167n38; evil and, 165n19; giving of the Torah, 68–69, 166n27; God as responsible for, 104, 164n17; occurrence of, 67–69, 163–64n12, 164n18; "three partners" tradition, 10, 67, 81, 107–11, 191n107, 191n108, 192n117
Esau: birth order, 103, 188n79; as both Christian and pagan, 62; as Christian Rome, 27, 47, 50, 59–61, 153n2; conflict with Jacob over religious values, 49, 153n8, 154n9; erasure of, 8, 57–58, 160n81; as filth, 57–58; as Israel's other, 55, 56; as pagan Rome, 48, 49, 50, 153n2; struggle with Jacob, 3, 27, 49, 55; as symbolic of the Jews and synagogue in patristic sources, 47, 56; as uncircumcised, 51, 155n27, 161n93; as wicked, 50, 51, 155n30
Exodus (Israelites' departure from Egypt): baptism represented by parting of the sea, 43; crossing of the sea, 7, 24, 26, 30, 32, 36–37, 43, 149n23; fetuses and babies at, 30; generational memory of, 36–38; Origen on, 42–43, 152n60; singing at, 7, 24, 26, 30, 32; as transhistorical event, 36–37, 42–44, 152n60

Feldman, David, 200n201
fetal formation and development: Greco-Roman sources on, 72, 74, 170n54; menstrual blood in, 94, 183n27, 187n67, 187n68; nine-month gestation period, 73, 76, 169n49; nonviability of the eighth-month child, 73, 74–76, 170n58, 171n63, 171n65; order of, 72, 168n41; in rabbinic tradition, 19, 145n110; relation of God and Israel, 68–72, 166n27, 167n33, 167n38; theology of, 69–70, 87; timing of, 166n30; two formations for, 75, 76, 170n59, 171n66; viable birth, 74–75, 170n52, 170n53, 170n54, 170n55
fetuses: abortion, 18, 19, 145n110; Christian traditions on, 147n138, 147n139; genealogical filiation of, 131, 203n22; God as protector of, 73, 93–96, 107, 183n27; as guarantors of the tradition, 30–33, 44–45, 205n33; inheritance of physical characteristics, 69–70, 78, 81–82, 166n27, 167n33, 167n35, 173n78, 177n105, 177n106, 177–78n109, 178–79n115; Israel identified as, 10, 14, 18–19, 29, 30, 41, 48, 142n71; as *pinaks* (folded writing tablet), 1, 5, 6, 16, 21, 28, 72, 137n5, 138n22, 168–69n45; rabbinization of, in Babylonian Talmud (the *Bavli*), 41, 151n50; sex determination, 77–80, 166n30, 173n78, 173n80, 174n84, 174n85, 174–75n86, 175n87, 175n90; singing at Red Sea crossing, 7, 24, 26, 30, 32, 36–37; terms for, 15–16, 17, 143n82, 143n84, 144n91, 144n92, 144n94, 144n97, 145n121; Torah study by, 35–36, 40–41, 49–50, 150n39, 151n51; on transmission of halakhah to, 41, 151n51; visualizations of, 16–17, 20, 143n81, 144n91. *See also* ensoulment; pregnancy; womb
folded writing tablet (*pinaks*), 1, 5, 6, 16, 21, 28, 72, 137n5, 138n22, 168–69n45
Fonrobert, Charlotte, 95, 183–84n36; on menstruation, 185n52, 202n8; on rabbinic engagement with cultural environment, 66; on Roman governmental decrees prohibiting religious practices, 38, 150n39
forty-day gestation period of embryo, 68–70, 71, 166n27, 167n33, 167n38, 167–68n39

Name and Subject Index   233

Frend, W. H. C., 203n20
Frymer-Kensky, Tikva, 189n88, 198n173, 198n174

Galen, 95, 110, 181n6, 183n27, 183n31, 193n129
Ginsburg, Faye, 128–29
God: and *'adam*, 10, 37, 74, 91, 92, 101, 139n44, 140n46, 149n31; births in the Bible, 66, 82, 104, 112–13, 162n3, 178n111, 178n114, 190n89, 190n90; breast milk production from menstrual blood, 76–77, 173n74; care of fetus by, 34–35, 73, 93–96, 107, 114–15, 183n27, 196n156; contributions to creation of humans, 67, 81, 191n102; and the creation of Israel, 23; facial features of fetus determined by, 69–70, 78, 81–82; fetuses as guarantors of the tradition, 30–31, 32, 44–45, 205n33; power over human and earthly fertility, 117–18; pregnancy and, 74, 102, 104–5, 120, 123, 180n132, 190n89, 190n90, 190n91, 191n102; role in ensoulment, 68–69; role in sex determination, 78–80; in "three partners" tradition, 10, 67, 81, 106–10, 191n107, 191n108, 192n117; viability of fetus, 76; women's role in procreation and, 92, 93–94, 98. *See also* Torah and Torah study
God-fearers, 12, 13, 141n57, 141–42n63, 142n67
Greco-Roman embryology: Aristotle, 110, 177n102, 177n103, 183n27, 187n67, 187n68, 193n122; biblical proof texts for, 68; on childbirth, 119, 199n188; duration of gestation for viable birth, 74, 170n54; on fetal development, 72, 168n41; on God's role in creating the embryo, 116–17; Hippocrates, 76, 169n48; menstrual blood in, 76–77, 94, 172n72, 172–73n73, 173n74; on pregnancy, 169n48; rabbinic embryology influenced by, 66–67, 162–63n7; sources of, 163n10, 163n12; theology in, 120; theory of resemblance, 177n102; "three partners" tradition and, 111. *See also* Antoninus-Rabbi tradition; fetal formation and development; fetuses; male seed
Green, William Scott, 7

Hadrian, 50, 154n19
halakhah, transmission of, 41, 151n51
Halfota, Yosi bar, R., 58, 103, 117, 189n82, 197n170
Hall, Jonathan, 139n38
Hartouni, Valerie, 127

Hasan-Rokem, Galit, 96
Hayes, Christine, 131, 203n22
Herr, Moshe, 4, 38–39, 150n39, 150–51n44
Himmelfarb, Martha, 204n26, 205n33
Hippocrates, 76, 169n48
Hirshman, Marc, 42–43, 47–48, 139n44, 139n45, 140n49, 191n105
Hoffman, Lawrence, 108
house metaphor for woman, 21, 95, 97, 183–84n36
Huna, R., 56–57, 74, 75, 139n44, 171n60

idolatry, 3, 56, 84
impurity, procreation and, 10, 123–24, 166n30, 185n52, 202n221
Isaac, 82, 103, 118, 178n111, 178n112, 190n30
Israel: collective memory of, 36–38; constructions of, 13, 142n66; determination of paternity, 82–83, 178–79n115; fetuses as guarantors of the tradition, 30–31, 32, 44–45, 205n33; fetus identified as, 10, 14, 18–19, 29–30, 41, 48, 142n71; Jacob identified as, 3, 5, 7, 41, 47, 48, 58, 61, 160n80; Jewishness, use of term, 129, 130, 131, 203n19; Judaism and Jewishness designations and, 129, 130, 131; prenatal election of, 54, 55; rabbinic construction of, 3; rabbinic identification of, 7; relations with Rome, 49, 50, 52, 154n10, 154–55n21; use of term, 129–30, 131

Jacob: in birth order, 103, 188n79; as born circumcised, 50, 154n10, 161n93; conflict with Esau over religious values, 49, 153n8, 154n9; as elder, 58, 103, 160n80, 160n83, 161n99, 188n79; as first born, 58, 103, 188n79; identification as Israel as biblical, 61; identified with the Church, 37, 53, 54, 56, 57; as only son, 57–58, 61; prenatal election of, 54, 55; as rabbinic Israel, 3, 5, 41, 47, 48, 55, 60, 160n80; Reuben compared with, 188n79; righteous of, 3, 41, 50–51, 52, 56, 57, 155n29; struggle with Esau, 3, 27, 49, 55; Torah study by, 41, 49–50
Jakobovits, Immanuel, 132, 204–5n29
Jesus, 121–22, 147n138
Jewishness, use of term, 129, 130, 131, 203n19
Julian of Eclanum, 119, 199n188

Kalmin, Richard, 4, 38, 40, 41, 150n39, 150n41, 151–52n53
Keller, Eve, 23, 143n81, 146n126

Name and Subject Index

Kessler, E., 158n60
King, Helen, 76, 95
Kottek, Samuel, 168n41, 187n70
Kristeva, Julia, 12

Latour, Bruno, 20–21
Levinson, Joshua, 11–13, 108–9, 142n71; on communal narratives, 14; God-fearers defined by, 13, 141n57; models of identity, 141n54
Levi-Strauss, Claude, 8

male seed: absent from biblical accounts, 112–13, 195n144, 195n147, 195n148; as curdling agent, 100, 101, 102, 187n67, 187n68; denial of women's seed, 99, 102–3, 188n80; determination of paternity, 82–83, 178n111, 178n112; God's use of, 92, 98; as necessary to creation of embryo, 108, 191n108; Philo on, 114; in Second Temple period sources, 113–14; *shikhvat zera'*, 113, 115, 124, 125, 195n148; soil imagery, 197n165; in "three partners" tradition, 108–10, 111, 191n108; transmission of sin, 119–20; as white drop, 92, 99, 100, 106, 107, 123, 124, 198n177, 201n218
Malkin, Irad, 8, 138n28
Margulies, M., 99, 186n65
Mary, virginity of, 188n75
Meir, R., 30, 32, 117, 148n8
menstrual blood: breast milk production from, 73, 76–77, 124, 172n71, 172n72; in embryo formation, 183n27; as female seed, 193n129; during gestation, 98–99, 100–101; nutritive value of, 94, 183n27; one-seed theory of procreation, 110; Philo on, 114; in Second Temple period sources, 113–14; semen comingling with, 124; as sinful, 98–99
menstruation: conception and, 98, 185n51, 185n53; and purity, 10, 166n30, 185n51, 185n52, 202n221; sexual intercourse during, 201n220; and sin, 98, 185n52
messianism, 101–2, 188n74
Midrash on the Ten Commandments, 30–31, 42, 44–45
miscarriages, 16, 144n87, 144n91, 144–45n103
Morgan, Lynn, 18, 19

Needham, Joseph, 163n7, 168n41
Neusner, Jacob, 7, 58–59, 62, 63, 140n49, 184n49

Newman, Karen, 20
Newmyer, Stephen, 181n6
nine-month gestation period, 73, 76, 169n49, 183n21
nonprocreative sexual activity, 117, 121, 123, 200n201

'olalim, 30, 148n5, 148n8
one-seed theory of procreation, 24, 94, 106–7, 110–11, 181n3, 193n122, 194n131
Origen, 27; on covenantal relationship between God and Israel, 42–43; dating of works of, 158n55; on the Decalogue, 42–43, 153n72; Esau as synagogue, 47, 56; on the Exodus, 42–43, 152n57, 152n60; interpretations of Jacob and Esau, 53–54, 60; Jews' familiarity with, 55, 158n60; on prenatal merit, 159n63
original sin, 98, 119, 121–22, 199n184, 199n186, 200n200

pagan Rome, 48, 49, 50, 60, 153n2
Pagels, Elaine, 116–17
paqad, 104, 190n91
Pardes, Ilana, 34, 43
Paul, on Red Sea crossing as baptism, 43, 149n23
Pelagian controversy, 119, 120, 199n186, 200n200
Petchesky, Rosalind, 20, 21, 127
physical characteristics, inheritance of, 68–70, 78, 81, 166n27, 167n33, 167n35, 173n78, 177n105, 177n106, 177–78n109
pinaks (folded writing tablet), 1, 5, 6, 16, 21, 28, 72, 137n5, 138n22, 168–69n45
Porton, Gary, 4, 142n69
position of the fetus, 1, 5, 6, 16, 21, 28, 72, 137n5, 138n22, 168–69n45
pregnancy: barrenness, 112, 190n89, 195n143; in the Bible, 82, 104, 112–13, 178n111, 178n114, 190n89, 190n90; changing experiences of, 128; conception, 98, 185n51, 185n53; divine conception, 104, 189n88, 190n89; duration of, 72–74, 170n52, 170n53, 170n54, 170n55; God as responsible for, 74, 102, 104–5, 120, 123, 180n132, 190n89, 190n90, 190n91, 191n102; house metaphor, 21, 95, 97, 183–84n36; miscarriages, 16, 144n87, 144n91, 144–45n103; of Rebekah, 50, 72–73; ritual immersion, 185n51; sexual intercourse during, 73, 169n48, 201n215;

superfetation, 169n48; theological aspects of, 73, 169n47
Preuss, Julius: on the expression "to sit on the *mashber*," 176n96; the fetus as common topic in Midrash, 29; on menstrual blood in embryo formation, 183n27, 193n129; on rabbinic constructions of the fetus, 132; on the theories of generation, 173n78; on women's influence on the child, 177n109
procreation: *'adam*, 10, 37, 74, 91, 92, 101, 139n44, 140n46, 149n31; agricultural metaphors for, 116–18; anxieties about sex, 122–23; barrenness, 112, 190n89, 195n143; birth order, 103, 188n79; bodily impurity, 123–24, 166n30, 185n52, 202n221; commandment to, 170n57; gender roles in, 24; God's role in, 92, 189n83; menstrual blood in, 94, 98–99; seed theories of, 24, 94, 110–11, 174n85, 181n3, 193n122, 194n131; sexual intercourse, 122–23, 201n215; *tazria'*, 35, 97, 104, 198–99n185; theologization of, 122–23; "three partners" tradition in, 10, 67, 81, 106–9, 191n107, 192n117; women displaced from care of fetus, 92, 114–15, 196n156

Rabbi. *See* Yehudah haNasi
rabbinic embryology: adultery, 69–70, 71, 166–67n31, 177n109; child's physical resemblance to parents, 81–82, 177n106, 178n109, 178–79n115; forty-day gestation period of embryo, 68–70, 71, 166n27, 167n33, 167n38, 167–68n39; influence of Greco-Roman embryology on, 66–67, 85, 162–63n7, 180n130. *See also* Antoninus-Rabbi tradition; ensoulment; fetal formation and development; fetuses; Origen; pregnancy; seed; womb
rabbinic Israel: absorption of contemporaneous cultural ideas, 84–85; agricultural imagery used by, 117; ancestral merit, 205n33; conversion, 4, 132, 203n22, 204n22; defining Israel, 7–8, 38–39, 150n41; dialectics of desire in, 122; Greco-Roman culture and, 66; Jacob identified with, 3, 5, 41, 47, 48, 55, 60, 61, 160n80; patristic sources and, 56–62, 160n80, 161n94, 161n99; righteousness in, 50–51, 155n29; Roman governmental prohibition against religious observances, 38–40, 150n39, 150n44, 154n10; sexual intercourse, 122–23, 201n215. *See also* fetal formation and development; Greco-Roman embryology; Torah and Torah study

Rebekah: barrenness of, 112, 118; pregnancy of, 50, 72–73; womb of, 63, 64, 157n48. *See also* Esau; Jacob
Red Sea crossing: as baptism, 43, 149n23; birth imagery of, 34, 149n24; fetuses' singing at, 7, 24, 26, 30, 32, 36–37
religion, definitions of, 141n53
resurrection, 101–2, 104, 188n74
Reuben (biblical figure), as first born, 103, 189n82
Revelation of Torah at Mount Sinai: Decalogue, 42–43, 44, 153n72; fetuses as guarantors of the tradition, 30–33, 44–45; generational memory of, 36–38; Origen on, 42–43; singing at, 2, 137n6; Torah study as, 37; women at, 21, 145n120
righteousness, attainment of, 50–52, 55, 155n29
Rome: Christian Rome, 59–60, 61, 140n49; Esau identified as, 48, 49, 159n67; genealogization of, 62, 63; pagan Rome, 48–50, 60, 153n2; prohibition against religious observances, 38–40, 49, 150n39, 150n44, 154n10; relations with Israel, 49, 50, 52, 154n10, 154–55n21
Rubenstein, Jeffrey, 40

Sarah (biblical figure), 82, 104, 112, 178n111, 178n114, 190n89, 190n90
Satlow, Michael, 113
Schwartz, Seth, 65–66, 84, 162n1, 162–63n7
Scott, James, 86
seed: emission of, 107, 174n84, 174n85, 174–75n86, 191n105; God's creating embryo with, 98; one-seed theory of procreation, 24, 181n3; sex determination, 174n84, 174n85, 174–75n86; two-seed theory of procreation, 24, 110, 111, 174n85; women's, 92, 97–99, 102–3, 110–11, 174–75n86, 183n27, 188n80, 191n108, 193n122
Segal, Alan, 62, 155n32
semen. *See* male seed
sex determination, 174n84, 174n85, 174–75n86; of Dinah (biblical figure), 9, 77, 79, 80, 173n72, 176n94; prayer for, 80–81, 176n94, 176n95; "three partners" tradition, 10, 67, 81, 106, 107–11, 191n107, 191n108, 192n117; timing of, 80, 176n94; women's involvement in, 175–76n92, 186n64

sexual intercourse: menstruation and, 201n220; nonprocreative sexual activity, 117, 121, 123, 200n201; during pregnancy, 73, 169n48, 196n156; procreation, 122–23, 201n215
shefir merukam, 16, 143n84, 144n91
shikhvat zera', 113, 115, 124, 125, 195n148
Sinaitic revelation. *See* Revelation of Torah at Mount Sinai
singing: David's singing in the womb, 41, 151n53; God's praises, 33–34; at Red Sea crossing, 7, 24, 26, 30, 32, 36–37
Smith, Richard, 201n216
Soranus, 111, 169n48, 172n72, 173n74, 183n28, 194n131
Stern, Sacha, 8
Stol, M., 167n33, 179n123, 187n72, 195n148
Stormer, Nathan, 22, 146n126
Synagogue, Church relations with, 37, 47, 53, 54, 56, 57

tazria', 35, 97, 104, 198–99n185
Ten Commandments, 42–43, 44, 153n72
theology, use of term, 203n11
"three partners" tradition, 10, 67, 81, 106–11, 191n107, 191n108, 192n117
Torah and Torah study: in the *Bavli* (Babylonian Talmud), 35, 40, 41–42, 150n39; ensoulment compared with giving of, 68–70, 71, 166n27, 167n33, 167n38; fetuses and, 35–36, 40–41, 44, 49–50, 150n39, 151n51; forty-day gestation period of embryo, 68–70, 71, 166n27, 167n33, 167n38, 167–68n39; Gentiles banned from studying, 139n45; Israel, identification with, 55; Jacob and, 41, 49–50; transmission of halakhah, 41, 151n51; universality of, 139n45. *See also* Revelation of Torah at Mount Sinai
Tropper, Amram, 205n32
twins. *See* Esau; Jacob
two-seed theory of procreation, 24, 110, 111, 174n85

Urbach, E. E., 191n108

valad (vlad), 17, 143n82, 144n94, 145n121
van der Horst, Pieter, 113–14
vataharvateled, 113, 196n150
vayitrotsatsu, 49

vayyitser, 75, 171n61
visibility of fetuses, 31, 128–29, 148n10
Visotzky, Burton: on anti-Christian polemics in *Leviticus Rabbah*, 121–22, 200n199; on *Gen. Rab.* 63:6-8, 53; on Judaism as Hellenistic religion, 162n1; on original sin, 199n184, 200n200; on structure of *Leviticus Rabbah*, 91, 183n26, 184n49

white drop, 92, 99, 100, 123, 124, 198n177, 201n218
womb: David's singing in, 41, 151n53; formation of embryo in, 16, 143n81; gender identity of, 25; as house of study, 41; insemination, 100; Jewish identity of, 25; midrashic imagery of, 34, 149n22; position of the fetus in, 1, 5, 6, 16, 21, 28, 72, 137n5, 138n22, 168–69n45; in rabbinic narrative, 146n126; shape of, 93; Torah study in, 35–36, 40–41, 150n39, 151n51; transparency of, 2, 3, 21, 31, 128–29, 148n10. *See also* conception; embryos; fetuses; menstrual blood; pregnancy; seed
women: bellies like glass, 2, 3, 21, 31, 129, 148n10; breasts, 30, 93, 95; components of the fetus contributed by, 101–2, 106, 186n60, 190n98, 191n102; facial features of children influenced by, 67, 81–82, 177–78n109; God's role in creating the embryo, 92, 93–94, 98; house metaphor for, 21, 95, 97, 183–84n36; involvement in sex determination, 186n64; as passive in procreation, 23, 95, 101–3, 117, 119–20; prominence of fetuses and absence of, 21–22, 145n119, 145n120, 146n124, 146n126; as receptacle for fetus, 21, 145n121; as receptacle for semen, 98, 104; red emissions (*mazra'at 'odem*), 106, 107; reproductive theology and, 101–2; seed production of, 92, 97–99, 102–3, 110–11, 174–75n86, 183n27, 188n80, 191n108, 193n122; tazria', 97, 104, 198–99n185, 335. *See also* menstrual blood; pregnancy; womb

Yehudah haNasi, R., 68, 80, 85, 86, 156n37, 165n19
Yohanan, R., 49, 99, 100, 185n51
Yosi the Galilean, 30, 148n8
Yuval, Israel, 53, 56, 154n21

Citation Index

Hebrew Bible

Gen.
1:28, 116, 170n57, 197n161
2:7, 74, 75, 101, 168n43, 171n61
2:19, 171n61
3:6, 74
3:15, 195n148
3:16, 74, 170n56
3:47, 183n30
4:1, 113
4:25, 195n148
6:4, 167–68n39, 178n109
6:12, 195n148
7:4, 71
11:30, 144n94
13:6, 112
15:3, 113
16:2, 190n89
16:4, 195n147
16:10, 112, 195n148
17:5, 141n55
19:32, 195n147
20:18, 112
21:1, 104, 112, 165n21, 190n91
21:1–2, 189n88, 190n89
21:2, 81–82, 170n56, 178–79n115, 190n90
21:12, 51
24:60, 195n148
25, 47
25:19, 178–79n115
25:20, 118
25:21, 112, 198n177
25:22, 3, 49, 54, 61, 147n138, 149n21, 154–55n21, 156n37
25:22–23, 47, 51, 52, 154–55n21, 156n37
25:23, 3, 8, 49–54, 56–57, 60, 61, 147n1, 151n51, 154n21, 155n31, 155–56n32, 156n37, 159n67, 160n80, 161n94
25:24, 51, 72–73
25:25, 57–58
25:26, 57
25:27, 155n27
25:29–34, 61, 160n83
25:30, 153n1
27, 47
27:36, 61
29:31, 112
30:2, 113, 144n92
30:5, 178n110
30:17, 178n110
30:22, 112, 118
30:24, 80
30:32–33, 113
30:35, 113
30:37, 178n109
30:39, 184n48
30:41, 184n48
31:10, 184n48
32:29, 137n10
33:4, 47
35:10, 137n10
36:1, 153n1
37:3, 177n106
38:8–9, 195n148
38:9, 195n148
38:18, 195n147
38:24, 180n132
49:3, 103

Exod.
1:13, 82
4:22, 58, 61
5, 43, 152n61
6, 152n60
8, 152n57
15:1, 152n60
15:1–2, 30
15:2, 2, 36
15:11, 2, 10, 26, 33, 139n43, 189n85
15:16, 181n6

19:1, 37
19:12, 32
19:15, 32, 170n55
19:17, 32, 148n15
19:18, 144n99
20:1–6, 152n57
20:2, 42
20:3, 43
20:12, 140n46
20:16, 32
21:22, 144n92
21:22–24, 166n25
21:22–25, 196n151
23:25–26, 117
23:26, 112
24:18, 69
34:28–29, 69

Lev.
12, 166n30
12:1–3, 10
12:2, 10, 27, 28, 35, 91–94, 97–100, 102–5, 107, 113, 115, 119, 120, 125, 149n31, 150n31, 174n85, 174n86, 175n90, 182n12, 182n14, 184n40, 189n85, 191n106, 198–99n185, 200n200
12:2–6, 202n221
12:3, 79, 175n90
12:4–6, 10
14:52, 185n51
15, 196–97n149, 201n220
15:16, 195n148
18:1–2, 9
18:3, 9, 70, 167n36
18:19, 201n220
19:3, 140n46
20:18, 201n220
114:2, 201n218

Num.
5:28, 104, 189n88
20, 153n1
23:10, 107
26:7, 179n115

Deut.
5:16, 140n46
6:13, 140n46
7:13, 117, 144n92
12:23, 191n102

14, 35
23:9, 173n81
27:9, 150n35
28:4, 144n92
28:12, 118
28:18, 144n92
29, 150n37
29:14, 37
32:9, 139n42
32:18, 9, 69, 71, 156n37
33:2, 161n98
33:4, 151n51
33:29, 26, 31, 33

Judg.
13:3, 112

1 Sam.
1:5, 195n144
1:19, 195n144
1:19–20, 112
1:20, 170n52
2:20, 195n144
2:20-21, 112
2:21, 165n21, 190n91

2 Sam.
6:23, 144n94
11:4, 195n147
12:24, 195n147

Isa.
44:2, 193n139
44:24, 193n139
49:5, 193n139
60:2, 147n1
66:7, 102, 188n75

Jer.
1:5, 49, 52, 55, 138n24, 154n15, 193n139
9:20, 148n8
16:14–15, 139n43
18:6, 9, 80

Hos.
9:11, 112
12:4, 156n33, 161n100

Joel
2:16, 30

Obad.
1, 153n1

Mal.
1:2, 50, 55, 138n24
1:(2–)3, 53, 55
1:2–3, 54, 158–59n62
1:3, 50, 52, 56, 138n24

Ps.
8:3, 30–33, 148n11
8:5, 148n12
22:11, 29
27:10, 97, 98, 184n49
29:11, 31, 148n17
51:4, 200n203
51:7, 97, 98–99, 121, 184n47, 184n48, 184n49, 185n51, 200n200, 200n203, 202n223
58:4, 49, 56, 154n11, 154n13
68:27, 30
103, 34
103:1, 34, 164n18
103:4, 34
104, 34
113:9, 112
127:3, 112, 173n81, 189n87
139, 144n88
139:3, 99, 107, 192n112
139:5, 92, 149n31, 182n15, 188n73
139:13, 72
139:13–16, 92, 162n3
139:16, 17, 72, 168n44
145:6, 198n174
145:16, 118

Prov.
3:9, 140n46
4:1–2, 35
4:4, 35, 149n29
21:8, 155n27
30:15–16, 149n22
31:26, 151n53

Job
3:16, 30
4:14, 172n71
9:10, 37, 150n37, 192n113
10, 72, 144n88
10:3, 71
10:8–12, 162n3
10:10–11, 101
10:10–12, 149n30
10:10–13, 187n69
10:11, 72
10:12, 68, 77, 93, 94, 101, 165n24, 168n44, 188n71
14:4, 124, 202n226
14:15, 140n48
24:15, 70
26:3, 182n17
27:3, 68
29:2–4, 149n29, 149n30
29:3, 93, 149n27
29:4, 35
31:15, 193n139
36:3, 92
38:8, 34, 95, 96
38:9, 96
38:10, 96
38:11, 96, 124, 184n40

Song of Songs
4:12, 82, 83

Ruth
4:13, 74, 112

Lam.
4, 153n1

Eccles.
11:2, 79
11:5, 79, 193n139, 200n214, 201n214, 201n218

Rabbinic Sources

Mishnah

m. Ber.
9:3, 80, 173n80, 176n94, 176n95

m. Pes.
10:5, 36, 139n44

m. Yev.
   5:2, 171n66
   12:6, 171n66

m. Kid.
   3:12, 144n94

m. Avot
   3:1, 103
   3:15, 181n7

m. Bek.
   8:1, 143n83, 145n103, 171n66

m. Ker.
   1:3, 143n83, 145n103

m. Nid.
   3:1–2, 144n87
   3:3, 143n83, 144n94, 168n44
   3:6, 144n94
   3:7, 10, 144n94, 165n23, 166n30

Tosefta

t. Shab.
   9:14, 148n7
   16:4, 171n66

t. Yev.
   6:1, 171n66
   12:5, 171n66

t. Sot.
   6:4, 147n4

t. Bek.
   1:5, 178n109
   6:2, 171n66

t. Shab.
   9:14, 148n7
   16:4, 171n66

t. Nid.
   2:1, 172n71, 183n29
   2:7, 197n168
   3:3(50d), 182n16
   4, 144n87
   4:10, 16, 137n2, 143n83, 144n90, 144n91, 149n30, 168n44
   4:12, 143n83
   4:14, 166n30

Palestinian Talmud (Yerushalmi)

y. Ber.
   9:5(14a), 146n134, 176n93, 176n98

y. Bik.
   1:4(64a), 141n55, 204n28

y. Shab.
   9:3(12a), 170n55

y. Yev.
   1:1, 117
   4:2, 171n60
   4:2(5c), 170n55
   4:2(5d), 170n59
   4:11(6a), 170n55
   9:3, 188n80
   34:11(6a), 170n55

y. Sot.
   4:4(19c), 172n71, 183n29
   5:6 (20c), 144n99, 147n4
   9:3[23c], 168n41

y. Kid.
   1:7(61b), 140n46, 191n104

y. Kel., 164n16
   8:3(31c), 67, 81, 175n87, 186n60, 188n76, 190n92, 192n116

Midrash

Avot d'Rabbi Natan
   16, 165n19, 188n81

Deut. Rab.
   7:6, 190n93

Eccles. Rab. (Qoh. Rab.)
   3:2, 149n22
   4:3, 155n24
   5:10, 81, 175n87, 190n92, 190n99, 191n105
   5:10.2, 67
   5:11, 149n22, 182–83n20, 200n218
   12:1, 188n81
   12:10, 169n49

Exod. Rab.
   5:9, 144n99
   28:2, 145n120
   28:6, 148n13, 150n37

Gen. Rab.
  1:1, 72, 147n140
  4:7, 102, 181n1
  8:1, 182n12, 182n15, 188n73
  14:2, 74, 170n59, 171n66, 171n613
  14:5, 72, 101, 102, 104, 144n89, 149n30,
    177n102, 181n2, 182n12, 187n68, 188n70,
    188n71
  14:8, 144n90, 176n101
  14:9, 164n13
  14:51, 168n43
  17:7, 182n18
  17:8, 165n20
  20:6, 74, 170n57, 170n59, 171n66
  26:4, 195n148
  26:7, 168n39, 178n109
  32:5, 71, 166n27, 168n40
  34:10, 67–68, 104, 165n23, 179n125
  45:4, 189n83
  45:5, 188n80, 195n147
  46:2, 103, 189n82
  51:9, 189n83
  53:6, 81–82, 104, 165n21, 169n49, 170n56,
    188n80, 189n88, 190n91
  53:8, 189n87, 190n91
  56:2, 165n21, 190n91
  60:13, 165n21, 190n91
  63, 59, 62, 63, 151n50, 155n30
  63:5, 118, 182n18, 198n177
  63:6, 41, 49, 54, 55, 138n24, 153n8, 154n10,
    154n16, 156n37, 160n81
  63:6–7, 50–51, 158n61
  63:6–8, 41, 48–53, 55, 56, 60, 61, 63, 64,
    137n11, 154n21, 155n30, 159n66
  63:6–9, 53
  63:7, 50, 53, 60, 138n24, 154n10, 154n16,
    160n72
  63:8, 51, 57, 58, 60, 61, 103, 154n16, 160n81,
    188n78, 189n82
  65:12, 175–76n92, 200n214, 201n214
  71:1, 189n87
  71:1–2, 190n91
  71:2, 189n87
  72:6, 9, 79–80, 81, 146n134, 165n21,
    176n101, 190n91
  73:1, 165n21, 190n91
  73:4, 190n93, 198n174
  73:10, 178n109
  78:9, 47
  82:7, 144n94
  84:4–5, 197n168
  84:8, 177n106, 178n112
  85:5, 177n106, 189n83, 195n148, 197n170
  86:6, 177n106
  87:14, 190n96
  94:9, 186n57, 189n83
  98:4, 117
  99:6, 103, 189n82

Lam. Rab.
  1:11, 169n49

Lev. Rab.
  1:2, 140n49
  1:11, 140n49
  1:11–13, 140n49
  4:7, 34, 41, 149n21
  8:1, 167n38
  14, 10, 27–28, 34, 97, 98, 105, 107, 120–21,
    140n47, 140n48, 172n71, 182n12, 183n21,
    184n49, 187n68
  14:1, 91–92, 93, 99, 182n12, 188n73
  14:1–4, 98
  14:2, 34, 92, 93, 97, 108, 149n22, 149n27,
    169n50, 173n75, 182n11, 198n177,
    200n218
  14:2–4, 77, 114–15
  14:2–6, 182n12
  14:3, 73, 76, 77, 93, 94–95, 97, 100, 101,
    182n11, 183n23, 183n29, 184n36, 184n48,
    192n113, 196n156
  14:4, 34, 95, 96, 97, 169n47, 182n11,
    183–84n36
  14:5, 97, 98, 100, 119, 121, 123, 185n52,
    192n112, 196n159, 199n194, 200n199,
    200n200, 202n223
  14:6, 97, 99, 107–8, 192n112, 198n179,
    199n193
  14:7, 79, 175n91, 186n64, 200n214
  14:8, 6, 16–17, 72, 137n2, 144n90, 174n85,
    174n86, 174–75n86, 175n90, 176n92,
    176n101, 182n16, 186n64, 196n156,
    205n35
  14:9, 72, 97, 99, 100, 101–2, 108, 114,
    144n89, 148n7, 149n30, 177n102, 181n2,
    182n12, 185n52, 187n68, 187–88n70,
    188n73, 188n74, 192n110
  14:18, 1
  15:5, 184n37
  18:1, 188n81
  23, 70
  23:12, 9, 69, 70, 71, 73, 81, 166–167n31,
    177n104, 177n105, 177n109, 191n103,

192n117
24:2, 73
25:5, 96
27:9, 188n81
30:13, 170n51
31:3, 140n48
31:8, 73, 149n27, 183n21

Mekhilta of Rabbi Ishmael (MRI) on

Bahodesh
8, 140n46, 191n104

B'shalakh
8, 81, 82, 104, 173n79, 177n104, 178n113, 182n10, 182n15, 189n85, 189n87, 190n94, 192n111, 200n218, 201n218

Shirata
1, 30, 147n4
3, 36, 148n19, 150n33
8, 139n43

Mekhilta of Rabbi Shimeon ben Yochai (MRS) on

B'shalakh, 182n10, 182n12, 183n20

Exod.
19:18, 144n99
15:11, 182n16
19:17, 32

Mid. HaGadol
19:18, 148n16

Mid. Mishle
6, 144n99, 148n16

Mid. Psalms on
Ps. 8:3, 33, 148n11
Ps. 8:4, 144n97, 148n18, 152n68
Ps. 8:5, 148n4, 148n12, 148n18
Ps. 18:26, 149n21
Ps. 68:14, 148n4
Ps. 103:3, 149n21

Mid. Tanhuma (Buber) on

Bereishit
31, 159n67

Nitsavim
8, 150n37

Tazria'
1, 144n97

2, 149n31
4, 144n97

Tetsaveh
5, 147n1

Vayishlakh
25, 178n111

Yitro, 150n35
11, 150n37

Mid. Tanhuma on

B'shalakh
11, 147–48n4

Exod.
19:1, 37

Naso
4, 166n31

Nitsavim
3, 150n37

Pekudei
3, 37, 126, 146n131, 150n37, 150n38, 192n109

Tazria', 42
1, 149n30, 149n31
2, 35, 149n31, 189n85
3, 174n86

Toldot
1, 82
6, 178–79n115

Vayegesh
2, 148n16

Vayyetze
8, 176n99

Num. Rab.
3:8, 173n81
5:4, 167n38
9:1, 166n31, 177n109
9:5, 177n109
9:34, 178n109
11:31, 169n49
15:7, 183n21
23:10, 186n57

Pesikta de Rav Kahana
3, 155n29, 155n30, 156n37
20:1, 189n87

Pesikta Rabbati
  42:2, 190n89
Pirkei Rabbi Eliezer
  29, 155n27
  40, 148n13, 150n37
Ruth Rab.
  7:14, 189n87
  proem 3, 154n10
Sifra, 164n16
  Qedoshim
    1:4–7, 164n15
    1:7, 140n46, 191n104
  Tazria'
    3:6, 148n7
Sifre
  Deut.
    1, 152n57
    41, 160n72
    319, 156n37
    343, 161n98
    Ki Tetse 43, 173n81
  Num.
    Naso, 190n91
    8, 169n49
    19, 165n21
Song of Songs Rab.
  1:4, 32
  2, 150n35
  4:12, 82–83
  on 1:4, 148n16, 148n17, 155n24
  on 1:4(1), 144n99
Tanna debe Eliyyahu Zuta
  19, 154n17

Babylonian Talmud (Bavli)
b. Ber.
  4a, 143n83, 151n53
  10a, 41, 149n21, 164n18, 189n85, 192n114, 198n178
  15b, 149n22
  57b, 156n37
  60a, 146n134, 165n23, 173–74n83, 175n87, 175n88, 176n93
b. Shev.
  18b, 175n90
  39a, 150n37
b. Shab.
  9:3(12a)86a, 170n55
  55b, 184n43
  118b, 197n170
  135b–136a, 171n68
  145b–146a, 142n71
b. Tan.
  2a, 190n93
  2b, 198n174
b. Meg.
  6a, 155n29
  11a, 155n29
  14a, 189n85, 192n114, 198n178
b. Yev.
  34b, 197n168
  35b, 171n66
  42a, 170n52
  47b, 204n22
  62b, 165n21
  64a, 198n176
  69b, 165n23
  77b, 173n81
  78a, 192n109
  98a, 188n78, 192n109
  100a, 171n66
b. Ket.
  7b, 148n4
  30a, 179n122
  39a, 172n71
  60a, 172n71
  60b, 183n29
b. Sot.
  2a, 167n38
  8b, 179n122
  10b, 151–52n53
  20b, 169n49
  27a, 192n109
  30b, 147n4, 148n10
  30b–31a, 148n12
  41b, 147n1, 151n50, 156n37
  45b, 168n41
  48b, 149n28
b. Kid.
  30b, 140n46, 164n15, 191n104

b. Bab. Kam.
92a, 195n145

b. Bab. Metz.
84a, 178n109
87a, 77, 82, 178n111

b. Bab. Bat.
15b, 149n28

b. Sanh.
22a, 167n38
36b, 192n109
39a, 182n18
39b, 155n29
56a, 179n122
59b, 155n27
91a–b, 147n1
91b, 41, 68, 150n38, 151n50, 165n21, 165n23, 179n125
92a, 149n22, 156n37
113a, 190n93

b. Shev.
39a, 150n37
18b, 175n90

b. Avod. Zar.
2b, 147n1
11a, 156n37
20a, 188n80, 188n81

b. Men.
99b, 68–69, 166n27, 168n40

b. Hull.
69a, 186n61
79a, 190n96

b. Bek.
6b–7a, 178n109
21b, 167n38
45a, 183n34, 183–84n36, 190n93

b. Nid.
8b, 171n66
9a, 124, 172n71, 186n56, 192n109
16b, 155n29, 165n21, 192n109
17b, 148n7
18a, 148n7
22a, 148n7
25a, 137n2, 144n90, 144n91, 149n30, 168n44, 182n16
25b, 174n83
30a–b, 166n30
30b, 10, 35, 137n3, 137n5, 149n22, 149n27, 149n30, 155n29, 164n15, 166n30, 169n50, 183n21, 183n23, 205n35
30b–31b, 181n8
31a, 1, 67, 79, 106, 107, 137n5, 165n20, 169n47, 169n48, 174n84, 174n85, 175n87, 181n9, 182n10, 182n16, 186n57, 186n59, 189n85, 190n92, 191n105, 191n108, 192n110, 196n156
31b, 183n24, 185n51, 185n52
38a, 170n55
38b, 170n52
41b, 148n7
70b–71a, 173n81, 174n83, 175n87, 175n88, 175n90
71a, 175n91

Second Temple Literature

2 Macc.
7:22–23, 188n72

4 Macc.
13:19, 114
13:20, 114

Philo

On the Creation of the World
67, 196n154
132, 196n154

De specialibus legibus
3.108–9, 166n25
111.108-9, 196n151

Quaestiones ad Genesim
3.47, 196n154

Wisd. of Sol.
7:1–2, 113–14

Old Testament Pseudepigrapha

4 Ezra
6:7–10, 154n17

Testaments of the Twelve Patriarchs
T. Reuv.
   5:1–7, 168n39

New Testament

1 Cor.
   10, 149n23
   10:1–2, 43

Gal.
   4:28–29, 156n33

Heb.
   11:11, 199n188
   12:16–17, 156n33

John
   3:5, 43

Rom.
   5:12, 119
   9, 27, 48, 53, 54, 55
   9-11, 156n34
   9:6–13, 51–55, 156n32
   9:8, 54
   9:10–13, 52
   9:11, 159n63
   9:11–13, 6, 53–54, 138n24, 155n25
   9:12, 54
   9:30, 55
   9:30–33, 52

Patristic Sources

Augustine

Contra Julian, 119
   2.56, 199n190
   2.83, 199n190
   2.179, 199n190
   3.85.3–4, 199n188
   3.85.4, 199n190
   3.88.3–4, 199n190
   5.34(8), 199n192
   6.59(19), 199n192
   34.12(2), 199n192

De nuptiis
   2.26(13), 199n187

Opus Imperfectum, 119
   2.56, 199n190
   2.83, 199n190
   2.179, 199n190
   3.85.4, 199n190
   3.88.3–4, 199n190

Clement of Alexandria

Paidogogos
   1.39.3, 172–73n73
   1.48.1–2, 181n2
   2.83, 116, 197n172
   2.83.3, 197n165
   2.93, 197n167

Strom.
   6.147.4, 197n163, 197n172

Origen

Comm., 55
   7:15, 159n63
   7:18, 158n58

Hom. Gen.
   12:1, 53–54, 159n63
   12:3, 54
   12:4, 158n52, 159n63

Hom. Lev.
   8:2(6), 200n200
   8:3(5), 200n200

Tertullian

De anima
   26, 157n48
   37, 170n58, 171n65

Greek Sources

Aristotle

Generation of Animals
   776a15–17, 173n74
   739b22, 187n67

    740b9–10, 168n41
History of Animals
    7.3.583b, 143–44n86
    522a4, 172n72
    581a8–10, 173n74
    583b, 166n30, 168n41, 170n54
    584a, 169n48
    584b, 169n48
    586a32, 168n41
    586b3–4, 169n45
    739b22, 181n2
    book 10, 193n126
Politics
    7.16, 177n10

Hippocrates
Diseases of Women
    1.25, 94

On the Nature of the Child
    15, 168n41
    18, 166n30
    19, 168n41
    28, 168–69n45
    29, 168n41
Nutriment
    4, 163n12
Regimen
    1.26, 166n30

Acknowledgments

I would like to express my gratitude to the series editors of Divinations: Rereading Late Ancient Religion at the University of Pennsylvania Press. In particular, I thank Derek Krueger for his suggestion that I submit my manuscript and his encouragement throughout the process. Virginia Burrus read the initial submitted draft and made numerous insightful comments; her feedback helped me improve this project in countless ways. Daniel Boyarin was a hovering presence throughout the writing of this book. My indebtedness to Daniel is palpable, and his scholarship has influenced, informed, and shaped my own on multiple levels. In the final stages of this book's coming into being, Daniel challenged me to clarify my ideas further, and I am grateful for his inspiration and his generosity. I also thank Jennifer Shenk, Erica Ginsburg, and Yumeko Kawano for their hard work ushering the manuscript through production. I extend heartfelt appreciation to Jerome Singerman for his unwavering attentiveness, encouragement, and understanding.

I have benefited greatly from many colleagues during the writing of this book. I thank Neil Danzig, Elliot Dorff, Patricia Cox Miller, and Menahem Schmelzer for their comments on a very early draft. Shaye J. D. Cohen, Alan Cooper, Charlotte Fonrobert, Stephen Garfinkel, Richard Kalmin, Seth Schwartz, and Andrea Sterk kindly shared their expertise in answer to my queries. I thank David Kraemer for pointing out to me my own interest in rabbinic theology—long before I fully embraced this aspect of what is now quite central to this book. I am lucky to count the following people as colleagues and friends, and I thank them for the various ways they helped me while I was writing this book: Kathryn Baker, Carol Bakhos, Richard I. Cohen, Shari Crandall, Mitchell Hart, Melila Hellner-Eshed, Todd Hasak-Lowy, Taal Hasak-Lowy, Shaya Isenberg, Robert Kawashima, Eric Kligerman, Jack Kugelmass, Sarra Lev, Jim Mueller, and Judy Page. I also thank the Panush Judaica Fund of the Center for Jewish Studies at the University of Florida for generously providing funds for the index.

I owe a special debt to Denise Kimber Buell. Denise was a consistent source of support; at a critical stage during revisions, she helped me uncover my voice and gave me the courage to use it. Nina Caputo provided enormous help; she read many chapters, often in more than one version, and her critical feedback and consistent encouragement were invaluable. Iscah Waldman, my hevruta and friend, was always ready to learn with me and then to argue with me; I learned a great deal both with her and from her. Alyssa Gray, my dear friend and colleague since graduate school, remains a beacon for me; I thank her for answering many questions and for being an endless source of profound intellectual and emotional encouragement and support. Stacey Langwick guided me through my readings in the anthropology of reproduction and, more important, she has been a beloved friend; I thank her for her companionship and for countless conversations over coffee about, well, fetuses and so much more. Leah Hochman has been a most cherished friend, confidante, and ally; I thank her too for countless conversations over coffee, and for much, much more. Finally, I am forever indebted to my dear friend and colleague Kim Emery. Kim read and reread numerous versions of each chapter of this book, and all of them are better for it. She provided a fresh set of eyes, lent her incredibly sharp mind, and poured her heart and soul into this book and its author, ultimately giving me the heart to finish this project.

I owe enormous thanks to my parents, Sharon and Mel Kessler, for their support and understanding, and for learning not to ask when the book would be finished. My mother's inquisitive, keen, and critical mind, and her pursuit of Jewish learning, remains a model, and inspiration, for me; I am forever grateful. I owe thanks to my brother, Alan Kessler, for his support and encouragement. I also take this opportunity to thank Elaine and Steve Cohen, Maya Orli Cohen, Ayelet Cohen, and Marc Margolius for their friendship and encouragement.

Finally, I thank my partner, Tamara Ruth Cohen, for her love and support over the past eleven years. Tamara has simultaneously waited patiently and refused to wait, so that during the writing of this book, in addition to being sustained and nurtured by her on a daily basis, I have also experienced the joys of a public celebration of our love and commitment and the birth and parenting of our child, Tobias Ezekiel Kessler-Cohen. I cannot thank Tamara enough for her companionship and wisdom and for the poetry she brings to my life. Although Toby is too young to know this, he has already provided me with enough love to fill a lifetime.

This book is dedicated to Burton L. Visotzky, my mentor, colleague and friend. Burt's enthusiasm for this project—from its conception—has been awe inspiring. His attentiveness to this book, and its author, has been above and beyond any expectations. What is mine, in many ways, is also his.